The Wills Eye Manual

**Office and Emergency Room
Diagnosis and Treatment of Eye Disease**
Third Edition

Contributors to the Third Edition

Christine W. Chung, M.D.
Brian P. Connolly, M.D.
Vincent A. Deramo, M.D.
Kammi B. Gunton, M.D.
Marlon Maus, M.D.
Medical Illustrator

Mark R. Miller, M.D.
Ralph E. Oursler III, M.D.
Mark F. Pyfer, M.D.
Douglas J. Rhee, M.D.
Jay C. Rudd, M.D.
Brian M. Sucheski, M.D.

Contributors to the Second Edition

Neal H. Atebara, M.D.
Medical Illustrator
Mark C. Austin, M.D.
Jerry R. Blair, M.D.
Benjamin Chang, M.D.
Mary Ellen Cullom, M.D.
R. Douglas Cullom, Jr., M.D.
Jack Dugan, M.D.
Forest J. Ellis, M.D.
C. Byron Faulkner, M.D.
Mary Elizabeth Gallivan, M.D.
J. William Harbour, M.D.
Paul M. Herring, M.D.
Allen Ho, M.D.
Carol J. Hoffman, M.D.

Thomas I. Margolis, M.D.
Mark L. Mayo, M.D.
Michele A. Miano, M.D.
Wynne A. Morley, M.D.
Timothy J. O'Brien, M.D.
Florentino E. Palmon, M.D.
William B. Phillips, M.D.
Tony Pruthi, M.D.
Carl D. Regillo, M.D.
Scott H. Smith, M.D.
Mark R. Stokes, M.D.
Janine G. Tabas, M.D.
John R. Trible, M.D.
Christopher Williams, M.D.

Contributors to the First Edition

Melissa M. Brown, M.D.
Catharine J. Crockett, M.D.
Bret L. Fisher, M.D.
Patrick M. Flaharty, M.D.
Mark A. Friedberg, M.D.
James T. Handa, M.D.
Victor A. Holmes, M.D.

Bruce J. Keyser, M.D.
Marlon Maus, M.D.
Medical Illustrator
Ronald L. McKey, M.D.
Christopher J. Rapuano, M.D.
Paul A. Raskauskas, M.D.
Eric P. Suan, M.D.

The Wills Eye Manual

Office and Emergency Room Diagnosis and Treatment of Eye Disease
Third Edition

Douglas J. Rhee, M.D.
Mark F. Pyfer, M.D.
Editors for the Third Edition

Mark A. Friedberg, M.D.
Christopher J. Rapuano, M.D.
Founding Editors

 LIPPINCOTT WILLIAMS & WILKINS
A **Wolters Kluwer** Company
Philadelphia · Baltimore · New York · London
Buenos Aires · Hong Kong · Sydney · Tokyo

Acquisitions Editor: Paula Callaghan
Developmental Editor: Michelle LaPlante
Manufacturing Manager: Tim Reynolds
Production Manager: Liane Carita
Production Editor: Patrick Carr
Cover Designer: Sandra Mohandru
Indexer: Mary Kidd
Compositor: Lippincott Williams & Wilkins Desktop Division
Printer: R. R. Donnelley, Crawfordsville

Printed in the United States of America

9 8 7 6 5 4 3 2

Library of Congress Cataloging-in-Publication Data
The Wills eye manual: office and emergency room diagnosis and treatment of eye disease. — 3rd ed. / Douglas J. Rhee, and Mark F. Pyfer, editors.
    p. cm.
Includes bibliographical references and index.
ISBN 0-7817-1602-0
1. Eye—Diseases—Handbooks, manuals, etc. 2. Ophthalmologic emergencies—Handbooks, manuals, etc. I. Rhee, Douglas J.   II. Pyfer, Mark F. III. Wills Eye Hospital (Philadelphia, Pa.)
    [DNLM: 1. Eye Diseases—diagnosis outlines. 2. Eye Diseases—therapy outlines. 3. Emergencies outlines.   WW 18.2 W741 1999]
RE48.9.W54 1999
617.7–dc21
DNLM/DLC
for Library of Congress   98-31758
                                                                                                                        CIP

Consultants

Cornea

Major Consultants

Elisabeth J. Cohen, M.D.
Christopher J. Rapuano, M.D.

Consultants

Peter R. Laibson, M.D.
Irving M. Raber, M.D.

Glaucoma

Major Consultant

George L. Spaeth, M.D.

Consultants

L. Jay Katz, M.D.
Marlene R. Moster, M.D.
Jonathan S. Myers, M.D.
Eliyathamby Sivalingam, M.D.
Louis W. Schwartz, M.D.
Annette K. Terebuh, M.D.
Richard P. Wilson, M.D.

Neuro-Ophthalmology

Consultants

Peter J. Savino, M.D.
Robert C. Sergott, M.D.

Oculo-Plastics

Consultants

Joseph C. Flanagan, M.D.
Marlon Maus, M.D.
Robert Penne, M.D.

Oncology

Consultants

James J. Augsburger, M.D.
Carol L. Shields, M.D.
Jerry A. Shields, M.D.

PEDIATRICS

Consultants

Joseph H. Calhoun, M.D.
Leonard B. Nelson, M.D.
Bruce M. Schnall, M.D.

GENERAL

Consultants

Edward A. Jaeger, M.D.
John B. Jeffers, M.D.
Richard Tipperman, M.D.

RETINA

Major Consultants

William E. Benson, M.D.
William Tasman, M.D.

Consultants

Jonathan B. Belmont, M.D.
Gary C. Brown, M.D.
David H. Fischer, M.D.
Mark A. Friedberg, M.D.
Joseph I. Maguire, M.D.
Arunan Sivalingam, M.D.
James F. Vander, M.D.
Tamara R. Vrabec, M.D.

FOREWORD

Nothing is as exciting as success. Since 1989, when the first edition of *The Wills Eye Manual* was published, we've enjoyed considerable success. Now our residents are presenting a third edition, which, as they point out in their preface, has been expanded where necessary but remains a concise, easily referenced volume.

The idea of a resident manual was conceived by Dr. Christopher Rapuano and Dr. Mark Friedberg while they were in training at our facility. Thanks to them and Dr. Edward Jaeger, who contacted Lippincott Williams & Wilkins, subsequent resident classes have had the opportunity to continue this venture and that is one of the reasons I feel particularly pleased to write this foreword to the third edition.

As we stand on the threshold of the next millennium, advances in medicine continue to increase at an exponential rate. We can only let our imaginations run wild when we speculate about what the future holds. It is our earnest hope that we will be able to continue publishing *The Wills Eye Manual* and that future editions will incorporate the latest developments in ophthalmology.

I would like to congratulate this year's editors, Dr. Douglas Rhee and Dr. Mark Pyfer, as well as the members of their class and other classes, who have worked long and hard to update a volume that I am sure residents and practitioners alike will find useful.

William Tasman, M.D.
Ophthalmologist-in-Chief
Department of Ophthalmology
Jefferson Medical College
Philadelphia, Pennsylvania

PREFACE

The first two editions of *The Wills Eye Manual: Office and Emergency Room Diagnosis and Treatment of Eye Disease* were an overwhelming success. We hope that this third edition will also be well received. As with the previous editions, our goal has been to provide a quick reference containing concise answers to diagnostic and therapeutic problems that span most of ophthalmology.

The Wills Eye Manual should continue to appeal to residents, comprehensive ophthalmologists, and even subspecialists who encounter problems outside their field of interest. In addition, emergency room physicians, primary care practitioners, and medical students will find that this book remains a useful resource when caring for patients with ocular complaints.

There have been many advances in ophthalmology over the past several years. Results of important collaborative clinical ophthalmic research trials, such as the Optic Neuritis Treatment Trial, Macular Photocoagulation Study, Endophthalmitis Vitrectomy Study, and the Herpetic Eye Disease Studies have altered the way we treat common ophthalmic disorders. The third edition of *The Wills Eye Manual* includes recent critically reviewed clinical data and new medications. All the sections have been updated wherever it was appropriate. We have consolidated some chapters, and, when necessary, expanded others. At the same time we have resisted unnecessarily expanding a manual that has been valued for its concise and accessible nature. In particular, there are new recommendations for hyphema, corneal ulcers, and eyelid trauma. The chapter on glaucoma and the acquired immunodeficiency syndrome (AIDS) sections have been completely rewritten. This edition also contains several new sections, including refractive surgery complications and diagnostic imaging in ophthalmology. Additionally, *The Wills Eye Manual* now has a pocket-sized companion, *The Wills Eye Drug Guide*, containing the newest treatment regimens and information on ocular pharmaceuticals.

Once again, as residents, we have consulted with our many mentors at the Wills Eye Hospital. They have assisted us in interpreting the changes in ophthalmology and in determining which studies have led to important modification of treatment regimens.

We hope this book continues to provide a quick and useful source of information for the diagnosis and treatment of eye disease.

Mark F. Pyfer, M.D.
Douglas J. Rhee, M.D.

PREFACE TO THE FIRST EDITION

Our goal has been to produce a concise book, providing essential diagnostic tips and specific therapeutic information pertaining to eye disease. We realized the need for this book while managing emergency room patients at one of the largest and busiest eye hospitals in the country. Until now, reliable information could only be obtained in unwieldy textbooks or inaccessible journals.

As residents at Wills Eye Hospital we have benefited from the input of some of the world-renowned ophthalmic experts in writing this book. More importantly, we are aware of the questions that the ophthalmology resident, the attending ophthalmologist, and the emergency room physician (not trained in ophthalmology) want answered immediately.

The book is written for the eye care provider who, in the midst of evaluating an eye problem, needs quick access to additional information. We try to be as specific as possible, describing the therapeutic modalities used at our institution. Many of these recommendations are, therefore, not the only manner in which to treat a particular disorder, but indicate personal preference. They are guidelines, not rules.

Because of the forever changing wealth of ophthalmic knowledge, omissions and errors are possible, particularly with regard to management. Drug dosages have been checked carefully, but the physician is urged to check the *Physicians Desk Reference* or *Facts and Comparisons* when prescribing unfamiliar medications. Not all contraindications and side effects are described.

We feel this book will make a welcome companion to the many physicians involved with treating eye problems. It is everything you wanted to know and nothing more.

Christopher J. Rapuano, M.D.
Mark A. Friedberg, M.D.

ACKNOWLEDGMENTS

We would like to thank the numerous residents of several residency classes who assisted us in updating this edition of *The Wills Eye Manual*. We are particularly grateful to the many Wills Eye Hospital attendings, without whose support and guidance this book would not have been possible.

CONTENTS

5 Conjunctiva/Sclera/External Disease   119

6 Eyelid   145

7 Orbit   167

11 NEURO-OPHTHALMOLOGY   273

12 RETINA   331

The Wills Eye Manual

**Office and Emergency Room
Diagnosis and Treatment of Eye Disease**
Third Edition

DIFFERENTIAL DIAGNOSIS OF OCULAR SYMPTOMS

Burning

More common   Blepharitis, dry-eye syndrome, conjunctivitis (discharge or eyelid sticking additionally).

Less common   Corneal problem (fluorescein staining of the cornea usually), inflamed pterygium/pinguecula, episcleritis, superior limbic keratoconjunctivitis.

Crossed Eyes in Children

See Esodeviations in Children (eyes turned in), Section 9.3, or Exodeviations in Children (eyes turned out), Section 9.4.

Decreased Vision

I. Transient visual loss (vision returns to normal within 24 hours, usually within 1 hour).

More common   Few seconds (usually bilateral): Papilledema.

Few minutes: Amaurosis fugax [transient ischemic attack (TIA); unilateral], vertebrobasilar artery insufficiency (bilateral).

10 to 60 minutes: Migraine (with or without a subsequent headache).

Less common   Impending central retinal vein occlusion, ischemic optic neuropathy, ocular ischemic syndrome (carotid occlusive disease), glaucoma, sudden change in blood pressure, central nervous system (CNS) lesion, optic disc drusen, giant cell arteritis.

II. Visual loss lasting longer than 24 hours.
   A. Sudden, painless loss.
      More common Retinal artery or vein occlusion, ischemic optic neuropathy, vitreous hemorrhage, retinal detachment, optic neuritis (usually pain with eye movements).
      Less common Other retinal or CNS disease.
   B. Gradual, painless loss (over weeks, months, or years).
      More common Cataract, refractive error, open-angle glaucoma, chronic retinal disease [e.g., age-related macular degeneration (ARMD), diabetic retinopathy].
      Less common Chronic corneal disease (e.g., corneal dystrophy), optic neuropathy/atrophy (e.g., CNS tumor).
   C. Painful loss: Acute angle-closure glaucoma, optic neuritis (pain with eye movements), uveitis, corneal hydrops (keratoconus).

❖ **Note** *Always remember nonphysiologic visual loss.*

Discharge

See Red Eye in this chapter.

Distortion (of Vision)

More common Refractive error, macular disease (e.g., central serous chorioretinopathy or ARMD), corneal irregularity.
Less common Cataract, topical eye drops (miotics), retinal detachment, migraine (transient), CNS abnormality.

Double Vision

I. Monocular (The double vision remains when the uninvolved eye is occluded.)
   More common Refractive error, corneal opacity or irregularity, cataract.
   Less common Dislocated natural lens or lens implant, extra pupillary openings, macular disease, retinal detachment, nonphysiologic.
II. Binocular (The double vision is eliminated when either eye is occluded.)
   A. Typically intermittent: Myasthenia gravis, intermittent decompensation of an existing phoria.
   B. Constant: Isolated sixth-, third-, or fourth-nerve palsy; orbital disease (e.g., thyroid eye disease, orbital inflammatory pseudotumor, tumor); cavernous sinus/superior orbital fissure syndrome; status post ocular surgery (e.g., residual anesthesia, displaced muscle);

status post trauma (e.g., orbital wall fracture with extraocular muscle entrapment, orbital edema); internuclear ophthalmoplegia, vertebrobasilar artery insufficiency, other CNS lesions, spectacle problem.

Dry Eyes

See Dry Eye Syndrome, Section 4.2.

Eyelid Crusting

More common   Blepharitis, meibomianitis, conjunctivitis.
Less common   Canaliculitis, nasolacrimal duct obstruction, dacryocystitis.

Eyelid Droop

See Ptosis and Pseudoptosis in Chapter 2.

Eyelid Swelling

A. Associated with inflammation (usually erythematous).
   More common   Hordeolum, blepharitis, conjunctivitis, preseptal or orbital cellulitis, trauma, contact dermatitis.
   Less common   Ectropion, corneal abnormality, urticaria/angioedema, insect bite, dacryoadenitis, erysipelas, eyelid or lacrimal gland mass.
B. Noninflammatory: Chalazion; prolapse of orbital fat (retropulsion of the globe increases the prolapse); laxity of the eyelid skin; cardiac, renal, or thyroid disease; eyelid or lacrimal gland mass.

Eyelid Twitch

Fatigue, lack of sleep, excess caffeine, habit, corneal or conjunctival irritation (especially from an eyelash or cyst), dry eye, blepharospasm (bilateral), hemifacial spasm, albinism (photosensitivity), a serum electrolyte abnormality, or anemia (rarely).

Flashes of Light

More common   Retinal break or detachment, posterior vitreous detachment, migraine, rapid eye movements (particularly in darkness).
Less common   CNS (particularly occipital lobe) disorders, retinitis, entopic phenomena.

Floaters

See Spots in Front of the Eyes in this chapter.

Foreign-Body Sensation

Dry-eye syndrome, blepharitis, conjunctivitis, trichiasis, corneal abnormality (e.g., corneal abrasion or foreign body, recurrent erosion, superficial punctate keratitis), contact lens–related problem, episcleritis, pterygium, or pinguecu-lum.

Halos Around Lights

Cataract, acute angle-closure glaucoma or corneal edema from another cause (e.g., corneal endothelial dystrophy, aphakic/pseudophakic bullous keratopa-thy), corneal haziness or mucus, drugs (e.g., digitalis, chloroquine).

Headache

See Headache, Section 15.3.

Itchy Eye

Conjunctivitis (especially viral, vernal, and allergic), blepharitis, dry-eye syn-drome, topical drug allergy or contact dermatitis, giant papillary conjunctivi-tis or another contact lens–related problem.

Light Sensitivity

See Photophobia in this chapter.

Night Blindness

More common Refractive error (especially undercorrected myopia), advanced glaucoma, small pupil (especially from miotic drops), retinitis pigmentosa, congenital stationary night blindness, drugs (e.g., pheno-thiazines, chloroquine, quinine).
Less common Vitamin A deficiency, gyrate atrophy, choroideremia.

Pain (Ocular)

Typically mild to moderate: Dry-eye syndrome, blepharitis, conjunctivitis, episcleritis, inflamed pingueculum or pterygium, foreign body (corneal or conjunctival), corneal disorder (e.g., superficial punctate keratitis), episcleritis, others.

Typically moderate to severe: Corneal disorder (abrasion, erosion, infiltrate/ulcer), anterior uveitis, scleritis, acute angle-closure glaucoma.

Pain (Orbital)

Sinusitis, dry eyes, orbital pseudotumor, optic neuritis, diabetic cranial nerve palsy.

Photophobia

More common Corneal abnormality (e.g., abrasion or edema) or anterior uveitis.

Less common Conjunctivitis (mild photophobia), posterior uveitis, albinism, total color blindness, aniridia.

With normal eye examination Migraine, meningitis, retrobulbar optic neuritis, subarachnoid hemorrhage, trigeminal neuralgia, or a lightly pigmented eye.

Proptosis

See Orbital Disease, Section 7.1.

Ptosis

See Ptosis and Pseudoptosis in Chapter 2.

Red Eye

I. Discharge present

  More common Conjunctivitis, ophthalmia neonatorum in infants, blepharitis.

  Less common Acute allergic reaction, dacryocystitis, canaliculitis.

II. No discharge present.

  A. Pain present: See Pain in this chapter.

  B. Minimal or no pain present.

  More common Subconjunctival hemorrhage, injected pterygium/pingueculum, blepharitis, dry-eye syndrome.

  Less common Conjunctival tumor.

Spots in Front of the Eyes

A. Transient: Migraine.

B. Permanent or long-standing.

  More common Posterior vitreous detachment, posterior uveitis, vitreous hemorrhage, vitreous condensations/debris.

  Less common Retinal detachment, corneal opacity.

❖ **Note** *Some patients are referring to a blind spot in their visual field caused by a retinal, optic nerve, or CNS disorder.*

Tearing

I. Adults.
   A. Pain present: Corneal abnormality (e.g., abrasion, foreign body/ rust ring, recurrent erosion, edema), anterior uveitis, eyelash (trichiasis, entropion), cyst, or foreign body rubbing against the cornea, conjunctival abnormality (e.g., foreign body, laceration).
   B. Minimal or no pain present: Dry eye-syndrome, blepharitis, naso-lacrimal duct obstruction, punctal occlusion or other tear drainage abnormality, ectropion, conjunctivitis (especially allergic and toxic), lacrimal sac mass or inflammation.
II. Children: Nasolacrimal duct obstruction, congenital glaucoma, corneal or conjunctival foreign body or other irritative disorder.

White Pupil

See Leukocoria, Section 9.1.

DIFFERENTIAL DIAGNOSIS OF OCULAR SIGNS

Anterior Chamber/Anterior Chamber Angle

Blood in Schlemm's Canal on Gonioscopy

Compression of episcleral vessels by a gonioprism (iatrogenic), Sturge–Weber syndrome, arteriovenous fistula (e.g., carotid–cavernous sinus fistula), superior vena cava obstruction, hypotony.

Hyphema

After trauma or intraocular surgery, bleeding from iris or corneal wound neovascularization, herpes simplex or zoster iritis, blood dyscrasia or clotting disorder (e.g., hemophilia), intraocular tumor (e.g., juvenile xanthogranuloma, retinoblastoma, leukemia).

Hypopyon

Infectious corneal ulcer, endophthalmitis, severe iritis, reaction to an intraocular lens or retained lens protein after cataract surgery, intraocular tumor necrosis [e.g., retinoblastoma (a pseudohypopyon)], a tight contact lens.

Cornea/Conjunctival Findings

Band Keratopathy

See Band Keratopathy, Section 4.11.

Corneal Crystals

Schnyder's crystalline dystrophy, multiple myeloma, cystinosis, gout, uremia, hypergammaglobulinemia, drugs (e.g., indomethacin, chloroquine), infectious crystalline keratopathy.

Corneal Edema

A. Congenital: Congenital glaucoma, congenital hereditary endothelial dystrophy, posterior polymorphous dystrophy (PPMD), birth trauma (forceps injury).

B. Acquired: Early postoperative, aphakic or pseudophakic bullous keratopathy, Fuchs' endothelial dystrophy, contact lens overwear, trauma, acute angle-closure glaucoma and other causes of acute increase in intraocular pressure, corneal hydrops (acute keratoconus), herpes simplex or zoster keratitis, iritis, failed corneal graft, iridocorneal endothelial (ICE) syndrome, PPMD.

Corneal Filaments

See Filamentary Keratopathy, Section 4.3.

Dilated Episcleral Vessels (in the Absence of Ocular Irritation or Pain)

Underlying uveal melanoma, arteriovenous fistula (e.g., carotid–cavernous fistula), polycythemia vera, leukemia, ophthalmic vein or cavernous sinus thrombosis.

Enlarged Corneal Nerves

Most important   Multiple endocrine neoplasia type IIb (medullary carcinoma of the thyroid gland, pheochromocytoma, mucosal neuromas; may have marfanoid habitus).

Others   Keratoconus, keratitis, neurofibromatosis, Fuchs' endothelial dystrophy, Refsum's syndrome, trauma, congenital glaucoma, failed corneal graft, leprosy.

Membranous Conjunctivitis

(Removal of the membrane is difficult and causes bleeding). Streptococci; pneumococci; chemical burn; ligneous conjunctivitis; *Corynebacterium diphtheriae*; adenovirus or herpes simplex virus. See also Pseudomembranous Conjunctivitis in this chapter.

Opacification of the Cornea in Infancy

Congenital glaucoma, birth trauma (forceps injury), congenital hereditary endothelial or stromal dystrophy (bilateral), PPMD, developmental abnormality of the anterior segment (especially Peter's anomaly), metabolic abnormalities (bilateral; e.g., mucopolysaccharidoses, mucolipidoses), interstitial keratitis, herpes simplex virus, corneal ulcer, corneal dermoid, sclerocornea.

Pannus (Superficial Vascular Invasion of the Cornea)

Rosacea, tight contact lens or contact lens overwear, phlyctenule, chlamydia (trachoma and inclusion conjunctivitis), superior limbic keratoconjunctivitis (micropannus only), staphylococcal hypersensitivity, vernal keratoconjunctivitis, herpes simplex virus, chemical burn, aniridia.

Large Papillae on the Superior Tarsus
Vernal or atopic conjunctivitis, giant papillary conjunctivitis, exposed suture, prosthesis-induced trachoma, superior limbic keratoconjunctivitis (fine papillae).

Pigmentation of the Conjunctiva
Racial pigmentation (perilimbal), nevus, primary acquired melanosis, melanoma, ocular and oculodermal melanocytosis (congenital, blue, episcleral, not conjunctival), Addison's disease, mascara, pregnancy, radiation, drug (e.g., chlorpromazine) or metal (e.g., argyrosis from silver).

Pseudomembranous Conjunctivitis
(Removal of the membrane is easy, and no bleeding results.) All of the causes of membranous conjunctivitis, as well as ocular cicatricial pemphigoid, Stevens–Johnson syndrome, superior limbic keratoconjunctivitis, gonococci, staphylococci, chlamydia in newborns, and others.

Symblepharon [Fusion of the Eyelid (Palpebral) Conjunctiva with the Conjunctiva Covering the Globe (Bulbar Conjunctiva)]
Ocular cicatricial pemphigoid, Stevens–Johnson syndrome, chemical burn, trauma, drugs, long-standing inflammation, epidemic keratoconjunctivitis, atopic conjunctivitis, radiation.

Whorl-like Opacity in the Corneal Epithelium
Amiodarone, chloroquine, Fabry's disease and carrier state, phenothiazines, indomethacin.

Eyelid Abnormalities

Eyelid Edema or Swelling
More common   Orbital fat herniation from aging, conjunctivitis, allergy, chalazion, orbital disease.
Less common   Cardiac disease, renal disease, urticaria/angioneurotic edema, dacryoadenitis, hypothyroidism, superior vena cava syndrome.

Eyelid Lesion
See Malignant Tumors of the Eyelid, Section 6.11.

Pseudoptosis
Dermatochalasis (laxity of the eyelid skin from old age), brow ptosis, enophthalmos (e.g., from a traumatic blow-out fracture), phthisis bulbi,

microphthalmia (small eye), chalazion or other eyelid tumor, eyelid edema, hypotropia (e.g., in double-elevator palsy) and retraction of the contralateral eyelid.

Ptosis

More common   Aging (e.g., levator dehiscence), following intraocular surgery or trauma, congenital.

Less common   Myasthenia gravis, Horner's syndrome, third-nerve palsy, chronic progressive external ophthalmoplegia, corneal or anterior segment disease (e.g., corneal abrasion), prolonged use of topical steroids, botulinum toxin or subtenons steroid injection.

Fundus Findings

Bone Spicules (Widespread Pigment Clumping)

More common   Retinitis pigmentosa and associated syndromes, disseminated chorioretinitis (especially old syphilis), trauma, pigmentary changes of aging.

Less common   Following spontaneous reattachment of a retinal detachment (e.g., toxemia of pregnancy, Harada's disease), Kearns–Sayre syndrome, abetalipoproteinemia, vitamin A deficiency, viral infections (e.g., rubella), drugs (e.g., thioridazine and other phenothiazines), retinopathy of prematurity (when seen years later as an adult), cystinosis, old vascular occlusions.

Bull's-Eye Macular Lesion

Age-related macular degeneration (ARMD), Stargardt's disease, cone dystrophy, chloroquine retinopathy, Spielmeyer–Vogt syndrome.

Choroidal Folds

Orbital or choroidal tumor, thyroid orbitopathy, orbital inflammatory pseudotumor, posterior scleritis, hypotony, retinal detachment, marked hyperopia, scleral laceration, papilledema.

Choroidal Neovascularization (Gray-Green Membrane or Blood Seen Deep to the Retina)

More common   ARMD, ocular histoplasmosis syndrome, high myopia, angioid streaks, choroidal rupture (trauma).

Less common   Drusen of the optic nerve head, tumors, following retinal laser photocoagulation, idiopathic.

Cotton-Wool Spots, Without Other Abnormalities (White Fluffy Lesions with Feathered Edges, Often Obscuring Retinal Vessels)

More common   Acquired immunodeficiency syndrome (AIDS) retinopathy, hypertension, diabetes, collagen–vascular disease (e.g., systemic lupus erythematosus), retinal artery/arteriole occlusion.

Less common   Retinal vein occlusion, cardiac valvular disease, carotid artery obstruction, chest trauma (Purtscher's retinopathy), anemia, leukemia, lymphoma.

Embolus
See Amaurosis Fugax, Section 12.6; Branch Retinal Artery Occlusion, Section 12.2; or Central Retinal Artery Occlusion, Section 12.1.

- Platelet-fibrin [dull gray and elongated (as opposed to round)]: Carotid disease.

❖ **Note** *Similar-appearing fibrin emboli also may arise from the heart.*

- Cholesterol (sparkling yellow, usually at an arterial bifurcation: Carotid disease).
- Calcium (dull white, typically around or on the disc: Cardiac disease).
- Cardiac myxoma (common in young patients, particularly in the left eye. Often occludes the ophthalmic or central retinal artery behind the globe and is not seen).
- Talc and cornstarch (small yellow–white glistening particles in macular arterioles. May produce peripheral retinal neovascularization: Intravenous (i.v.) drug abuse).
- Lipid or air [cotton-wool spots, not emboli, are often seen. Results from chest trauma (Purtscher's retinopathy) and fracture of long bones].
- Others (tumors, parasites, other foreign bodies).

Macular Exudates
More common   Diabetes, choroidal (subretinal) neovascular membrane, hypertension.
Less common   Macroaneurysm, Coats' disease (children), peripheral retinal capillary hemangioma, retinal vein occlusion, papilledema, radiation.

Normal Fundus in the Presence of Decreased Vision
Retrobulbar optic neuritis, cone degenerations, Stargardt's disease/fundus flavimaculatus, other optic neuropathy (e.g., tumor, alcohol/tobacco), rod monochromatism, amblyopia, nonphysiologic visual loss.

Optociliary Shunt Vessels on the Disc
Orbital or intracranial tumor (especially meningioma), status post central retinal vein occlusion, chronic papilledema (e.g., pseudotumor cerebri), chronic open-angle glaucoma, optic nerve glioma.

Retinal Neovascularization
A. Posterior pole: Diabetes, following central retinal vein occlusion.
B. Peripheral: Sickle cell retinopathy, following branch retinal vein occlusion, diabetes, sarcoidosis, retinopathy of prematurity, emboliza-

tion from i.v. drug abuse, chronic uveitis, others (e.g., leukemia, anemia, Eales' disease).

Roth's Spots (Hemorrhages with White Centers)

More common   Leukemia, septic chorioretinitis (e.g., secondary to subacute bacterial endocarditis), diabetes.

Less common   Pernicious anemia (and rarely other forms of anemia), sickle-cell disease, scurvy, systemic lupus erythematosus, other collagen–vascular diseases.

Sheathing of Retinal Veins (Periphlebitis)

More common   Syphilis, sarcoidosis, pars planitis, sickle-cell disease.

Less common   Tuberculosis, multiple sclerosis, Eales' disease, viral retinitis [e.g., human immunodeficiency virus (HIV), herpes], Behçet's disease, fungal retinitis, septicemia, or bacteremia.

Tumor

See Malignant Melanoma of the Choroid, Section 8.3.

Glaucoma

Acute Increase in Intraocular Pressure

Acute angle-closure glaucoma, glaucomatocyclitic crisis (Posner–Schlossman syndrome), inflammatory open-angle glaucoma, malignant glaucoma, postoperative glaucoma, suprachoroidal hemorrhage, retrobulbar hemorrhage.

Iris

Iris Heterochromia (Irides of Different Colors)

A. Involved iris is lighter than normal: Congenital Horner's syndrome, Fuchs' heterochromic iridocyclitis (most), chronic uveitis, juvenile xanthogranuloma, metastatic carcinoma, Waardenburg's syndrome (white forelock, decreased hearing, telecanthus).

B. Involved iris is darker than normal: Ocular melanocytosis or oculodermal melanocytosis, hemosiderosis, siderosis, retained intraocular foreign body, ocular malignant melanoma, diffuse iris nevus, retinoblastoma, leukemia, lymphoma, ICE syndrome, Fuchs' heterochromic iridocyclitis (some).

Iris Lesion

A. Melanotic (brown): Nevus, melanoma, adenoma, or adenocarcinoma of the iris pigment epithelium.

❖ **Note** *In heavily pigmented irides, cysts, foreign bodies, neurofibromas, and other lesions may appear pigmented.*

B. Amelanotic (white, yellow, or orange): Amelanotic melanoma, inflammatory nodule or granuloma (sarcoidosis, tuberculosis, leprosy, other granulomatous disease), neurofibroma, patchy hyperemia of syphilis, juvenile xanthogranuloma, foreign body, cyst, leiomyoma, seeding from a posterior segment tumor.

Neovascularization of the Iris
Diabetic retinopathy, central retinal vein or artery occlusion, branch retinal vein occlusion, ocular ischemic syndrome (carotid occlusive disease), chronic uveitis, chronic retinal detachment, intraocular tumor (e.g., retinoblastoma), other retinal vascular disease.

Lens

Iridescent Lens Particles
Drugs, hypocalcemia, myotonic dystrophy, familial, idiopathic.

Lenticonus
A. Anterior (marked convexity of the anterior lens): Rule out Alport's syndrome (hereditary nephritis).
B. Posterior (marked concavity of the posterior lens surface): Usually idiopathic; may be associated with persistent hyperplastic primary vitreous.

Neuroophthalmic Abnormalities

Afferent Pupillary Defect
A. Severe (2 to 3+): Optic nerve disease (e.g., ischemic optic neuropathy, optic neuritis, tumor, glaucoma); central retinal artery or vein occlusion; less commonly, a lesion of the optic chiasm/tract.
B. Mild (1+): Any of the above, amblyopia, vitreous hemorrhage, macular degeneration, branch retinal vein or artery occlusion, retinal detachment, or other retinal disease.

Anisocoria (Pupils of Different Sizes)
See Anisocoria, Section 11.1.

Limitation of Ocular Motility
A. With exophthalmos and resistance to retropulsion: See Orbital Disease, Section 7.1.

B. Without exophthalmos and resistance to retropulsion: Isolated third-, fourth-, or sixth-nerve palsy; multiple ocular motor nerve palsies (see Cavernous Sinus/Superior Orbital Fissure Syndrome, Section 11.9); myasthenia gravis; chronic progressive external ophthalmoplegia; orbital blow-out fracture with muscle entrapment; ophthalmoplegic migraine; Duane's syndrome; other central nervous system (CNS) disorders.

Optic Disc Atrophy

More common   Glaucoma; following central retinal vein or artery occlusion; ischemic optic neuropathy; chronic optic neuritis; chronic papilledema; compression of the optic nerve, chiasm, or tract by a tumor or aneurysm; traumatic optic neuropathy.

Less common   Syphilis, retinal degeneration (e.g., retinitis pigmentosa), toxic/metabolic optic neuropathy, Leber's optic atrophy, Leber's congenital amaurosis, retinal storage disease (e.g., Tay–Sachs), radiation neuropathy, other forms of congenital or hereditary optic atrophy (nystagmus almost always present in the congenital forms).

Optic Disc Swelling (Edema)

See Papilledema, Section 11.13.

Optociliary Shunt Vessels

See Fundus Findings in this chapter.

Paradoxic Pupillary Reaction (Pupil Dilates in Light and Constricts in Darkness)

Congenital stationary night blindness, cone dystrophy, optic neuritis, dominant optic atrophy. Rarely, amblyopia and strabismus.

Orbit

Extraocular Muscle Thickening on Computed Tomography Scan

More common   Thyroid orbitopathy, orbital inflammatory pseudotumor.

Less common   Tumor (especially lymphoma, metastasis, or spread of lacrimal gland tumor to muscle), carotid–cavernous fistula, cavernous hemangioma (usually appears in the muscle cone without muscle thickening), rhabdomyosarcoma (children).

Lacrimal Gland Lesions

See Lacrimal Gland Mass/Chronic Dacryoadenitis, Section 7.7.

Optic Nerve Lesion (Isolated)

More common   Optic nerve glioma (especially children), optic nerve meningioma (especially adults).

Less common   Metastasis, leukemia, orbital inflammatory pseudotumor, sarcoidosis, increased intracranial pressure with secondary optic nerve swelling.

Orbital Lesions/Proptosis
See Orbital Disease, Section 7.1.

Pediatrics

Leukocoria (White Pupillary Reflex)
See Leukocoria, Section 9.1.

Nystagmus in Infancy (See Section 11.19)
Congenital nystagmus, albinism, Leber's congenital amaurosis, CNS (thalamic) injury, spasmus nutans, optic nerve or chiasmal glioma, optic nerve hypoplasia, congenital cataracts, aniridia, congenital corneal opacities.

Postoperative Problems

Shallow Anterior Chamber
  A. Accompanied by increased intraocular pressure: Pupillary block glaucoma, suprachoroidal hemorrhage, malignant glaucoma.
  B. Accompanied by decreased intraocular pressure: Wound leak, choroidal detachment.

Hypotony
Wound leak, choroidal detachment, cyclodialysis cleft, retinal detachment, ciliary body shutdown, aqueous suppression caused by medication.

Refractive Problems

Progressive Hyperopia
Orbital tumor pressing on the posterior surface of the eye, serous elevation of the retina (e.g., central serous chorioretinopathy), posterior scleritis, presbyopia, hypoglycemia, cataracts.

Progressive Myopia
High (pathologic) myopia, diabetes, cataract, use of miotic drops, staphyloma and elongation of the globe, medications (e.g., sulfa drugs, tetracycline), childhood (physiologic).

Visual Field Abnormalities

Altitudinal Field Defect
  More common   Ischemic optic neuropathy, hemibranch retinal artery or vein occlusion.

Less common   Glaucoma, optic nerve or chiasmal lesion, optic nerve coloboma.

Arcuate Scotoma

More common   Glaucoma.

Less common   Ischemic optic neuropathy (especially nonarteritic), optic disc drusen, high myopia.

Binasal Field Defect

More common   Glaucoma, bitemporal retinal disease (e.g., retinitis pigmentosa).

Rare   Bilateral occipital disease, tumor or aneurysm compressing both optic nerves or chiasm.

Bitemporal Hemianopsia

More common   Chiasmal lesion (e.g., pituitary adenoma, meningioma, craniopharyngioma, aneurysm, glioma).

Less common   Tilted optic discs.

Rare   Nasal retinitis pigmentosa.

Blind-Spot Enlargement

Papilledema, glaucoma, optic nerve drusen, optic nerve coloboma, medullated nerve fibers off the disc, drugs, myopic disc with a crescent, others.

Central Scotoma

Macular disease; optic neuritis; ischemic optic neuropathy (more typically produces an altitudinal field defect); optic atrophy (e.g., from tumor compressing the nerve, toxic/metabolic disease); rarely, an occipital cortex lesion.

Homonymous Hemianopsia

Optic tract or lateral geniculate body lesion; temporal, parietal, or occipital lobe lesion of the brain (stroke and tumor more common; aneurysm and trauma less common). Migraine may cause a transient homonymous hemianopsia.

Constriction of the Peripheral Fields Leaving Only a Small Residual Central Field

Glaucoma; retinitis pigmentosa or some other peripheral retinal disorder; chronic papilledema; after panretinal photocoagulation; central retinal artery occlusion with cilioretinal artery sparing; bilateral occipital lobe infarction with macular sparing; nonphysiologic visual loss; carcinoma-associated retinopathy; rarely, drugs.

Vitreous

Vitreous Opacities

Asteroid hyalosis; synchysis scintillans; vitreous hemorrhage; inflammatory cells in vitritis or posterior uveitis; snowball opacities of pars planitis or sarcoidosis; normal vitreous strands from age-related vitreous degeneration; tumor cells; rarely, amyloidosis or Whipple's disease.

TRAUMA

3.1 CHEMICAL BURN

Treatment should be instituted IMMEDIATELY, even before testing vision.

❖ **Note** *This includes alkali (e.g., lye, cements, plasters), acids, solvents, detergents, and irritants (e.g., mace).*

Emergency Treatment
1. Copious irrigation of the eyes, preferably with saline or Ringer's lactate solution, for at least 30 minutes. However, if nonsterile water is the only liquid available, it should be used. Do not use acidic solutions to neutralize alkalis or vice versa. It is helpful to place an eyelid speculum and topical anesthetic (e.g., proparacaine) in the eye before irrigation. Pull down the lower eyelid and evert the upper eyelid, if possible, to irrigate the fornices. Manual use of intravenous (i.v.) tubing connected to an irrigation solution facilitates the irrigation process.
2. Five to ten minutes after ceasing irrigation (to allow equilibration), litmus paper should to touched to the inferior cul-de-sac. Irrigation should be continued until neutral pH is reached (i.e., 7.0).
3. Sweeping the conjunctival fornices with a moistened cotton-tipped applicator or glass rod for crystallized particles should be performed for a persistently elevated pH. Double eversion of eyelids with a Desmarres eyelid retractor may aid in removing particles in the deep fornix.

❖ **Note** *The volume of irrigation fluid required to reach neutral pH will vary with the chemical and with the duration of the chemical exposure. The vol-*

ume required may range from a few liters to several liters (>8–10). As stated earlier, irrigation should be continued until neutral pH is reached.

A. Mild-to-Moderate Burns

Critical Signs
Corneal epithelial defects range from scattered superficial punctate keratitis (SPK) to focal epithelial loss to sloughing of the entire epithelium. No significant areas of perilimbal ischemia are seen (no sign of interrupted blood flow through the conjunctival or episcleral vessels).

Other Signs
Focal areas of conjunctival chemosis, hyperemia, hemorrhages, or a combination of these; mild eyelid edema; mild anterior-chamber (AC) reaction; first- and second-degree burns of the periocular skin.

Workup
1. History: Time of injury? Chemical to which the patient was exposed? Duration of the exposure until irrigation was started? Duration of the irrigation?
2. Slit-lamp examination with fluorescein staining. Evert the eyelids to search for foreign bodies. Check the intraocular pressure (IOP).

❖ **Note** *In the presence of a distorted cornea, IOP may be most accurately measured with a Tono–pen or McKay–Marg tonometer.*

Treatment During and After Irrigation
1. Fornices should be thoroughly searched, including a sweep with a moistened cotton-tipped applicator or glass rod to remove any sequestered particles of caustic material and necrotic conjunctiva, which may contain residual chemicals. Calcium hydroxide particles may be more easily removed with a cotton-tipped applicator soaked in sodium ethylenediamine tetraacetic acid (EDTA).
2. Cycloplegic (e.g., scopolamine, 0.25%). Avoid phenylephrine because of its vasoconstrictive properties.
3. Topical antibiotic ointment (e.g., erythromycin) every 1–2 hours while awake or pressure patch for 24 hours.
4. Oral pain medication (e.g., acetaminophen with or without codeine) as needed. If IOP is increased, acetazolamide (e.g., Diamox) 250 mg p.o., q.i.d., or 500 mg sequel p.o., b.i.d., or methazolamide (e.g., Neptazane) 25–50 mg p.o., b.i.d.–t.i.d., may be given. Add a topical β-blocker (e.g., timolol, 0.5% b.i.d., or levobunolol 0.5% b.i.d.) if additional IOP control is required.

5. Frequent use of preservative-free artificial tears (e.g., q 1 h while awake) if not pressure patched.

Follow-up

Recheck and treat with antibiotic ointment plus a cycloplegic drop and repatching if desired every day until the corneal defect is healed. Watch for corneal ulceration and infection.

B. Severe Burns

Critical Signs

Pronounced chemosis and conjunctival blanching; corneal edema and opacification, sometimes with little to no view of the AC, iris, or lens; a moderate-to-severe AC reaction (may not be appreciated if the cornea is opaque).

Other Signs

Increased IOP, second- and third-degree burns of the surrounding skin, and local necrotic retinopathy as a result of direct penetration of alkali through the sclera.

❖ **Note** *If you suspect an epithelial defect but do not see one on fluorescein staining, repeat the fluorescein application to the eye. Sometimes the defect is slow to take up the dye. Occasionally the whole epithelium may slough off, leaving only Bowman's membrane, which may take up fluorescein poorly.*

Workup

Same as for mild-to-moderate burns (A).

Treatment After Irrigation

1. Admission to the hospital may be necessary for close monitoring of IOP and corneal healing.
2. Debride necrotic tissue containing foreign matter.
3. Cycloplegic (e.g., scopolamine, 0.25%, or atropine, 1%, 3–4 times per day). Avoid topical phenylephrine as it is a vasoconstrictor.
4. Topical antibiotic [e.g., trimethoprim/polymyxin (Polytrim) drops 4 times per day, erythromycin ointment 2–4 times per day].
5. Topical steroid (e.g., prednisolone acetate, 1%, or dexamethasone, 0.1%, 4–9 times per day) if significant inflammation of the AC or cornea is present. May use a combination antibiotic–steroid such as tobramycin–dexamethasone q 1–2 h.
6. Pressure patch between drops/ointment.

7. Antiglaucoma medications if the IOP is increased or cannot be determined. See the antiglaucoma recommendations earlier.
8. Lysis of conjunctival adhesions by using a glass rod or end of a thermometer covered with an antibiotic ointment, sweeping the fornices b.i.d. If symblepharons begin to form despite attempted lysis, consider using a scleral shell or ring to maintain the fornices.
    - Consider a therapeutic soft contact lens, collagen shield, or tarsorrhaphy (usually used if healing is delayed beyond 2 weeks).
    - If any melting of the cornea occurs, collagenase inhibitors may be used [e.g., acetylcysteine, 10–20% (Mucomyst) q 4 h].
    - If the melting progresses (or the cornea perforates), consider cyanoacrylate tissue adhesive. An emergency patch graft or corneal transplant may be necessary; however, the prognosis is better if this procedure is performed 12–18 months after the injury.
9. Frequent use of preservative-free artificial tears (e.g., q 1 h while awake).

Follow-up
These patients need to be monitored closely, either in the hospital or daily as outpatients. Topical steroids must be tapered after 7–10 days because they can promote corneal melting. Long-term use of artificial tears and lubricating ointment (e.g., Refresh Plus, q 1–6 h, and Refresh PM ointment, 1–4 times per day) may be required. A severely dry eye may require a tarsorrhaphy, conjunctival flap, or mucous membrane graft. A conjunctival transplant may be performed in unilateral injuries that fail to heal within several weeks to several months.

C. Super Glue

Rapid-setting super glues harden quickly on contact with moisture.

Treatment
1. Treat acid or basic pH as described earlier.
2. If the eyelids are glued together, they can be separated with gentle traction. Lashes may need to be cut to separate the eyelids. Misdirected lashes or hardened glue mechanically rubbing the cornea, as well as glue adherent to the cornea, should be carefully removed with fine forceps.
3 Resulting epithelial defects are treated as corneal abrasions (see Section 3.2, Corneal Abrasion).
4. Warm compresses q.i.d. may help remove any remaining glue stuck in the lashes that did not require removal.

Follow-up
Daily until corneal epithelial defects are healed.

3.2 Corneal Abrasion

Symptoms

Sharp pain, photophobia, foreign-body sensation, tearing, history of scratching the eye.

Critical Sign

Epithelial staining defect with fluorescein.

Other Signs

Conjunctival injection, swollen eyelid, mild anterior-chamber (AC) reaction.

Differential Diagnosis

- Recurrent erosion syndrome (See Recurrent Corneal Erosion, Section 4.6).
- Herpes simplex keratitis (See Herpes Simplex Virus, Section 4.15).

Workup

1. Slit-lamp examination: Use fluorescein, measure the size of the abrasion, diagram its location, and evaluate for an AC reaction. Evaluate for infiltrate, corneal laceration, or penetrating trauma.
2. Evert the eyelids to make certain no foreign body is present.

Treatment

1. Antibiotic
   a. Non–contact lens wearer: Antibiotic ointment (e.g., erythromycin or bacitracin, q 2–4 h) or antibiotic drops (e.g., polymyxin B/trimethoprim, q.i.d.)
   b. Contact lens wearer: must have antipseudomonal coverage. May use antibiotic ointment (e.g., tobramycin, q 2–4 h) or antibiotic drops (e.g., tobramycin, ofloxacin, or ciprofloxacin, q.i.d.).

❖ **Note** *Decision to use drop versus ointment depends on needs of the patient. Ointments offer better barrier function between eyelid and abrasion but tend to blur vision (not an issue if pain in so intense that the patient cannot open his or her eye). We prefer frequent ointments.*

2. Cycloplegic agent (e.g., cyclopentolate, 1% to 2%) for comfort from traumatic iritis, which may develop 24 to 72 hours after trauma. Avoid steroid use for iritis because it may retard epithelial healing and increase the risk of infection. Avoid use of long-acting cycloplegics for small abrasions.

3. Consider patching for comfort but do NOT patch if mechanism of injury involves vegetable matter, false fingernails, or if the patient wears contact lenses. We generally avoid patching, but encourage patients to keep eyes shut.
4. Consider topical nonsteroidal antiinflammatory drug (NSAID) drops (e.g., ketorolac, q.i.d., for 3 days) for pain control.
5. Consider debriding loose or hanging epithelium because it may inhibit healing.
6. NO contact lens wear. Some clinicians use bandage contact lenses for therapy. We do not.

Follow-up
A. Non–contact lens wearer
   1. If patched, patient should return in 24 hours for reevaluation or sooner if the symptoms worsen.
   2. Central or large corneal abrasion: Return the next day to determine if the epithelial defect is improving. If the abrasion is healing, may see 2 to 3 days later. Instruct the patient to return sooner if symptoms worsen. Revisit every 3 to 5 days until healed.
   3. Peripheral or small abrasion: Return 2 to 5 days later. Instruct the patient to return sooner if symptoms worsen. Revisit every 3 to 5 days until healed.
B. Contact lens wearer
   Have the patient return every day until the epithelial defect resolves, and then treat with topical tobramycin, ofloxacin, or ciprofloxacin drops for 1 to 2 additional days. The patient may resume contact lens wear after the eye feels perfectly normal for a week without medication (also examine the lens for tears, scratches, protein build-up, and other defects).

❖ **Note** *If at any time a corneal infiltrate is observed, appropriate smears and cultures should be obtained, and more aggressive antibiotic therapy instituted (see Section 4.12, Infectious Corneal Infiltrate/Ulcer).*

3.3 CORNEAL AND CONJUNCTIVAL FOREIGN BODIES

Symptoms
Foreign-body sensation, tearing, history of a trauma.

Critical Sign
Conjunctival or corneal foreign body with or without rust ring.

Other Signs

Conjunctival injection, eyelid edema, mild anterior-chamber (AC) reaction, and superficial punctate keratitis (SPK). A small infiltrate may surround a corneal foreign body. This infiltrate is usually sterile. Linear, vertically oriented corneal scratches may indicate a foreign body under the upper eyelid.

Workup

1. History: Determine the mechanism of injury. Was the patient wearing safety goggles? Did the foreign body arise from metal striking metal, which may suggest an intraocular foreign body?
2. Document visual acuity before any procedure is performed. One or two drops of topical anesthesia may be necessary to control blepharospasm and pain.
3. Slit-lamp examination: Locate and assess the depth of the foreign body. Rule out self-sealing lacerations, iris tears, lens opacities, AC shallowing, and asymmetrically low intraocular pressure (IOP) in the involved eye. If there is no evidence of perforation, evert the eyelids and inspect the fornices for additional foreign bodies. Double everting the upper eyelid with a Desmarres lid retractor may be necessary. Carefully inspect a conjunctival laceration to rule out a scleral laceration or perforation. Measure the dimensions of any infiltrate, the degree of any AC reaction, and the IOP.
4. Dilate the eye and examine the vitreous and retina for a possible intraocular foreign body.
5. Consider a B-scan ultrasound, a computed tomography (CT) scan of the orbit (axial and coronal views, 1-mm cuts), and/or ultrasound biomicroscopy to exclude an intraocular or intraorbital foreign body. Avoid magnetic resonance imaging (MRI) if there is a history of possible metallic foreign body.

Treatment

A. Corneal Foreign Body
1. Apply topical anesthetic (e.g., proparacaine). Remove the corneal foreign body with a foreign-body spud or a 25-gauge needle at a slit lamp. Multiple superficial foreign bodies may be more easily removed by irrigation.
2. Remove the rust ring. This may require an ophthalmic drill. It is sometimes safer to leave a deep, central rust ring to allow time for the rust to migrate to the corneal surface, at which point, it can be more easily removed.
3. Measure the size of the resultant corneal epithelial defect.
4. Treat as for corneal abrasion (see Corneal Abrasion, Section 3.2).

B. Conjunctival Foreign Body
   1. Remove foreign body under topical anesthesia.
      a. Multiple or loose foreign bodies can often be removed with saline irrigation.
      b. A foreign body can be removed with a cotton-tipped applicator soaked in topical anesthetic or with fine forceps. For deeply embedded foreign bodies, consider pretreatment with a cotton-tipped applicator soaked in phenylephrine (e.g., Neo-Synephrine), 2.5%, to reduce conjunctival bleeding.
      c. Small, relatively inaccessible, buried subconjunctival foreign bodies may sometimes be left in the eye without harm. Occasionally they will surface with time, at which point they may be removed more easily.
   2. Sweep the conjunctival fornices with a glass rod or cotton-tipped applicator soaked with a topical anesthetic to catch any remaining pieces.

See Section 3.4 if there is a significant conjunctival laceration. If no laceration is noted:

   3. A topical antibiotic [e.g., erythromycin or bacitracin ointment, b.i.d., or trimethoprim/polymyxin (Polytrim) drops, q.i.d.] may be used.
   4. Artificial tears (Refresh, q.i.d. for 2 days) may be given for a mildly irritated eye.

Follow-up
   A. Corneal foreign body: Follow up as with corneal abrasion (see Corneal Abrasion, Section 3.2). If residual rust ring remains, reevaluate in 24 hours.
   B. Conjunctival foreign body: Follow up as needed, or in 1 week if residual foreign bodies were left in the conjunctiva.

❖ **Note** *An infiltrate accompanied by a significant AC reaction, purulent discharge, or extreme redness and pain should be cultured to rule out an infection and treated with antibiotics more aggressively (see Infectious Corneal Infiltrate/Ulcer Section 4.12).*

3.4 CONJUNCTIVAL LACERATION

Symptoms
Mild pain, red eye, foreign-body sensation; usually, a history of ocular trauma.

Signs

Fluorescein staining of the conjunctiva, noted on examination of the eye with the cobalt blue light. With the white light, the conjunctiva can be seen to be torn and rolled up on itself; the exposed white sclera may be noted. Conjunctival and subconjunctival hemorrhages are often present.

Workup

1. History: Determine the nature of the trauma and whether a ruptured globe or intraocular or intraorbital foreign body may be present (e.g., metal striking metal or BB-gun injuries).
2. Complete ocular examination, including a careful exploration of the sclera [after topical anesthesia (e.g., proparacaine)] in the region of the conjunctival laceration to rule out a scleral laceration or a subconjunctival foreign body. The entire area of sclera under the conjunctival laceration must be inspected. Use a proparacaine-soaked sterile cotton-top applicator to manipulate the conjunctiva to rule out underlying scleral injury. Dilated fundus examination, especially the area underlying the conjunctival injury, must be carefully evaluated by indirect ophthalmoscopy.
3. Consider a computed tomography (CT) scan of the orbit (axial and coronal views, 1- to 3-mm cuts) to exclude an intraocular or intraorbital foreign body or a ruptured globe. A B-scan ultrasound or ultrasound biomicroscope may additionally be helpful.
4. Exploration of the site in the operating room under general anesthesia may be necessary when a ruptured globe is suspected.
5. Children often do not give an accurate history of trauma, and they must be questioned and examined carefully.

Treatment

In case of ruptured globe or penetrating ocular injury, see "Ruptured Globe and Penetrating Ocular Injury," Section 3.14.

1. Antibiotic ointment (e.g., erythromycin) t.i.d. for 4 to 7 days. A pressure patch can be used for the first 24 hours.
2. Large lacerations (> 1 to 1.5 cm) may be sutured [e.g., with 8-0 polyglactin 910 (e.g., Vicryl)], but most lacerations heal without surgical repair. When suturing, it is important not to bury folds of conjunctiva (e.g., by not correctly suturing the edges of the conjunctiva) nor to incorporate the tenons capsule in the wound. Additionally, avoid suturing the plica semilunaris or caruncle to the conjunctiva.

Follow-up

If there is no concomitant ocular damage, patients with large conjunctival lacerations are reexamined within 1 week; patients with small injuries are seen only as needed.

3.5 EYELID LACERATION

Symptoms
  Mild periorbital pain, epiphora.

Signs
  Superficial laceration/abrasion that may indicate a deep laceration.

Workup
  1. History: Determine mechanism of injury: bite, object with potential to leave a foreign body.
  2. Complete ocular examination including dilated fundus evaluation. Make sure there is no injury to the globe.
  3. Determination of the depth of the laceration, which can look deceptively superficial. We recommend using toothed forceps gently to pull open one edge of the wound to determine depth of penetration.
  4. Computed tomography (CT) scan of brain and orbit (axial and coronal views, 1- to 3-mm cuts) should be obtained when a foreign body or ruptured globe is suspected.
  5. If laceration is nasal to either upper or lower eyelid punctum, even if not obviously through the canalicular system (i.e., seems very superficial), perform punctal dilation and irrigation of canalicular system to exclude canalicular involvement.
  6. With uncooperative children, conscious sedation or an examination under anesthesia (EUA) may be necessary to fully examine the eyelids and globe.

Treatment
  Consider tetanus prophylaxis (see Appendix 10 for indications).

  A. Assess eyelid laceration. The following lacerations require repair in the operating room and are beyond the scope of this book.
     • Those associated with ocular trauma requiring surgery (e.g., ruptured globe or intraorbital foreign body).
     • Those involving the lacrimal drainage apparatus (i.e., punctum, canaliculus, common duct, or lacrimal sac), except when uncomplicated and near the punctum.
     • Those involving the levator aponeurosis of the upper eyelid (producing ptosis) or the superior rectus muscle; orbital fat is often exposed.
     • Those in which the medial canthal tendon is avulsed (exhibits a displaced medial canthus or abnormal laxity of the medial canthus).
     • Those that cause extensive tissue loss (especially more than one third of the eyelid) or severe distortion of anatomy.

B. Eyelid lacerations reparable in the office or emergency room.
1. Clean the area of injury and surrounding skin [e.g., povidone–iodine (Betadine)].
2. Give local subcutaneous anesthetic (e.g., 2% lidocaine with epinephrine).
3. Irrigate the wound thoroughly with saline in a syringe.
4. Search the wound carefully for foreign bodies, and remove them.

❖ **Note** *Lacerations resulting from human or animal bites or those otherwise with significant risk of contamination may require minimal debridement of necrotic tissue. Contaminated wounds may be left open for delayed repair, although some believe that the excellent blood supply of the eyelid allows primary repair. If electing primary repair, proceed to the subsequent steps.*

5. Isolate the surgical field with a sterile eye drape.
6. Place a drop of topical anesthetic (e.g., proparacaine) into the eye and a protective eye shell over the eye before suturing.
7. Lacerations involving the eyelid margin: Repair by using one of many methods. Figure 3-1 illustrates the method described.
   a. Place a 5-0 polyglactin 910 (e.g., Vicryl) suture on a spatulated needle through the tarsus on one side of the laceration, entering 3- to 4-mm deep to the eyelid margin; exit next to the eyelid margin. Enter the tarsus on the opposite side of the laceration next to the eyelid margin, and exit in the same vertical plane, 3- to 4-mm deep to the eyelid margin. Tie the suture. If the margin is well aligned, proceed to 7c.
   b. If the eyelid margin is not aligned after tying the suture, place a 6-0 silk vertical mattress suture (near-to-near, far-to-far) just anterior to the gray line. Near-to-near: enter the eyelid margin 1 mm from one edge of the laceration, exiting 1 mm from the edge of the laceration. Far-to-far: reenter the eyelid margin 2 to 3 mm from one edge of the laceration, and exit through the opposite side of the laceration 2 to 3 mm from the edge. Tie the suture, leaving the ends long, and incorporate the ends into the skin suture closest to the eyelid margin (see 7d).
   c. Use 5-0 polyglactin 910 sutures to close the subcutaneous tissues and remaining tarsus along the length of the laceration. Take a partial-thickness bite through tarsus on one side. Enter the tarsus on the opposite side of the laceration at the corresponding point, and exit in the same horizontal plane slightly anterior to the tarsus. Tie the suture, and repeat until the laceration is closed.

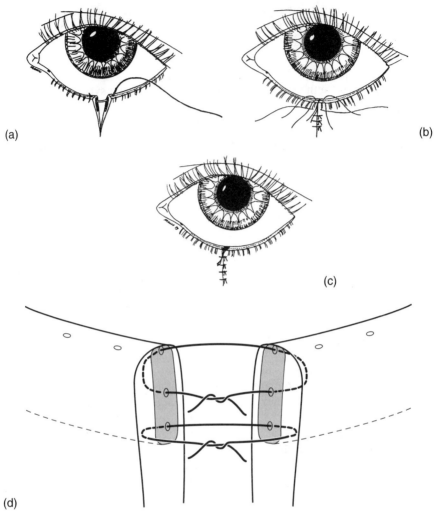

(a)

(b)

(c)

(d)

Figure 3-1.
Eyelid-margin repair. a: Suture 1 (see text). **b, c:** At the conclusion of the repair, the eyelid-margin sutures are tied under the knot of the skin suture closest to the eyelid margin. **d:** Eyelid margin repair (preferred method). See text.

d. Over the nonmarginal aspect of the laceration, close the skin with interrupted 6-0 plain gut suture.

8. Lacerations of the eyelid not involving the eyelid margin.
   a. If they are deep, place buried subcutaneous sutures by using 5-0 polyglactin 910. Take them from deep to superficial first, and then from superficial to deep on the opposite side.
   b. Close the skin, as in 7d.

9. Remove the protective eye shell.

10. Apply antibiotic ointment to the wound, b.i.d. (e.g., bacitracin).

11. Give systemic antibiotics if contamination is suspected [e.g., dicloxacillin or cephalexin, 250 to 500 mg, p.o., q.i.d. (adults); 25 to 50 mg/kg/day divided into four doses (children); for human or animal bites, consider penicillin V (same dose as dicloxacillin)]. Continue for 2- to 5-day course. In animal bites, also consider rabies prophylaxis if indicated.

❖ **Note** *Do not shave the eyebrow if it has been lacerated; in some cases, the hair will not grow back or will do so irregularly.*

Follow-up

The methods described use mostly absorbable sutures (except for the optional silk eyelid-margin suture described in 7b). If nonabsorbable sutures are used, eyelid-margin sutures should be left in place for 10 to 14 days, and other superficial sutures for 4 to 7 days.

3.6 TRAUMATIC IRITIS

Symptoms

Dull aching/throbbing pain, photophobia, tearing, onset of symptoms within 3 days of trauma.

Critical Signs

White blood cells and flare in the anterior chamber (AC) (seen under high-power magnification by focusing into the AC with a small, bright beam from the slit lamp).

Other Signs

Pain in the traumatized eye when a light is shined in either the nontraumatized or traumatized eye; lower (although sometimes higher) intraocular pressure (IOP), smaller pupil (which dilates poorly) or larger pupil (caused by iris sphincter tears) in the traumatized eye; perilimbal conjunctival injection; and sometimes, decreased vision.

Differential Diagnosis
- Traumatic corneal abrasion (Corneal epithelial defect that stains with fluorescein. May have an accompanying AC reaction. See Corneal Abrasion, Section 3.2).
- Traumatic microhyphema (Red blood cells suspended in the AC. Often accompanied by iritis. See Hyphema and Microhyphema, Section 3.7).
- Traumatic retinal detachment (May produce an AC reaction. May also see pigment in the anterior vitreous. A detachment is seen on dilated fundus examination. See Retinal Detachment, Section 12.19).
- Nongranulomatous anterior uveitis (No history of trauma, or the degree of trauma is not consistent with level of inflammation. See Anterior Uveitis, Section 13.1).

Workup
Complete ophthalmic examination, including IOP measurement and dilated fundus examination.

Treatment
Cycloplegic agent (e.g., cyclopentolate, 2%, q.i.d., or scopolamine, 0.25%, t.i.d.).

❖ **Note** *Some physicians also give a steroid drop (e.g., prednisolone acetate, 0.125% to 1%, q.i.d.); initially, we do not. Avoid steroid use if an epithelial defect is present.*

Follow-up
- Recheck in 5 to 7 days.
- If there is no improvement after 5 to 7 days, a steroid drop (e.g., prednisolone acetate, 1%, q.i.d.) may be given in addition to the cycloplegic agent.
- If resolved, the cycloplegic agent is discontinued.
- One month after trauma, examine the AC angle in both eyes by gonioscopy to look for angle recession. Also perform indirect ophthalmoscopy with scleral depression to detect retinal breaks or detachment.

3.7 HYPHEMA AND MICROHYPHEMA

Symptoms
Pain, blurred vision, history of blunt trauma.

Critical Signs

Blood in the anterior chamber (AC)

Hyphema: Layering or clot or both, usually visible grossly (without a slit lamp). A total (100%) hyphema may be black or red: when black, it is called an 8-ball or black hyphema; when red, the blood may settle out to be less than a 100% hyphema.

Microhyphema: Suspended red blood cells (RBCs) only, generally visible only with a slit lamp. Sometimes there may be enough suspended RBCs to see a haziness of the AC without a slit lamp—in these cases, the RBCs may settle out as a hyphema.

Workup

1. History: Mechanism (including force and direction) and exact time of injury; time of visual loss, if any. (Usually the visual loss occurs at the time of injury; decreasing vision over time suggests a rebleed or continued bleed.)
2. Complete ocular examination, first ruling out a ruptured globe (see Ruptured Globe and Penetrating Ocular Injury, Section 3.14). External and periocular examinations should be performed, evaluating for other traumatic injuries. Quantitate (percentage) and draw the extent and location of any clot; measure the intraocular pressure (IOP) and perform a dilated retinal evaluation, if possible. Do not perform scleral depression. Avoid gonioscopy unless intractable IOP increase develops. (If gonioscopy is necessary, use a Zeiss lens gently.) Consider a B-scan if a retinal detachment cannot be ruled out because of a poor view of the fundus. Also consider ultrasound biomicroscopy (UBM) to evaluate anterior segment/lens, if lens capsule rupture, foreign bodies, or other anterior segment abnormalities are suspected but not clearly visible.
3. Consider a computed tomography (CT) scan of the orbits and brain (axial and coronal views, with 1-mm cuts through the orbits), when indicated.
4. Black and Mediterranean patients should be screened for sickle cell trait or disease (order Sickledex; if necessary, may check hemoglobin electrophoresis).

Treatment

Many aspects remain controversial, including whether hospitalization and absolute bedrest are necessary. Consider hospitalization for noncompliant microhyphema patients, hyphema patients at high risk for secondary hemorrhage, and patients with other severe ocular or orbital injuries. In addition, consider hospitalization and generally more aggressive treatment for children, especially those at risk of amblyopia. Some studies suggested that the following are associated with a higher risk of poor outcome:

1. Poor visual acuity at presentation (worse than 20/200).
2. Sickle cell disease/trait with increased IOP.

3. Medically uncontrollable increased IOP.
4. Large initial hyphema size (>1/3 to 1/2).
5. Recent aspirin or nonsteroidal antiinflammatory drug (NSAID) use, especially in large amounts.
6. Delayed presentation to the ophthalmologist (often represents delayed visual deterioration or pain, as may occur with rebleeding or increased IOP).

For ALL PATIENTS
1. Confine either to bedrest with bathroom privileges or to limited activity. Elevate head 30 degrees (use pillows if not in hospital using an adjustable bed). No strenuous activity allowed.
2. Place a shield (metal or clear plastic) over the involved eye at all times. No eye patch because it prevents recognition of sudden visual loss in the event of a rebleed.
3. Atropine, 1% drops, 3 times a day, for hyphema patients, 1 to 2 times a day for microhyphema patients.
4. No aspirin-containing products or NSAIDs.
5. Mild analgesics only (e.g., acetaminophen). Avoid sedatives.
6. To prevent heavy, fibrinous AC reaction, or if the eye becomes photophobic, consider a topical steroid (e.g., prednisolone acetate, 1%, 4 to 8 times per day). Traumatic iritis symptoms and itching often develop 2 to 3 days after trauma.
7. For increased IOP:

❖ **Note** *Increased IOP, especially soon after trauma, may be transient, secondary to acute mechanical plugging of the trabecular meshwork. Elevating the patient's head may decrease the IOP by causing RBCs to settle inferiorly.*

Non–sickle cell disease/trait: (>30 mm Hg)
a. Start with β-blocker (e.g., timolol or levobunolol, 0.5%, b.i.d.).
b. If that is unsuccessful, add topical α-agonist (e.g., apraclonidine, 0.5%, or brimonidine, 0.2%, t.i.d.) or topical carbonic anhydrase inhibitor (e.g., dorzolamide, 2%, or brinzolamide, 1%, t.i.d.).
c. If still unsuccessful, add p.o. acetazolamide, 500 mg, q12 h, or mannitol, 1 to 2 g/kg i.v. over 45 minutes q24 h. (If mannitol is necessary to control the IOP, surgical evacuation may be an imminent necessity.)
Sickle cell disease/trait: (>24 mm Hg)
d. Start with β-blocker (e.g., timolol or levobunolol, 0.5%, b.i.d). All other agents must be used with extreme caution: topical dorzolamide and brinzolamide may reduce AC pH and induce sickling; topical α-agonists (e.g., brimonidine or apraclonidine) may affect iris vasculature; miotics and epinephrine are vasoactive and may

promote inflammation. Avoid latanaprost because it may promote inflammation.
  e. Try to avoid systemic diuretics as they promote sickling because of systemic acidosis and volume contraction. If a carbonic anhydrase inhibitor is necessary, use methazolamide, 50 mg, p.o. q8 h instead of acetazolamide, although this is also controversial. If mannitol is necessary to control the IOP, surgical evacuation may be an imminent necessity.
  f. AC paracentesis is safe and effective if IOP cannot be safely medically lowered. See Central Retinal Artery Occlusion, Section 12.1. This procedure is often only a temporizing measure, when the need for surgical evacuation is anticipated.
8. If admitting patient, see the following for hospitalized patients; for outpatients, see later for nonhospitalized patients.

For Hospitalized Patients
All previously mentioned treatment as well as:

1. Aminocaproic acid, 50 mg/kg, p.o., q4 h (maximum, 30 g per day). Aminocaproic acid may cause postural hypotension during the first 24 hours. It should not be used in pregnant patients or those with coagulopathies or renal disease, and it should be used with caution in patients with hepatic, cardiovascular, or cerebrovascular disease. [Pending Food and Drug administration (FDA) approval, aminocaproic topical gel may soon be available as an alternative that appears to have comparable efficacy and fewer side effects compared with the oral form, and which could be used on an outpatient basis.]
2. Antiemetics (e.g., prochlorperazine, 10 mg, i.m., q8 h or 25 mg, q12 h prn; under 12 years old, trimethobenzamide suppositories, 100 mg, q6 h prn.)
3. In hospital, check visual acuity and IOP, and perform a slit-lamp examination b.i.d. Look for new bleeding, increased IOP, corneal stromal blood staining, and other intraocular pathology as the blood clears (e.g., iridodialysis). Hemolysis, which may appear as bright red fluid, should be distinguished from a rebleed, which forms a new clot. If the IOP is increased, treat as previously described (see For All Patients), depending on the patient's age and the status of the optic nerve.
4. If a rebleed does not occur:
  a. Posttrauma day 2: decrease the dose of aminocaproic acid by one-half.

❖ **Note** *When the aminocaproic acid is decreased, fibrinolysis increases over the next 48 to 72 hours, which may result in increased IOP.*

Allow gradual increase in activity level (e.g., walking).

    b. Posttrauma day 3: discontinue oral aminocaproic acid and discharge if stable.
5. If there is a rebleed, continue the aminocaproic acid for an additional day. Check coagulation profile and aminocaproic acid dose. Patients rarely rebleed on the appropriate dose.
6. Surgical evacuation of hyphema may be indicated for the following: corneal stromal blood staining (surgery should be done urgently), significant visual deterioration, total filling of AC with blood, persistent clot packed in the angle for 7 days, or IOP increase despite maximal medical therapy (IOP, >50 for 5 days or >35 for 7 days).
7. On discharge, maintain patients with atropine, topical steroid, and any antiglaucoma medications, as listed, if needed. Instructions regarding activity should be given (see Follow-up).

For Nonhospitalized Patients
1. The patient should return daily for 3 days after initial trauma to check visual acuity and IOP, and for a slit-lamp examination. Look for new bleeding, increased IOP, corneal blood staining, and other intraocular pathology as the blood clears. Hemolysis, which may appear as bright red fluid, should be distinguished from a rebleed, which forms a new clot. If the IOP is increased, treat as described earlier (see For All Patients), depending on the patient's age and the status of the optic nerve.
2. The patient should be instructed to return immediately for reevaluation if a sudden increase in pain or decrease in vision is noted (which may be symptoms of a rebleed or secondary glaucoma).
3. If a rebleed or an intractable IOP increase occurs, the patient should be hospitalized.
4. After this initial close follow-up period, may maintain patient on atropine, 1% drops, 1 to 2 times a day, depending on severity of condition. Other instructions should be given as follows.
5. Prednisolone, 1%, q.i.d., if symptoms of traumatic uveitis exist.

Follow-up (Hospitalized and Nonhospitalized Patients)
1. Glasses or eye shield during the day and eye shield at night for 2 weeks following trauma, after which the patient should wear protective eyewear (polycarbonate lenses) any time the potential of an eye injury exists.
2. Have the patient refrain from strenuous physical activities (including bearing down or Valsalva maneuvers) for 2 weeks after the initial injury. The patient may resume normal activities after the initial 2 weeks from the date of injury.
3. Outpatient examinations after discharge (or after initial daily follow-up, for outpatients).

a. For hospitalized patients, 2 to 3 days after discharge; for non-hospitalized patients, several days to 1 week after initial daily follow-up period, depending on severity of condition (amount of blood, potential for IOP increases, other ocular or orbital pathology).
b. Two to four weeks after trauma for gonioscopy and dilated fundus examination with scleral depression for all patients.
c. Yearly because of the potential of developing angle-recession glaucoma.
d. If any complications arise, more frequent follow-up is required.
e. If filtering surgery was performed, the patient may be advised to refrain from strenuous physical activity for 4 to 8 weeks.

Nontraumatic (Spontaneous) and Postsurgical Hyphema or Microhyphema

Symptoms
May be seen as decreased vision or as transient visual loss (intermittent bleeding may cloud vision temporarily).

Etiology (of Spontaneous Hyphema or Microhyphema)
Must exclude the possibility of occult trauma.

- Neovascularization of the iris or AC angle (e.g. from diabetes, old central retinal vein occlusion, ocular ischemic syndrome, chronic uveitis).
- Blood dyscrasia.
- Iris–intraocular lens chafing.
- Other (e.g., leukemia, retinoblastoma, juvenile xanthogranuloma, child abuse).

Workup
1. Gonioscopy.
2. For spontaneous hemorrhages, may consider additional studies.
   a. Consider checking prothrombin time/partial thromboplastin time (PT/PTT), complete blood count (CBC) with platelet count, bleeding time, proteins C and S.
   b. Consider intravenous fluorescein angiogram (IVFA) of iris.

Treatment
Consider atropine, 1% drops, 1 to 3 times a day, limited activity, elevation of head of bed, avoidance of aspirin or NSAIDs. May recommend protective plastic or metal shield if etiology unclear. Monitor IOP. Postsurgical hyphemas and microhyphemas are usually self-limited and often require observation only, with close attention to IOP.

3.8 COMMOTIO RETINAE

Symptoms
Decreased vision or asymptomatic; history of recent ocular trauma.

Critical Signs
Confluent area of retinal whitening.

Other Signs
The retinal blood vessels are undisturbed in the area of retinal whitening. Other signs of ocular trauma may be noted.

Differential Diagnosis
- Retinal detachment (retinal vessels can be seen to rise upward with the detached retina. A retinal break or dialysis, anterior vitreous pigment, and an anterior-chamber (AC) reaction may be seen. See Retinal Detachment, Section 12.19).
- Branch retinal artery occlusion (Rarely follows trauma. Whitening of the retina with edema occurs along the distribution of an artery; cotton-wool spots, narrowed arterioles, and sludging of blood in the affected vessels may be seen. See Branch Retinal Artery Occlusion, Section 12.2).
- White without pressure (A common retinal anomaly unrelated to trauma. A prominent vitreous base is seen in the peripheral retina, often bilaterally).

Workup
Complete ophthalmic examination, including dilated fundus examination. Scleral depression is performed except when a hyphema, microhyphema, or iritis is present.

Treatment
No treatment is required, as this condition usually clears without therapy.

Follow-up
A dilated fundus examination is repeated in 1 to 2 weeks. Patients are instructed to return sooner if retinal-detachment symptoms are experienced (see Retinal Detachment, Section 12.19).

3.9 TRAUMATIC CHOROIDAL RUPTURE

Symptoms

Decreased vision or asymptomatic; history of ocular trauma.

Critical Signs

A yellow or white crescent-shaped subretinal streak, usually concentric to the optic disc. It may be single or multiple. Often the rupture cannot be seen until several days or weeks after trauma, as it may be obscured by overlying blood.

Other Signs

Rarely the rupture may be radially oriented. A choroidal neovascular membrane (CNVM) may later develop.

Differential Diagnosis

- Lacquer cracks of high myopia (Often bilateral. A tilted disc, a scleral crescent adjacent to the disc, or a posterior staphyloma also may be seen. A CNVM also may develop in this condition. See High Myopia, Section 12.12).
- Angioid streaks (Bilateral reddish brown or gray subretinal streaks that radiate out from the optic disc, sometimes associated with a CNVM. See Angioid Streaks, Section 12.13).

Workup

1. Complete ocular examination, including dilated fundus evaluation to detect a traumatic choroidal rupture. A CNVM is best seen with slit-lamp biomicroscopy with either a fundus contact or 60- or 90-diopter lens.
2. Consider fluorescein angiography to confirm the presence of a choroidal rupture or to delineate a CNVM.

Treatment

Laser therapy should be considered when a CNVM >200 μm from the center of the fovea is detected. Treatment should be applied within 72 hours of obtaining the fluorescein angiogram.

Follow-up

After ocular trauma, patients with hemorrhage obscuring the underlying choroid are reevaluated every 1 to 2 weeks until the choroid can be well visualized. If a choroidal rupture is present, patients are instructed in the use of an Amsler grid and asked to test themselves daily and return immediately if a change in the appearance of the grid is noted (see Appendix 3). Fundus examinations are performed every 6 to 12 months. Patients treated for a CNVM must be followed closely after treatment; watch for a persistent or new CNVM (see Age-Related Macular Degeneration, Section 12.10, for further follow-up guidelines).

3.10 ORBITAL BLOW-OUT FRACTURE

Symptoms

Pain (especially on attempted vertical eye movement), local tenderness, binocular double vision (the double vision disappears when one eye is covered), eyelid swelling and crepitus after nose blowing, recent history of trauma.

Critical Signs

Restricted eye movement (especially in upward or lateral gaze or both), subcutaneous or conjunctival emphysema, hypesthesia in the distribution of the infraorbital nerve (ipsilateral cheek and upper lip), palpable step-off along the orbital rim, point tenderness, enophthalmos (may initially be masked by orbital edema).

Other Signs

Nosebleed, eyelid edema and ecchymosis, and superior rim and orbital roof fractures may show hypesthesia in the distribution of the supratrochlear or supraorbital nerve (ipsilateral forehead), ptosis, point tenderness.

Differential Diagnosis

- Orbital edema and hemorrhage without a blow-out fracture (May have limitation of ocular movement, periorbital swelling, and ecchymosis, but these resolve over 7 to 10 days).
- Cranial-nerve palsy (Limitation of ocular movement, but no restriction on forced-duction testing).

Workup

1. Complete ophthalmologic examination, including measurement of extraocular movements and globe displacement. Compare the sensation of the affected cheek with that on the contralateral side; palpate the eyelids for crepitus (subcutaneous emphysema); and evaluate the globe carefully for a rupture, hyphema or microhyphema, traumatic iritis, and retinal or choroidal damage. Intraocular pressure (IOP) should be measured.
2. Forced-duction testing is performed if restriction of eye movement persists beyond 1 week (see Appendix 5).

3. Computed tomography (CT) scan of the orbits and brain (axial and coronal views, 3-mm cuts) is obtained if the diagnosis is uncertain, if surgical repair is being considered, or if an orbital roof fracture is suspected (upward-moving trauma).

Treatment

1. Nasal decongestants [e.g., pseudoephedrine (Afrin) nasal spray, b.i.d.] for 10 to 14 days.
2. Broad-spectrum oral antibiotics [e.g., cephalexin (Keflex) 250 to 500 mg, p.o., q.i.d., or erythromycin, 250 to 500 mg, p.o., q.i.d.] for 10 to 14 days.
3. Instruct the patient not to blow his or her nose.
4. Ice packs to the orbit for the first 24 to 48 hours.
5. Surgical repair at 7 to 14 days after trauma is undertaken if the patient has persistent diplopia when looking straight ahead or attempting to read, if he or she has cosmetically unacceptable enophthalmos, if a large fracture is present, or if the fracture is part of a complex trauma involving rim or zygomatic arch with displacement.
6. Neurosurgical consultation is recommended for most orbital roof fractures.

❖ **Note** *Some physicians use oral steroids initially to decrease the inflammatory reaction; generally, we do not. Some prefer immediate repair; we do not.*

Follow-up

Patients should be seen at 1 and 2 weeks after trauma and evaluated for persistent diplopia or enophthalmos after the acute orbital edema has subsided. The presence of these findings may indicate entrapment of the orbital contents or a large displaced fracture and the need for surgical repair. Patients should also be monitored for the development of associated ocular injuries (e.g, orbital cellulitis, angle-recession glaucoma, and retinal detachment). Gonioscopy of the anterior chamber (AC) angle and dilated retinal examination with scleral depression is performed 3 to 4 weeks after trauma. Warning symptoms of retinal detachment and orbital cellulitis are explained to the patient.

3.11 TRAUMATIC RETROBULBAR HEMORRHAGE

Symptoms

Pain, decreased vision, recent history of trauma or surgery to the eye or orbit.

Critical Signs

Proptosis with resistance to retropulsion, diffuse subconjunctival hemorrhage extending posteriorly.

Other Signs

Eyelid ecchymosis, chemosis, congested conjunctival vessels, increased intraocular pressure (IOP); sometimes, limited extraocular motility in any or all fields of gaze.

Differential Diagnosis

- Orbital cellulitis (Fever, proptosis, chemosis, limitation of eye movements with pain on motion; also may follow trauma, but generally not so acute. See Orbital Cellulitis, Section 7.4).
- Orbital fracture (blow-out, medial wall, or tripod fracture). (Limited extraocular motility, infraorbital hypesthesia, and crepitus. Enophthalmos, not proptosis, may be present. See Section 3.10).
- Ruptured globe (Subconjunctival edema and hemorrhage may mask a ruptured globe. A shallow or deep anterior chamber (as compared to the other eye), hyphema, and limitation of ocular motility are often present. Intraocular pressure (IOP) is commonly low, and there is usually no proptosis. See Ruptured Globe and Penetrating Ocular Injury, Section 3.14).
- Carotid–cavernous fistula (May follow trauma; pulsating exophthalmos, ocular bruit, corkscrew-arterialized conjunctival vessels, chemosis. IOP may be increased. Often bilateral involvement because of venous communications. See Cavernous Sinus/Superior Orbital Fissure Syndrome, Section 11.9).
- Varix (Increased proptosis with Valsalva maneuver. Is not usually seen acutely, and there is usually no history of trauma or surgery).

Workup

1. Complete ophthalmic examination; check specifically for an afferent pupillary defect, loss of color vision (color plates), increased or decreased IOP, pulsations of the central retinal artery, and choroidal folds (signs that vision is threatened). Pulsations of the central retinal artery often precede a central retinal artery occlusion.
2. Computed tomography (CT) scan of the orbit (axial and coronal views). The CT scan should be delayed until treatment has been instituted in cases in which vision is threatened.

Treatment

If IOP is increased (e.g., >30 mm Hg in a patient with a normal optic nerve or >20 mm Hg in a patient whose optic cup is very large and who normally has a lower IOP), any or all of the following methods are used to reduce the IOP. When vision is threatened, all of them are instituted immediately.

1. Oral carbonic anhydrase inhibitor (e.g., acetazolamide, 250 mg, p.o. ×2, simultaneously).
2. Topical β-blocker (e.g., timolol or levobunolol, 0.5%, q30 minutes ×2), α-agonist (e.g., brimonidine, 0.2%, q30 min ×2 doses), and/or topical carbonic anhydrase inhibitor (e.g., dorzolamide, 2%, or brinzolamide, 1%, q30 min ×2 doses).
3. Hyperosmotic agent (e.g., mannitol, 20%, 1 to 2 g/kg, i.v., over 45 minutes).

❖ **Note** *A 500-ml bag of mannitol, 20%, contains 100 g of mannitol.*

4. Lateral canthotomy and cantholysis (see Fig. 3-2). After local injection with xylocaine, 2%, with epinephrine, a hemostat is placed horizontally over the lateral canthus and clamped for 1 minute to compress the tissues and reduce bleeding. (a) The clamp is released, and sterile scissors are used to make a horizontal incision ~1 cm into the tissue compressed by the hemostat. (b) The skin and conjunctiva in the area of the incision are separated, and the scissors are placed between them to cut the inferior arm of the lateral canthal tendon. (c) Hemostasis is generally achieved with pressure. A sterile dressing is placed over the wound.

If IOP is not reduced or if vision is still threatened after this treatment, hospitalization is indicated. Emergency orbital decompression surgery may be required if the optic nerve becomes compromised, visual acuity decreases, or color vision is lost.

Follow-up
In cases in which vision is threatened, monitor the patient daily until stable. After the acute episode has resolved, reexamination should be performed every few weeks at first; watch for infection and abscess formation. Fibrosis may develop later, limiting extraocular motility.

3.12 INTRAORBITAL FOREIGN BODY

Symptoms
Decreased vision, pain, double vision, or may be asymptomatic; history of trauma (can be years before presentation).

Critical Signs
Orbital foreign body identified by radiograph, computed tomography (CT) scan, orbital ultrasound, or a combination of these.

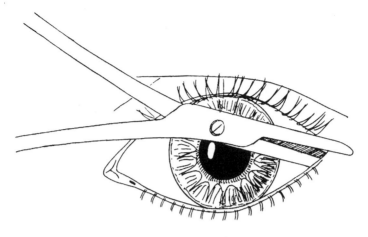

(a)

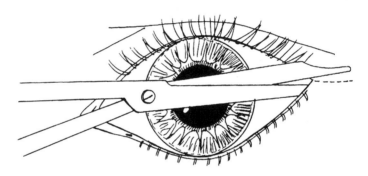

(b)

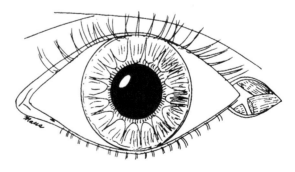

(c)

Figure 3-2.
a–b. Lateral canthotomy and cantholysis. See text.

Other Signs

A palpable orbital mass, limitation of ocular motility, proptosis; an eyelid or conjunctival laceration erythema, edema, or ecchymosis of eyelids. The presence of an afferent pupillary defect may indicate a traumatic optic neuropathy.

Types of Foreign Bodies

1. Poorly tolerated (often lead to inflammation): Organic (e.g., wood and vegetable matter) and sometimes copper foreign bodies.
2. Fairly well tolerated (typically produce a chronic low-grade inflammatory reaction): Copper alloys <85% copper (e.g., brass, bronze).
3. Well tolerated (inert): Stone, glass, plastic, iron, lead, steel, aluminum, and most other metals.

❖ **Note** *BBs and shotgun pellets are typically made of 80-90% lead and 10-20% iron.*

Workup

1. History: Determine the nature of the injury and the foreign body.
2. Complete ocular and periorbital examination, with special attention to pupillary reaction, intraocular pressure (IOP), and retinal evaluation. Examine carefully for an entry wound.
3. CT scan of the orbit and brain (axial and coronal views, 1-mm cuts of the orbit). Rule out a ruptured globe, determine the location of the intraorbital foreign body, and rule out optic nerve or CNS involvement. Magnetic resonance imaging (MRI) is contraindicated if a metal foreign body is suspected or cannot be excluded.
4. B-scan orbital ultrasound if a foreign body is suspected but not detected by CT scan.
5. Culture any drainage sites.

Indications for Surgical Exploration and Attempted Extraction of Foreign Body

1. Signs of infection (e.g., fever, proptosis, restricted motility, severe chemosis, a palpable orbital mass, an abscess on CT scan).
2. Fistula formation.
3. Signs of optic nerve compression.
4. The presence of a poorly tolerated intraorbital foreign body (see earlier) when it can be well localized.
5. A large or sharp-edged foreign body (independent of composition) that can be easily extracted.

Treatment

1. Tetanus toxoid prn (see Appendix 10).
2. Consider hospitalization, especially if surgery is contemplated. Management in the hospital:

    a. Administer systemic antibiotics promptly; suggest cefazolin, 1 g, i.v. q8 h for clean inert objects. If the object is contaminated, treat as orbital cellulitis (see Orbital Cellulitis, Section 7.4).

    b. Follow vision, assess degree (if any) of an afferent pupillary defect; evaluate motility, proptosis, and eye discomfort daily.

    c. Surgical exploration and removal of the foreign body when indicated.

    d. If the decision is made to leave the foreign body in place, discharge when stable with oral antibiotics (e.g., amoxicillin–clavulanate, 250 to 500 mg, p.o., q8 h) to complete a 10- to 14-day course.

3. Patients with small nonorganic foreign bodies not requiring surgical intervention may be discharged without hospitalization with oral antibiotics for 10- to 14-day course. Daily follow-up as described for hospitalized patients until stable.

Follow-up

After hospitalization or when stable, the patient is told to return in 1 week, or sooner if the condition worsens.

See Ruptured Globe and Penetrating Ocular Injury and Traumatic Optic Neuropathy, in this chapter, and Orbital Cellulitis, Section 7.4, as needed.

3.13 CORNEAL LACERATION

A. Partial-Thickness Laceration

The anterior chamber (AC) is not entered and, therefore, the cornea is not perforated.

Workup

1. Complete ocular examination; use a slit lamp carefully to exclude ocular penetration. Carefully inspect the cornea, conjunctiva, and sclera. Make sure the AC is deep and does not contain blood. Measure the intraocular pressure (IOP) by applanation tonometry only if the laceration site can be avoided (otherwise, use a Tono-pen or gently assess IOP with your fingers).

2. Seidel test (see Appendix 4). If Seidel's test is positive, a full-thickness laceration is present; see (B).

Treatment

1. A cycloplegic (e.g., scopolamine, 0.25%), and antibiotic (e.g., erythromycin ointment or gentamicin or ofloxacin drop), and a pressure patch.
2. Occasionally a bandage soft contact lens is used with an antibiotic drop (e.g., ofloxacin or gentamicin, q.i.d.) after cycloplegia, as described previously.
3. When a moderate-to-deep corneal laceration is accompanied by wound gape, it is often best to suture the wound closed in the operating room to avoid excessive scarring and corneal irregularity, especially in the visual axis.

Follow-up

Reevaluate daily, as described previously, until the epithelium heals.

B. Full-Thickness Laceration

See Ruptured Globe and Penetrating Ocular Injury, Section 3.14.

3.14 RUPTURED GLOBE AND PENETRATING OCULAR INJURY

Symptoms

Pain, decreased vision, history of trauma.

Critical Signs

1. Ruptured globe: Severe subconjunctival hemorrhage (often involves 360 degrees of bulbar conjunctiva), a deep or shallow anterior chamber (AC) compared with the contralateral eye, hyphema (often with clotted blood), limitation of extraocular motility (greatest in the direction of rupture), intraocular contents may be outside of the globe.
2. Penetrating injury: Full-thickness scleral or corneal laceration accompanying signs of a ruptured globe, history of a sharp object entering the globe.

Other Signs

Low intraocular pressure (IOP) (although it may be normal or increased), irregular pupil, iridodialysis, cyclodialysis, periorbital ecchymosis, dislocated or subluxed lens, commotio retinae, choroidal rupture, retinal breaks, vitreous hemorrhage, or traumatic optic neuropathy.

Workup/Treatment

Once the diagnosis of a ruptured globe or penetrating ocular injury is made by penlight or, if possible, by slit-lamp examination, further examination should be deferred until the time of surgical repair in the operating room to avoid placing any pressure on the globe and risking extrusion of the intraocular contents. The following measures should be taken:

1. Protect the eye with a shield.
2. No food or drink (NPO).
3. Systemic antibiotics [e.g., cefazolin, 1 g i.v., q8 h, and ciprofloxacin, 200 to 400 mg p.o./i.v., b.i.d. (adults); cefazolin, 25 to 50 mg/kg/day, i.v., in three divided doses, and gentamicin, 2 mg/kg i.v., q8 h (children)].*
4. Tetanus toxoid prn (see Appendix 10).
5. Antiemetic [e.g., prochlorperazine (Compazine), 10 mg, i.m., q8 h] prn to prevent Valsalva.
6. Bedrest with bathroom privileges.
7. Determine when the patient had his last meal. The timing of surgical repair is often influenced by this information.
8. Computed tomography (CT) scan (axial and coronal views) of the orbits and brain. B-scan ultrasound may be needed to localize the rupture site(s) and to rule out an intraocular or intraorbital foreign body. Ultrasound biomicroscopy may be helpful in some cases.
9. Arrange for surgical repair to be done as soon as possible.

❖ **Note** *In any severely traumatized eye in which there is no chance of restoring vision, enucleation should be considered initially or within 7 to 14 days after the trauma to prevent the rare occurrence of sympathetic ophthalmia.*

3.15 INTRAOCULAR FOREIGN BODY

Symptoms

Eye pain, decreased vision, or may be asymptomatic; often suggestive history (e.g., ocular foreign body after hammering metal).

Critical Signs

May have a clinically detectable corneal or scleral perforation site or an intraocular foreign body. Intraocular foreign bodies are usually seen on computed tomography (CT) scan, B-scan ultrasound, or both.

---

*Antibiotic doses may need to be reduced if renal function is impaired. Gentamicin peak and trough levels are obtained one-half hour before and after the fifth dose, and blood urea nitrogen and creatinine levels are evaluated every other day.

Other Signs

Microcystic (epithelial) edema of the peripheral cornea (a clue that a foreign body may be hidden in the anterior chamber (AC) angle in the same sector of the eye), an iris transillumination defect (see Workup), an irregular pupil, anterior or posterior segment inflammation or both, vitreous hemorrhage, decreased intraocular pressure (IOP). Long-standing iron-containing intraocular foreign bodies may cause siderosis, manifesting as anisocoria, heterochromia, corneal endothelial and epithelial deposits, anterior subcapsular cataracts, lens dislocation, and optic atrophy.

Types of Foreign Bodies

A. Frequently Produce Severe Inflammatory Reactions
   1. Magnetic: Iron and steel.
   2. Nonmagnetic: Copper and vegetable matter.
B. Typically Produce Mild Inflammatory Reactions When Left in the Eye
   1. Magnetic: Nickel.
   2. Nonmagnetic: Aluminum, mercury, and zinc.
C. Inert foreign bodies: Carbon, coal, glass, lead, plaster, platinum, porcelain, rubber, silver, and stone.

❖ **Notes** *Even inert foreign bodies can be toxic to the eye because of a coating or chemical additive. Most BBs and gunshot pellets are made of 80% to 90% lead and 10% to 20% iron.*

Workup

1. History: Composition of foreign body and time of last meal.
2. Ocular examination, including visual-acuity assessment and careful evaluation of whether the globe is intact. If there is an obvious perforation site, the remainder of the examination may be deferred until surgery. If there does not appear to be a risk of extrusion of the intraocular contents, the globe is inspected gently to localize the site of perforation and detect the foreign body.
   a. Slit-lamp examination; search the anterior chamber (AC) and iris for a foreign body and look for an iris transillumination defect (direct a small beam of light directly through the pupil and look at the iris for a red reflex penetrating through it). Examine the lens for disruption, cataract, or embedded foreign body. Check the IOP.
   b. Consider gonioscopy of the AC angle if no wound leak can be detected and the globe appears intact.
   c. Dilated retinal examination using indirect ophthalmoscopy.
3. Obtain a CT scan of the orbit and brain (coronal and axial views; magnetic resonance imaging (MRI) is contraindicated in the presence of a

metallic foreign body). It may be difficult to visualize wood, glass, or plastic on a CT scan.

4. B-scan ultrasound of the globe and orbit. (Note that intraocular air can mimic a foreign body).
5. Culture the object from which the foreign body arose, if possible. Culture the wound site, if it appears infected.
6. Determine whether the foreign body is magnetic (e.g., examine material from which the foreign body came).

Treatment
1. Hospitalization.
2. No food or drink (NPO).
3. Place a protective shield over the involved eye.
4. Tetanus prophylaxis as needed (see Appendix 10).
5. Antibiotics (e.g., vancomycin, 1 g i.v., q12 h, and ceftazidime, 1 g i.v., q12 h or ciprofloxacin, 750 mg p.o., q12 h.).*
6. Cycloplegic (e.g., atropine, 1%, t.i.d.) for posterior segment foreign bodies.
7. Surgical removal of an acute intraocular foreign body is usually advisable. For some metallic foreign bodies, a magnet may be useful during surgical extraction. Copper or contaminated foreign bodies may require especially urgent removal. A long-standing intraocular foreign body may require removal if associated with severe recurrent inflammation or if in the visual axis.

Follow-up
Observe the patient closely in the hospital for signs of inflammation or infection. Periodic follow-up for years is required; watch for a delayed inflammatory reaction. When an intraocular foreign body is left in place, an electroretinogram (ERG) should be obtained as soon as it can be done safely, and the patient should have serial ERGs performed to look for toxic retinal metallosis. If found, this retinal toxicity often reverses after the foreign body is removed.

3.16 TRAUMATIC OPTIC NEUROPATHY

Symptoms
Decreased vision after a traumatic injury to the eye or periocular area; other trauma symptoms (e.g., pain).

---

*Ciprofloxacin is contraindicated in children and pregnant women.

Critical Signs

A new afferent pupillary defect in a traumatized eye that cannot be accounted for by retinal or other ocular pathology (which would have to be severe).

Other Signs

Decreased color vision in the affected eye, a visual field defect, and other signs of trauma. Optic disc acutely appears normal in most cases.

❖ **Note** *Optic disc pallor usually does not appear for weeks after a traumatic optic nerve injury. If pallor is present immediately after trauma, a preexisting optic neuropathy should be suspected.*

Etiology

Shearing injury from blunt trauma; compression of the nerve by bone, hemorrhage, or perineural edema; laceration of the nerve by bone or an intraorbital foreign body (which may or may not still be present in the orbit).

Differential Diagnosis

(Other causes of a traumatic afferent pupillary defect)

- Severe retinal trauma (Retinal pathology evident on examination).
- Traumatic vitreous hemorrhage (Obscured retinal view on dilated fundus examination. The relative afferent pupillary defect is mild).
- Intracranial trauma with asymmetric damage to the optic chiasm.
- Functional/nonphysiologic visual loss (No afferent pupillary defect, must be a diagnosis of exclusion. See Section 11.22).

Workup

1. Complete ocular examination if a penetrating injury or ruptured globe is ruled out, and it is determined to be safe to examine the globe without risking extrusion of the intraocular contents. A pupillary evaluation is essential to diagnose a traumatic optic neuropathy.
2. Color vision testing in each eye (color plates).
3. Visual fields by confrontation. Formal visual-field testing may be deferred.
4. Computed tomography (CT) scan of the head and orbit (coronal and axial views) to rule out an intraorbital foreign body or a fracture through the optic canal. Thin cuts through the optic canal should be obtained.
5. B-scan ultrasound when a foreign body is suspected but not discovered by CT scan.

Treatment

1. Consider hospitalization in acute cases.
2. Systemic antibiotics in the presence of a sinus wall fracture or penetrating orbital injury (e.g., gentamicin, 2.0 mg/kg, i.v. load, and then 1

mg/kg, i.v., q8 h, and cefazolin, 1 g, i.v., q8 h, or clindamycin, 600 mg, i.v., q8 h).
- Consider i.v. steroids (e.g., methylprednisolone, 250 mg, i.v., q6 h for 12 doses, or megadose if vision is decreased significantly; loading dose is 30 mg/kg and then 5.4 mg/kg, q6 h for 48 hours) plus an H_2 antagonist (e.g., ranitidine, 150 mg, p.o., b.i.d.).
- Surgical intervention is indicated if vision is decreasing and there is an optic nerve canal fracture seen on CT scan. Endoscopic canal decompression is performed by an otorhinolaryngologist (ENT specialist).

Follow-up

Daily evaluate vision, pupillary reactions, and color vision. If vision deteriorates after discontinuing steroids, they should be reinstituted as previously described. If visual deterioration occurs despite steroids, surgery may be considered (controversial).

CORNEA

4.1 SUPERFICIAL PUNCTATE KERATITIS (SPK)

Symptoms
Pain, photophobia, red eye, foreign-body sensation.

Critical Signs
Pinpoint corneal epithelial defects (stain with fluorescein): may be confluent if severe.

Other Signs
Conjunctival injection, watery or mucoid discharge.

Etiology
SPK is nonspecific but is most commonly seen with the following disorders:

- Dry-eye syndrome (Poor tear lake or a decreased tear break-up time. See Section 4.2, Dry-Eye Syndrome)
- Blepharitis (Erythema, telangiectasias, and/or crusting of the eyelid margins, Meibomian gland dysfunction. See Section 5.10, Blepharitis/Meibomianitis)
- Trauma (Can occur from relatively mild trauma, such as chronic eye rubbing)
- Exposure keratopathy (Poor eyelid closure with failure to cover the entire globe. See Section 4.4, Exposure Keratopathy)
- Topical drug toxicity (e.g., neomycin, gentamicin, or any drops with preservatives, including artificial tears)
- Ultraviolet burn/photokeratopathy (Often in welders or from sun lamps. See Section 4.7, Thermal/Ultraviolet Keratopathy)
- Mild chemical injury (See Section 3.1, Chemical Burn)

- Contact lens–related disorder (e.g., chemical toxicity, tight-lens syndrome, contact lens overwear syndrome, giant papillary conjunctivitis. See Section 4.17, Contact Lens–Related Problems)
- Thygeson's SPK (Bilateral, recurrent SPK without conjunctival injection. See Section 4.8, Thygeson's Superficial Punctate Keratopathy)
- Foreign body under the upper eyelid (Typically linear SPK, fine scratches arranged vertically)
- Conjunctivitis (Discharge, conjunctival injection, eyelids stuck together on awakening. See Sections 5.1, Acute Conjunctivitis; 5.2, Chronic Conjunctivitis)
- Trichiasis/distichiasis (One or more eyelashes rubbing on the cornea. See Section 6.4, Trichiasis)
- Entropion or ectropion (Eyelid margin turned in or out. Area of SPK is superior or inferior. See Sections 6.2, Ectropion; 6.3, Entropion)
- Floppy eyelid syndrome (Extremely loose eyelids that pull away from the eye very easily. See Section 6.5, Floppy Eyelid Syndrome)

Workup

1. History: Trauma? Contact lens wear? Eyedrops? Discharge or eyelid matting? Chemical or UV exposure?
2. Evaluate the cornea and tear film. Evert the upper and lower eyelids, and look for a foreign body. Check eyelid closure and eyelid laxity, and look for inward-growing lashes.
3. Inspect contact lenses for fit (if still in the eye) and for the presence of deposits, sharp edges, and cracks.

❖ **Note** *A soft contact lens should be removed before placing fluorescein in the eye.*

Treatment

See the appropriate section to treat the underlying disorder. SPK is often treated nonspecifically as follows:

A. Non–contact lens wearer with a small amount of SPK
  1. Artificial tears q.i.d., preferably nonpreserved (e.g., Refresh Plus or Theratears) or neutral preservative (e.g., GenTeal or Refresh Tears).
  2. Can add a lubricating ointment qhs (e.g., Refresh PM).
B. Non–contact lens wearer with a large amount of SPK
  1. Antibiotic [e.g., erythromycin ointment 2 to 3 times per day or trimethoprim/polymyxin (e.g., Polytrim) drops q.i.d.] for 3 to 5 days.
  2. Consider a cycloplegic drop (e.g., cyclopentolate, 2%, or scopolamine, 0.25%) for relief of pain and photophobia.
  3. Optionally, pressure patch for the first 24 hours, after applying cycloplegic drop and antibiotic ointment.*

*Note: Although patching has not been shown in general to influence healing rate, it does prevent eye rubbing and increase comfort in some patients.

C. Contact lens wearer with a small amount of SPK
1. Artificial tears 4 to 6 times per day, preferably nonpreserved (e.g., Refresh Plus or Theratears).
2. Lenses may or may not be worn, depending on the symptoms and the degree of SPK.
D. Contact lens wearer with a large amount of SPK
1. Discontinue contact lens wear.
2. Fluoroquinolone [e.g., ofloxacin (e.g., Ocuflox), ciprofloxacin (e.g., Ciloxan)] or tobramycin drops 4 to 6 times per day, and tobramycin or ciprofloxacin ointment qhs.
3. Consider a cycloplegic drop (e.g., cyclopentolate, 2%, or scopolamine, 0.25%) for relief of pain and photophobia.

❖ **Note** *DO NOT patch contact lens–related epithelial defects.*

Follow-up
A. Non–contact lens wearers with SPK (especially traumatic SPK) are not seen again solely for the SPK unless the patient is a child or is unreliable. Reliable patients are told to return if their symptoms worsen or do not improve. When underlying ocular pathology is responsible for the SPK, follow-up is in accordance with the guidelines for the underlying problem (see the specific section).
B. Contact lens wearers with a large amount of SPK are seen every day until significant improvement is demonstrated. Contact lenses are not to be worn until the condition clears. The antibiotic may be discontinued when the SPK resolves. The patient's contact lens regimen (e.g., wearing time, cleaning routine) is corrected and/or the contact lenses are changed if either is thought to be responsible (see Section 4.17, Contact Lens–Related Problems). Contact lens wearers with a small amount of SPK are rechecked in several days to 1 week, depending on their symptoms and degree of SPK.

❖ **Note** *In general, contact lens wearers should not wear their lenses when their eyes feel irritated.*

4.2 DRY-EYE SYNDROME

Symptoms
Burning or foreign-body sensation, may have excess tearing, often exacerbated by smoke, wind, heat, low humidity, or prolonged use of the eye. Usually bilateral and chronic (although patients sometimes are seen with

recent onset in one eye). Often causes more discomfort than the clinical signs would suggest.

Critical Signs
(Either or both may be present.)

- Scanty tear meniscus seen at the inferior eyelid margin. The normal meniscus should be at least 1 mm in height and have a convex shape.
- Decreased tear break-up time (measured from a blink to the appearance of a tear film defect, by using fluorescein stain). Normally should be longer than 10 seconds.

Other Signs
Punctate corneal and/or conjunctival fluorescein or rose bengal staining, usually inferiorly or in the interpalpebral area. Excess mucus or debris in the tear film and filaments on the cornea may be found.

Differential Diagnosis
- Blepharitis (Eyelid margin crusting, thickening, erythema, and telangiectasias, often seen in combination with dry eyes. See Section 5.10, Blepharitis/Meibomianitis. May be associated with ocular rosacea. See Section 5.8, Ocular Rosacea.)
- Eyelid abnormality leading to exposure (exposure keratopathy). (Often secondary to a seventh-nerve palsy, trauma, a chemical or thermal burn, a congenital anomaly, senile ectropion, or other causes. See Section 4.4, Exposure Keratopathy.)
- Nocturnal lagophthalmos (Eyelids remain partially open while asleep.)

Etiology
- Idiopathic
- Collagen–vascular diseases (e.g., Sjögren's syndrome, rheumatoid arthritis, Wegener's granulomatosis, systemic lupus erythematosus)
- Conjunctival scarring (e.g., ocular cicatricial pemphigoid, Stevens–Johnson syndrome, trachoma, chemical burn)
- Drugs (e.g., oral contraceptives, antihistamines, β-blockers, phenothiazines, atropine)
- Infiltration of the lacrimal glands (e.g., sarcoidosis, tumor)
- Postradiation fibrosis of the lacrimal glands
- Vitamin A deficiency (Usually from malnutrition or intestinal malabsorption. See Section 14.10, Vitamin A Deficiency.)

Workup
1. History and external examination to detect underlying etiology.
2. Slit-lamp examination with fluorescein stain to examine the tear meniscus and tear break-up time. Use rose bengal or lissamine green stain to examine the cornea and conjunctiva.

3. Schirmer's test. Technique: Schirmer filter paper is placed at the junction of the middle and lateral one third of the lower eyelid in each eye for 5 minutes, after drying the eye of excess tears.
   a. Unanesthetized: Measures basal and reflex tearing. Normal, wetting of ≥ 15 mm in 5 minutes.
   b. Anesthetized: Topical anesthetic (e.g., proparacaine) is applied before drying the eye and placing filter paper. Measures basal tearing only. Normal, wetting of ≥ 10 mm in 5 minutes. We prefer the anesthetized method.

Treatment

MILD

Artificial tears q.i.d. (e.g., Refresh Tears, GenTeal, Hypo tears, Tears Naturale II)

MODERATE

1. Increase frequency of artificial tear application up to every 1 to 2 hours; use preservative-free artificial tears (e.g., Refresh Plus, Aquasite, Bion tears, Celluvisc).
2. Can add a lubricating ointment at bedtime (e.g., Refresh PM, Lacri-lube).
3. If these measures are inadequate or impractical, consider punctal occlusion with collagen inserts (temporary) or silicone plugs (reversible), occasionally followed by thermal punctal cautery (permanent) after a successful trial of the former.

SEVERE

1. Punctal occlusion, as described earlier (both lower and upper puncta if necessary) with preservative-free artificial tears up to every 1 to 2 hours as needed.
2. Add lubricating ointment (e.g., Refresh PM) 2 to 3 times per day during the daytime if needed.
3. Patch or moist chamber (plastic film sealed at orbital rim) with lubrication at night (may need to patch during the day pending more definitive treatment).
4. If mucus strands or filaments are present, remove with forceps and consider 10% acetylcysteine (e.g., Mucomyst) q.i.d.
5. Consider a lateral tarsorrhaphy if all of the previous measures fail. A temporary adhesive-tape tarsorrhaphy (to tape the lateral one third of the eyelid closed) can also be used, pending a surgical tarsorrhaphy.

❖ **Notes**
1. *In addition to treating the dry eye, treatment for contributing disorders (e.g., blepharitis, exposure keratopathy) should be instituted if these conditions are present.*

2. *Always use preservative-free artificial tears if using them more frequently than every 4 hours to prevent preservative toxicity.*
3. *If the history suggests the presence of a previously undiagnosed collagen–vascular disease (e.g., history of arthritic pain), referral should be made to an internist or rheumatologist for further evaluation.*

Follow-up
In days to weeks, depending on the severity of the drying changes and the symptoms. Anyone with severe dry eyes caused by an underlying chronic systemic disease (e.g., rheumatoid arthritis, sarcoidosis, ocular pemphigoid) may need to be monitored more closely.

❖ **Note** *Patients with significant dry eye should be discouraged from contact lens wear. Patients with Sjögren's syndrome have an increased incidence of lymphoma and mucous-membrane problems and may require internal medicine, rheumatologic, dental, and gynecologic follow-up.*

4.3 FILAMENTARY KERATOPATHY

Symptoms
Moderate-to-severe pain, red eye, foreign-body sensation, photophobia.

Critical Signs
Short strands of epithelial cells and mucus attached to the anterior surface of the cornea at one end of the strand. The strands stain with fluorescein.

Other Signs
Conjunctival injection, poor tear film, punctate epithelial defects.

Etiology
- Dry-eye syndrome (Most common cause. Can be associated with an autoimmune collagen–vascular disease such as Sjögren's syndrome. See Section 4.2, Dry-Eye Syndrome.)
- Superior limbic keratoconjunctivitis (Superior conjunctival injection and fluorescein staining, superior corneal pannus. See Section 5.5, Superior Limbic Keratoconjunctivitis.)
- Recurrent corneal erosions (Recurrent spontaneous corneal abrasions often occurring upon awakening. See Section 4.6, Recurrent Corneal Erosion.)
- Patching (e.g., postoperative, after corneal abrasions)

- Neurotrophic keratopathy (See Section 4.5, Neurotrophic Keratopathy)
- Chronic bullous keratopathy (See Section 4.28, Aphakic Bullous Keratopathy/Pseudophakic Bullous Keratopathy)

Workup
1. History, especially for the previously mentioned conditions.
2. Slit-lamp examination with fluorescein staining.

Treatment
1. Treat the underlying condition (see the specific sections).
2. Consider debridement of the filaments: After applying topical anesthesia (e.g., proparacaine), gently remove filaments at their base with fine forceps or a cotton-tipped applicator.
3. Lubrication with one of the following regimens
   a. Artificial tears (e.g., Refresh Plus or Theratears) 4 to 8 times per day and artificial-tear ointment (e.g., Refresh PM) qhs.
   b. Sodium chloride, 5%: drops q.i.d. and ointment qhs.
   c. Acetylcysteine, 10% (e.g., Mucomyst), q.i.d.
4. If the symptoms are severe or this treatment fails, then consider a bandage soft contact lens, unless the patient has severe dry eyes. Extended-wear bandage soft contact lenses may need to be worn for months.

Follow-up
In 1 to 4 weeks. If the condition is not improved, then consider or repeat the filament removal and/or apply a bandage soft contact lens if not yet tried. Lubrication must be maintained over the long term if the underlying condition cannot be eliminated.

4.4 EXPOSURE KERATOPATHY

Symptoms
Ocular irritation, burning, foreign-body sensation, and redness of one or both eyes. Usually worse in the morning.

Critical Signs
Inadequate blinking or closure of the eyelids, leading to corneal drying. Punctate epithelial defects are found on the lower one third of the cornea or as a horizontal band in the region of the palpebral fissure.

Other Signs
Conjunctival injection, corneal erosion, infiltrate or ulcer, eyelid deformity, or abnormal eyelid closure.

Etiology
- Seventh-nerve palsy [Orbicularis oculi weakness (e.g., Bell's palsy). See Section 11.8, Isolated Seventh-Nerve Palsy.]
- Eyelid deformity (e.g., ectropion or eyelid scarring from trauma, chemical burn, or herpes zoster ophthalmicus.)
- Nocturnal lagophthalmos (Failure to close the eyes during sleep.)
- Proptosis (e.g., due to an orbital process, such as thyroid eye disease. See Section 7.1, Orbital Disease.)
- After ptosis repair or blepharoplasty procedures.
- Floppy eyelid syndrome (See Section 6.5, Floppy Eyelid Syndrome)

Differential Diagnosis
See Section 4.1, Superficial Punctate Keratitis.

Workup
1. History: Previous Bell's palsy or eyelid surgery? Thyroid disease?
2. Evaluate eyelid closure and corneal exposure. Ask the patient to close his or her eyes gently (as if sleeping). Assess Bell's phenomenon. Check for eyelid laxity.
3. Slit-lamp examination: Evaluate the tear film and corneal integrity with fluorescein dye. Look for signs of secondary infection (corneal infiltrate, anterior-chamber reaction, severe conjunctival injection).
4. Investigate any underlying disorder (e.g., etiology of seventh-nerve palsy).

Treatment
In the presence of secondary corneal infection, see Section 4.12, Infectious Corneal Infiltrate/Ulcer.

1. Correct any underlying disorder.
2. Artificial tears (e.g., Refresh Plus, Theratears, or Celluvisc) q 1 to 6 h.
3. Lubricating ointment (e.g., Refresh PM) qhs or q.i.d.
4. Consider eyelid taping or patching at bedtime to maintain the eyelids in the closed position. If severe, consider taping the lateral one third of the eyelids closed (leaving the visual axis open) during the day. (Taping is rarely a definitive therapy, but may be tried when the underlying disorder is thought to be temporary.)
5. When maximal medical therapy fails to prevent progressive corneal deterioration, one of the following surgical procedures may be beneficial:

a. Eyelid reconstruction (e.g., for ectropion).
b. Tarsorrhaphy or eyelid gold-weight implant.
c. Orbital decompression (e.g., for proptosis).
d. Conjunctival flap (for severe corneal decompensation if above fail).

Follow-up
Reevaluate every 1 to 2 days in the presence of corneal ulceration. Less frequent examinations (e.g., in weeks to months) are required for less severe corneal pathology.

4.5 NEUROTROPHIC KERATOPATHY

Symptoms
Red eye, foreign-body sensation, swollen eyelid.

Critical Signs
Loss of corneal sensation, epithelial defects with fluorescein staining.

Other Signs
Early Perilimbal injection progressing to corneal punctate epithelial defects.
Late Corneal ulcer with associated iritis. The ulcer often has a gray, heaped-up border, tends to be in the lower one half of the cornea, and is oval.

Etiology
- Post infection with varicella-zoster or herpes simplex virus (HSV)
- Stroke
- Complication of trigeminal nerve surgery
- Complication of irradiation to the eye or an adnexal structure
- Tumor (especially an acoustic neuroma)

Differential Diagnosis
See Section 4.1, Superficial Punctate Keratitis.

Workup
1. History: Previous episodes of a red and painful eye (herpes)? Previous surgery, irradiation, stroke, or hearing problem?
2. Test corneal sensation bilaterally with a sterile cotton wisp (before topical anesthesia).
3. Slit-lamp examination with fluorescein staining.

4. Check the skin for herpetic lesions or scars from a previous herpes zoster infection.
5. Look for signs of a corneal exposure problem (e.g., inability to close an eyelid, seventh-nerve palsy, absent Bell's phenomenon).
6. If suspicious of a central nervous system (CNS) lesion, obtain a computed tomography (CT) scan (axial and coronal views) of the brain.

Treatment

Mild to moderate punctate epithelial staining   Artificial tears (e.g., Refresh Plus, Theratears, or Celluvisc) q 1 to 6 h and artificial-tear ointment (e.g., Refresh PM) qhs.

Small corneal epithelial defect   Antibiotic ointment (erythromycin or bacitracin) q.i.d. for 3 to 5 days or until resolved. Optional pressure patch for first day. Usually requires prolonged artificial-tear treatment, as described above.

Corneal ulcer   See Section 4.12 (Infectious Corneal Infiltrate/Ulcer) for the work-up and treatment of an infected ulcer. If the ulcer is sterile, then apply antibiotic ointment, cycloplegic drop, pressure patch, and reevaluate in 24 hours. Repeat procedure daily until healed. (Alternatively, antibiotic ointment every 2 hours without patching may be used.) A tarsorrhaphy, bandage soft contact lens, or conjunctival flap may be required.

❖ **Note** *Patients with neurotrophic keratopathy and corneal exposure often will not respond to treatment unless a tarsorrhaphy is performed (eyelids partly sewn together). A temporary adhesive-tape tarsorrhaphy (the lateral one third of the eyelid is taped closed) may be beneficial, pending more definitive treatment.*

Follow-up

Mild to moderate epithelial staining   In 3 to 7 days.

Corneal epithelial defect   Every 1 to 2 days until improvement demonstrated, and then every 3 to 5 days until resolved.

Corneal ulcer   Daily until significant improvement is demonstrated. Hospitalization is required for severe ulcers (see Section 4.12, Infectious Corneal Infiltrate/Ulcer).

4.6 Recurrent Corneal Erosion

Symptoms

Recurrent attacks of acute ocular pain, photophobia, and tearing, often at the time of awakening or during sleep when the eyelids are rubbed or opened; often a history of a prior corneal abrasion in the involved eye.

Critical Signs

Localized roughening of the corneal epithelium (fluorescein dye may lightly outline the area) or a corneal abrasion. Epithelial changes may resolve within hours of the onset of symptoms so that no abnormality is present when the patient is examined.

Other Signs

Corneal epithelial dots or small cysts (microcysts), a fingerprint pattern, or maplike lines may be seen in both eyes if anterior basement membrane (map–dot–fingerprint) dystrophy is the underlying problem.

Etiology

Damage to the corneal epithelium or epithelial basement membrane from one of the following:

- Anterior corneal dystrophy [e.g., anterior basement membrane (most common), Meesmann's, and Reis–Bückler's dystrophies]
- Previous traumatic corneal abrasion
- Stromal corneal dystrophy (Lattice, granular, and macular dystrophies)
- Keratorefractive, corneal transplant, or cataract surgery

Workup

1. History: Recent trauma? Previous corneal abrasion? Ocular surgery? Family history? (Corneal dystrophy)
2. Slit-lamp examination with fluorescein staining.

Treatment

1. Acute episode: A cycloplegic drop (e.g., cyclopentolate, 2%, or homatropine, 2%) is applied, and antibiotic ointment (e.g., erythromycin) is used 3 to 4 times per day. If the defect is large, a pressure patch may be placed.
2. After epithelial healing is complete: Artificial tears (e.g., Refresh Plus, Theratears, or Celluvisc) 4 to 8 times per day and artificial-tear ointment (e.g., Refresh PM) qhs for at least 3 months, or 5% sodium chloride drops 4 to 8 times per day and 5% sodium chloride ointment at bedtime for at least 3 months.
3. If the corneal epithelium is loose and heaped and is not healing, consider debridement of the abnormal epithelium. Apply a topical anesthetic (e.g., proparacaine), and use a sterile cotton-tipped applicator gently to remove the loose epithelium.
4. Erosions not responsive to the above treatment:
   a. Consider an extended-wear bandage soft contact lens for several months.
   b. Consider anterior stromal puncture (See Fig. 4-1). Generally used in extremely symptomatic, refractory cases, with erosions outside the visual axis. It can be performed with or without an intact

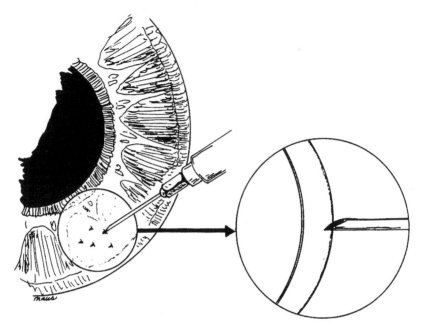

Figure 4-1
Anterior stromal puncture. In the area of the erosion, multiple superficial corneal punctures are made to the depth illustrated.

epithelium. The patient must be very cooperative. This treatment causes small permanent corneal scars.

Technique: Anesthetize the eye with a topical anesthetic (e.g., proparacaine). At the slit lamp, use a bent 25-gauge needle to perform multiple punctures into the superficial cornea through Bowman's membrane, just into the anterior stroma. Depending on the size of the erosion, between 20 and 150 punctures are placed close together until the entire area of the erosion has been punctured. A cycloplegic drop, antibiotic ointment, and optional pressure patch, as described earlier, are placed onto the eye after the procedure, and the patient is reexamined in 24 hours.

c. Epithelial debridement with diamond burr polishing of Bowman's membrane. Effective for large areas of epithelial irregularity and lesions in the visual axis.

d. Phototherapeutic keratectomy (PTK): Excimer laser ablation of the superficial stroma is successful in up to 90% of patients with recurrent erosions from corneal dystrophies.

Follow-up

Every 1 to 2 days until the epithelium has healed, and then every 1 to 6 months, depending on the severity and frequency of the episodes.

4.7 THERMAL/ULTRAVIOLET KERATOPATHY

Symptoms

Moderate-to-severe ocular pain, foreign-body sensation, red eye, tearing, photophobia, blurred vision; often a history of welding or using a sunlamp without protective eyewear. The symptoms are typically worst 6 to 12 hours after the exposure.

Critical Sign

Confluent punctate epithelial defects in an interpalpebral distribution seen with fluorescein staining.

Other Signs

Conjunctival injection, mild-to-moderate eyelid edema, mild-to-no corneal edema, and relatively miotic pupils that react sluggishly.

Differential Diagnosis

- Toxic epithelial keratopathy from exposure to a chemical (e.g., solvents, alcohol) or drug (e.g., neomycin, gentamicin, antiviral agents)
- Exposure keratopathy (Poor eyelid closure. See Section 4.4, Exposure Keratopathy)
- Nocturnal lagophthalmos (Eyelids remain partially open while asleep.)
- Floppy eyelid syndrome (Loose upper eyelids that evert easily during sleep. See Section 6.5, Floppy Eyelid Syndrome)

Workup

1. History: Welding? Sunlamp use? Topical medications? Chemical exposure? Prior episodes?
2. Slit-lamp examination: Use fluorescein stain. Evert the eyelids to search for a foreign body.
3. If chemical exposure suspected, check pH of tear lake in lower conjunctival fornix. If not neutral (6.8 to 7.5), treat as chemical burn (See Section 3.1, Chemical Burn).

Treatment

1. Cycloplegic drop (e.g., cyclopentolate, 2%, or scopolamine, 0.25%).
2. Antibiotic ointment (e.g., erythromycin or bacitracin) 3 to 4 times per day.
3. Optional pressure patch for 24 hours on the more severely affected eye.
4. Oral analgesics (e.g., acetaminophen with or without codeine) as needed.

Follow-up

Reliable patients are asked to assess their own symptoms after 24 hours (if a patch was placed, it is removed at this time).

- If much improved, the patient continues with topical antibiotics [e.g., erythromycin or bacitracin ointment 2 to 3 times per day, or trimethoprim/polymyxin (e.g., Polytrim) drops q.i.d. for 3 to 4 days.]
- If still significantly symptomatic, the patient should return for reevaluation. If significant punctate staining is still present, the patient is retreated with a cycloplegic, antibiotic, and possible pressure patch, as discussed previously.

Unreliable patients or those with an unclear etiology should be reexamined in 24 to 48 hours.

4.8 THYGESON'S SUPERFICIAL PUNCTATE KERATOPATHY

Symptoms

Foreign-body sensation, photophobia, tearing; no history of recent conjunctivitis. The disease is usually bilateral and has a chronic course with exacerbations and remissions.

Critical Sign

Coarse punctate to stellate gray–white corneal epithelial opacities, often central and slightly elevated with minimal-to-no staining with fluorescein.

Other Signs

No conjunctival injection, corneal edema, anterior-chamber reaction, or eyelid abnormalities.

Differential Diagnosis

See Section 4.1, Superficial Punctate Keratitis.

Treatment

MILD

1. Artificial tears (e.g., Refresh Tears, Refresh Plus, GenTeal, or Theratears) 4 to 8 times per day.
2. Artificial-tear ointment (e.g., Refresh PM) qhs.

1. Mild topical steroid (e.g., fluorometholone, 0.1%, q.i.d.) for 1 week. Then taper very slowly. May need prolonged low-dose topical steroid therapy.
2. If no improvement with topical steroids, a therapeutic soft contact lens can be tried.

Follow-up

Every week during an exacerbation, then every 3 to 12 months. Patients receiving topical steroids require periodic intraocular pressure checks.

4.9 PHLYCTENULOSIS

Symptoms

Tearing, irritation, pain, mild-to-severe photophobia; history of similar episodes. Corneal phlyctenules cause more severe symptoms than conjunctival phlyctenules.

Critical Signs

Conjunctival phlyctenule   A small, white nodule on the bulbar conjunctiva in the center of a hyperemic area. Often occurs at the limbus.

Corneal phlyctenule   A small, white nodule, initially at the limbus, with dilated conjunctival blood vessels bordering it. The phlyctenule may migrate toward the center of the cornea, producing wedge-shaped corneal neovascularization and ulceration behind the leading edge of the lesion. Can be bilateral.

Other Signs

Conjunctival injection, blepharitis, corneal scarring.

Etiology

Delayed hypersensitivity reaction usually as a result of one of the following:

- Staphylococcus (Often related to blepharitis. See Section 4.22, Staphylococcal Hypersensitivity.)
- Tuberculosis (TB)
- Rarely, another infectious agent (e.g., coccidioidomycosis, candidiasis, lymphogranuloma venereum)

Differential Diagnosis

- Inflamed pingueculum (Located within the palpebral fissure. Connective tissue is often seen to extend from the lesion to the limbus. Usually bilateral. See Section 4.10, Pterygium/Pingueculum.)
- Infectious corneal ulcer [Corneal phlyctenules that migrate from the limbus toward the center of the cornea may produce a sterile ulcer surrounded by a white infiltrate. When an infectious ulcer is suspected (e.g., increased pain, anterior-chamber reaction), appropriate diagnostic smears and cultures are necessary. See Section 4.12, Infectious Corneal Infiltrate/Ulcer.]
- Ocular rosacea (Corneal neovascularization with thinning and subepithelial infiltration may develop in an eye with rosacea. Telangiectasias, erythema, and/or pustules are found on the cheeks, nose, forehead, and eyelid margins. See Section 5.8, Ocular Rosacea.)
- Herpes simplex keratitis (May produce corneal neovascularization running into a stromal infiltrate. A history of recurrent herpes is often elicited. Usually unilateral. See Section 4.15, Herpes Simplex Virus.)

Workup

1. History: TB or recent infection?
2. Slit-lamp examination: Inspect the eyelid margin for signs of blepharitis and rosacea.
3. PPD (tuberculin skin test) with anergy panel in patients without blepharitis who have not had a positive PPD in the past.

❖ **Note** *The PPD should be read between 48 and 72 hours after placement. A positive reaction is defined as an area of skin induration (not just erythema) of more than a predetermined diameter (usually 10 mm). See Appendix 12.*

4. Chest x-ray if the PPD is positive or TB is suspected.

Treatment

Indicated for symptomatic patients.

1. Topical steroid (e.g., prednisolone acetate, 1%, 4 to 8 times per day, depending on severity of symptoms).
2. Eyelid hygiene 2 to 3 times per day for blepharitis (see Section 5.10, Blepharitis/Meibomianitis).
3. Artificial tears (e.g., Refresh Plus or Theratears) 4 to 6 times per day.
4. Antibiotic ointment at bedtime (e.g., bacitracin or erythromycin ointment).
5. In severe cases of blepharitis, use doxycycline, 100 mg p.o., b.i.d., or erythromycin, 250 mg p.o., q.i.d. (see Section 5.10, Blepharitis/Meibomianitis).

6. If the PPD or chest x-ray is positive for TB, then refer the patient to a medical internist or infectious disease specialist for appropriate treatment.
7. Penetrating keratoplasty may benefit patients with central corneal scarring from previous phlyctenules.

Follow-up

Recheck in several days. Healing occurs usually over a 10- to 14-day period with residual stromal scar. When the symptoms have significantly improved, start tapering the steroid. Maintain the antibiotic ointment as long as steroids are being used and for at least 2 to 3 weeks. Continue eyelid hygiene indefinitely and artificial tears as needed.

4.10 PTERYGIUM/PINGUECULUM

Symptoms

Irritation, redness, decreased vision; may be asymptomatic.

Critical Signs

Pterygium Wing-shaped fold of fibrovascular tissue arising from the interpalpebral conjunctiva and extending onto the cornea.

Pingueculum Yellow–white flat or slightly raised conjunctival lesion, usually in the interpalpebral fissure adjacent to the limbus, but not involving the cornea.

Other Signs

Either lesion may be highly vascularized and injected or may be associated with superficial punctate keratitis or dellen (thinning of the cornea secondary to drying). An iron line (Stocker's line) may be seen in the cornea central to a pterygium.

Etiology

Elastotic degeneration of deep conjunctival layers, possibly related to sunlight exposure and chronic irritation. More common in individuals from equatorial regions.

Differential Diagnosis

• Conjunctival intraepithelial neoplasia [Unilateral jellylike, velvety, or leukoplakic (white) mass, often elevated, vascularized, and not in a wing-shaped configuration. See Section 8.1, Conjuctival Tumors.]

- Limbal dermoid (Congenital rounded white lesion, usually at the infer-otemporal limbus. May be a manifestation of Goldenhar's syndrome if accompanied by preauricular skin tags and/or vertebral skeletal defects. See Section 8.1, Conjunctival Tumors.)
- Other conjunctival tumors (e.g., papilloma, nevus, melanoma. See Section 8.1, Conjunctival Tumors.)
- Pannus (Blood vessels growing into the cornea, often secondary to contact lens wear, blepharitis, ocular rosacea, herpes keratitis, phlyctenular keratitis, atopic disease, trachoma, and others. Usually at the level of Bowman's membrane with minimal to no elevation.)

Workup

Slit-lamp examination to identify the lesion and evaluate the adjacent corneal integrity and thickness.

Treatment

1. Protect the eyes from sun, dust, and wind (e.g., sunglasses or goggles if appropriate).
2. Lubrication with artificial tears (e.g., Refresh Plus or Theratears 4 to 8 times per day) to reduce ocular irritation.
3. For an inflamed pingueculum:
   a. Mild: A mild topical vasoconstrictor (e.g., naphazoline up to 3 to 4 times per day).
   b. Moderate-to-severe: A mild topical steroid (e.g., fluorometholone, 0.1%, 3 to 4 times per day). A topical nonsteroidal antiinflammatory medication [ketorolac (e.g., Acular) q.i.d.] can be added.
3. If a delle is present, then apply artificial-tear ointment (e.g., Refresh PM) and patch the eye for 24 hours.
4. Surgical removal is indicated when:
   a. The lesion is interfering with contact lens wear.
   b. The patient is experiencing excessive irritation not relieved by the previously mentioned treatment.
   c. The pterygium encroaches on the visual axis.

❖ **Note** *Pterygia frequently recur after surgical excision. Bare sclera dissection with a conjunctival autograft reduces the recurrence rate.*

Follow-up

Asymptomatic patients may be checked every 1 to 2 years.

- If treating with a topical vasoconstrictor, then the patient should be checked in 2 weeks. The vasoconstrictor drops should be tapered quickly when the inflammation has subsided.

- If treating with a topical steroid, then check every 1 to 2 weeks to monitor inflammation and intraocular pressure. Taper and discontinue the steroid drop over several weeks once the inflammation has abated. The nonsteroidal may be continued longer to help prevent recurrent inflammation.

4.11 BAND KERATOPATHY

Symptoms
Decreased vision, foreign-body sensation, white spot on the cornea; may be asymptomatic.

Critical Signs
Anterior corneal plaque of calcium at the level of Bowman's membrane within the interpalpebral fissure, separated from the limbus by clear cornea. Holes are often present in the plaque, giving it a Swiss-cheese appearance. The plaque usually begins at the 3- and 9-o'clock positions, adjacent to the limbus, and can extend across the cornea.

Other Signs
May have other signs of chronic eye disease.

Etiology
More common   Chronic uveitis (e.g., juvenile rheumatoid arthritis), interstitial keratitis, corneal edema, phthisis bulbi, long-standing glaucoma.

Less common   Hypercalcemia (may result from hyperparathyroidism, sarcoidosis, Paget's disease, vitamin D intoxication, and others), gout, corneal dystrophy, long-term exposure to irritants (e.g., mercury fumes), renal failure, and others.

Workup
1. History: Chronic eye disease? Chronic exposure to environmental irritants? Systemic disease?
2. Slit-lamp examination, intraocular pressure measurement, and optic-nerve evaluation.
3. If no signs of chronic anterior-segment disease or long-standing glaucoma are present and the band keratopathy cannot be accounted for, then consider the following work-up:
   a. Serum calcium, albumin, magnesium, phosphorus levels, blood urea nitrogen, and creatinine.
   b. Uric acid level if gout is suspected.

Treatment

MILD (I.E., FOREIGN-BODY SENSATION)

Artificial tears (e.g., Refresh Plus, Theratears, or Celluvisc) 4 to 6 times per day and artificial-tear ointment (e.g., Refresh PM) qhs.

SEVERE (E.G., OBSTRUCTION OF VISION, IRRITATION UNRELIEVED WITH LUBRICANTS, COSMETIC PROBLEM):

Remove the calcium at the slit lamp.

1. Dilute a solution of 15% disodium ethylenediamine tetraacetic acid (EDTA; e.g., Endrate) by mixing 2 ml of disodium EDTA with 8 ml of normal saline (0.9% NaCl). This gives a 3% mixture.
2. Anesthetize the eye with a topical anesthetic (e.g., cocaine 4% or proparacaine) and place an eyelid speculum.
3. Debride the corneal epithelium with a sterile scalpel or a sterile cotton-tipped applicator dipped in topical anesthetic.
4. Wipe a cellulose sponge or cotton swab saturated with the 3% disodium EDTA solution over the band keratopathy until the calcium clears (which may take 10 to 30 minutes).
5. Place an antibiotic ointment (e.g., erythromycin), a cycloplegic drop (e.g., cyclopentolate, 1% to 2%), and a pressure patch on the eye for 24 hours.
6. Consider giving the patient an analgesic (e.g., acetaminophen with or without codeine).

Follow-up
1. If surgical removal has been performed, then the patient should be examined every day with repatching (optional), an antibiotic, and a cycloplegic until the epithelial defect heals.
2. Residual anterior stromal scarring may be amenable to excimer laser phototherapeutic keratectomy.
3. The patient should be checked every 3 to 12 months, depending on the severity of symptoms. Surgical removal can be repeated if the band keratopathy recurs.

4.12 INFECTIOUS CORNEAL INFILTRATE/ULCER

Symptoms
Red eye, mild-to-severe ocular pain, photophobia, decreased vision, discharge.

Critical Signs

Focal white opacity (infiltrate) in the corneal stroma. An ulcer exists if there is also stromal loss with an overlying epithelial defect that stains with fluorescein.

❖ **Note** *An examiner using a slit beam cannot see through an infiltrate/ulcer to the iris, whereas stromal edema and inflammation are more transparent.*

Other Signs

Conjunctival injection, corneal thinning, stromal edema and inflammation surrounding the infiltrate, folds in Descemet's membrane, anterior-chamber reaction, hypopyon, mucopurulent discharge, upper eyelid edema. Posterior synechiae, hyphema, and glaucoma may occur in severe cases.

Etiology

- Bacterial (Most common infectious etiology. In general, corneal infections are assumed to be bacterial until proven otherwise by laboratory studies or until a therapeutic trial is unsuccessful.)
- Fungal [Must be considered after any traumatic corneal injury, particularly from vegetable matter (e.g., a tree branch). Infiltrates commonly have feathery borders and may be surrounded by satellite lesions. Candida infections tend to occur in diseased eyes. Hyphae or yeast may be evident on Giemsa stain, although they are also seen with Gomori methenamine silver stain. Most fungi grow on Sabouraud's dextrose agar. See Section 4.13, Fungal Keratitis.]
- Acanthamoeba [An extremely painful stromal infiltrate usually in a soft contact lens wearer who practices poor lens hygiene or has a history of swimming while wearing contact lenses. In the late stages, the infiltrate becomes ring-shaped. Acanthamoeba cysts may be seen with periodic acid–Schiff (PAS), Giemsa stain, or calcofluor white. This fastidious organism requires nonnutrient agar with *Escherichia coli* overlay for culture. See Section 4.14, Acanthamoeba.]
- Herpes simplex virus (HSV) (May have eyelid vesicles or corneal epithelial dendrites. A history of recurrent eye disease or known ocular herpes is common. Patients with chronic herpes simplex keratitis may develop bacterial superinfections. See Section 4.15, Herpes Simplex Virus.)
- Atypical mycobacteria (Usually follows ocular injuries or corneal grafts. Culture plates must be kept for 8 weeks.)

Differential Diagnosis

- Sterile ulcer (Not infectious; dry-eye syndrome, rheumatoid arthritis or other collagen-vascular diseases, vernal keratoconjunctivitis, neu-

rotrophic keratopathy, vitamin A deficiency, others. Cultures are negative, anterior-chamber inflammation is minimal to none, and the eye may be white and comfortable.)
- Staphylococcal hypersensitivity [Peripheral corneal infiltrate(s), sometimes with an overlying epithelial defect, usually multiple, often bilateral, with a clear space between the infiltrate and the limbus. There is minimal-to-no anterior-chamber reaction. Often with coexisting blepharitis. See Section 4.22, Staphylococcal Hypersensitivity.]
- Sterile corneal infiltrates from an immune reaction to contact lenses or solutions (Generally, multiple, small subepithelial infiltrates with an intact overlying epithelium and minimal-to-no anterior-chamber reaction. Usually a diagnosis of exclusion after ruling out an infectious process.)
- Residual corneal foreign body or rust ring (May be accompanied by corneal stromal inflammation, edema, and sometimes, a sterile infiltrate. There may be a mild anterior-chamber reaction. The infiltrate and inflammation generally clear after the foreign body is removed.)

Workup

1. History: Contact lens wear and lens-care regimen? Swim with lenses? Trauma or corneal foreign body? Eye care before visit (e.g., antibiotics or topical steroids)? Previous corneal disease? Systemic illness?
2. Slit-lamp examination: Stain with fluorescein to determine if there is epithelial loss overlying the infiltrate; document the size, depth, and location of the corneal infiltrate; assess the anterior-chamber reaction; and measure the intraocular pressure (IOP).
3. Corneal scrapings for smears and cultures are performed as described later for infiltrates considered to be infectious and for all ulcers. Small, nonstaining infiltrates are sometimes treated empirically with regular-strength broad-spectrum antibiotics without prior scraping.
4. In contact lens wearers suspected of having an infectious ulcer, the contact lenses and case are cultured if at all possible. Explain to the patient that the cultured contact lenses can never be worn again.

Culture Procedure

EQUIPMENT

Slit lamp; sterile Kimura spatula, knife blade, or moistened calcium alginate swab (i.e., with thioglycolate or trypticase soy broth); culture media; microscopy slides; alcohol lamp.

PROCEDURE

- Anesthetize the cornea with topical drops (proparacaine is best, as it appears to be less bacteriocidal than others.)
- At the slit lamp, scrape the base and the leading edge of the infiltrate firmly with the spatula, blade, or swab, and place the specimen on the

culture medium or slide. Sterilize the spatula over the flame of the alcohol lamp between each separate culture or slide. Be certain that the spatula-tip temperature has returned to normal before touching the cornea again.

MEDIA

Routine:

1. Blood agar (most bacteria)
2. Sabouraud's dextrose agar without cyclohexamide; place at room temperature (fungi)
3. Thioglycolate broth (aerobic and anaerobic bacteria)
4. Chocolate agar; place into a CO_2 jar (*Haemophilus* species, *Neisseria gonorrhoeae*)

Optional:

- Lowenstein–Jensen medium (mycobacteria, *Nocardia* species)
- Nonnutrient agar with *E. coli* overlay (acanthamoeba)
- Trypticase soy broth

SLIDES

Routine:

1. Gram's stain (bacteria, fungi)
2. Giemsa stain (bacteria, fungi, acanthamoeba)

Optional:

- Gomori methenamine silver stain, PAS stain (acanthamoeba, fungi)
- Acid-fast stain (mycobacteria, *Nocardia* species)
- Calcofluor white; a fluorescent microscope is needed (acanthamoeba, fungi)

❖ **Note** *When a fungal infection is suspected, deep scrapings into the base of the ulcer are essential. Sometimes a corneal biopsy is necessary to obtain diagnostic information.*

Treatment

As mentioned earlier, ulcers and infiltrates are generally treated as bacterial initially unless there is a high index of suspicion of another form of infection (see Fungal Keratitis, Section 4.13; Acanthamoeba, Section 4.14; and Herpes Simplex Virus, Section 4.15).

1. Cycloplegic (e.g., scopolamine, 0.25%, t.i.d., or atropine, 1%, t.i.d.).
2. Topical antibiotics according to the following algorithm:
    a. *Low risk of visual loss*
       Small nonstaining peripheral infiltrate with at most minimal anterior-chamber reaction and minimal discharge:

Non–contact lens wearer Broad-spectrum topical antibiotics (e.g., polymyxin B/bacitracin ointment q.i.d. or fluoroquinolone [ciprofloxacin or ofloxacin] drops q 2 to 6 h).

Contact lens wearer Tobramycin or fluoroquinolone (ciprofloxacin or ofloxacin) drops q 2 to 6 h; can add tobramycin or ciprofloxacin ointment qhs.

b. *Borderline risk*

Medium (1- to 1.5-mm diameter) peripheral infiltrate, or any smaller infiltrate with an associated epithelial defect, mild anterior chamber reaction, or moderate discharge:

Fluoroquinolone (ciprofloxacin or ofloxacin) every hour around the clock.

c. *Vision threatening*

Large (>1.5-mm diameter) staining infiltrate/ulcer, or any infiltrate with moderate-to-severe anterior-chamber reaction, purulent discharge, or involving the visual axis:

Fortified tobramycin or gentamicin (15 mg/ml) every hour alternating with fortified cefazolin (50 mg/ml) or vancomycin (25 mg/ml) every hour. (This means that the patient will be placing a drop in the eye every one-half hour around the clock.) (See Appendix 9 for directions on making fortified antibiotics.)

An alternative choice for smaller (<1.5 mm), peripheral staining infiltrates/ulcers is intensive topical fluoroquinolone therapy (ciprofloxacin or ofloxacin) 1 drop every 5 minutes for 3 doses, then every 15 minutes for 2 to 6 hours, then every 30 minutes around the clock.

3. Consider subconjunctival antibiotics [e.g., gentamicin (20 to 40 mg) and cefazolin (100 mg) or vancomycin (25 mg)] in very severe cases or when fortified antibiotics cannot be started within a short time. (See Appendix 7 for the injection technique.)

4. Eyes with corneal thinning should be protected by a shield without a patch (a patch is *never* placed over an eye thought to have an infection).

5. No contact lens wear.

6. Oral pain medication as needed (e.g., acetaminophen with or without codeine).

7. Oral fluoroquinolones (e.g., ciprofloxacin, 500 mg p.o., b.i.d.) penetrate the cornea well, and these may have added benefit for patients with scleral extension of infection or extremely deep ulcerations.

8. Admission to the hospital may be necessary if:
   • There is a sight-threatening infection.
   • The patient is unable to give him or herself the antibiotics at that frequency without difficulty.
   • There is a likelihood of noncompliance.

- The patient is unable or unwilling to return daily.
- Systemic antibiotics are needed (e.g., corneal perforation, scleral extension of the infection, gonococcal or *Haemophilus* infection)

9. For atypical mycobacteria, consider amikacin, 10 mg/ml drops, q 2 h for 1 week and then q.i.d. for 2 months (kanamycin or cefoxitin may be substituted).

Follow-up
- Daily evaluation at first, including repeated measurements of the size of the infiltrate and ulcer. The most important criteria in evaluating the response to treatment include the degree of eye pain, the size of the epithelial defect over the infiltrate, the size and depth of the infiltrate, and the anterior-chamber reaction. Less pain, a smaller epithelial defect and infiltrate, and a less-inflamed eye are all favorable responses. The IOP must be checked and glaucoma treated if present (see Section 10.4, Inflammatory Open-Angle Glaucoma).
- If the ulcer is improving, the antibiotic regimen is gradually tapered. Otherwise, the antibiotic regimen is adjusted according to the culture and sensitivity results.
- If the infiltrate or ulcer was not cultured originally and subsequently worsens, cultures, stains, and treatment with fortified antibiotics are needed. Hospitalization is considered.
- Reculture the ulcer (with the addition of optional media and stains) if it does not seem to be responding to the current antibiotic regimen and the original cultures are negative.
- A corneal biopsy may be required if the condition is worsening and infection is still suspected despite negative cultures.
- In an impending or completed corneal perforation, a corneal transplant or patch graft is considered. Cyanoacrylate tissue glue may also work in a treated corneal ulcer.

❖ **Note** *Outpatients are told to return immediately if the pain increases or the vision decreases.*

4.13 FUNGAL KERATITIS

Symptoms
Pain, photophobia, red eye, tearing, discharge, foreign-body sensation; a history of trauma, particularly with vegetable matter (e.g., a tree branch), or chronic eye disease.

Critical Signs

Corneal stromal gray–white opacity (infiltrate) with a feathery border. The epithelium over the infiltrate may be elevated above the remainder of the corneal surface, or there may be an epithelial defect with stromal thinning (ulcer).

Other Signs

Satellite lesions surrounding the primary infiltrate, conjunctival injection, mucopurulent discharge, anterior-chamber reaction, hypopyon.

Etiology

- Nonfilamentous fungi (typically *Candida* species). (Usually in previously unhealthy eyes.)
- Filamentous fungi (typically *Fusarium* or *Aspergillus* species). (Usually from trauma with vegetable matter.)

Differential Diagnosis

See Section 4.12, Infectious Corneal Infiltrate/Ulcer.

Workup

See Section 4.12 for complete work-up and culture procedure.

❖ Notes

1. *Be certain to obtain a Giemsa stain when a fungus is suspected (periodic acid-Schiff, Gomori methenamine silver, and calcofluor white stains also can be used), and scrape deep into the base of the ulcer for material.*
2. *If all cultures are negative, yet an infectious etiology is still suspected, consider a corneal biopsy to obtain further diagnostic information.*
3. *Consider irrigation of the lacrimal sac with culture of any reflux to rule out fungal dacryocystitis. If positive, a therapeutic dacryocystorhinostomy (DCR) may be required.*

Treatment

In general, corneal infiltrates and ulcers of unknown etiology are treated as bacterial until proven otherwise by laboratory studies (see Section 4.12, Infectious Corneal Infiltrate/Ulcer). If the stains and/or cultures indicate a fungal keratitis, institute the following measures:

1. Admission to the hospital is usually necessary, unless the patient is very reliable. It may take weeks to achieve complete healing.
2. Natamycin, 5% (50 mg/ml) drops, q 1 to 2 h while awake, q 2 h at night.
3. Cycloplegic (e.g., scopolamine, 0.25%, t.i.d.).
4. Treat glaucoma if present (see Section 10.4, Inflammatory Open-Angle Glaucoma).

5. No topical steroids. If the patient is currently taking steroids, they should be tapered rapidly.
6. No eye patch.
7. An eye shield, without a patch, may be advisable when the cornea is thinned.

If the infection involves the deep corneal stroma or is worsening despite appropriate treatment, one or more of the following medications may be added:

    a. Amphotericin B, 0.15% (1.5 mg/ml) drops q 1 h. (May be especially effective in *Candida* infections.)

    b. Itraconazole, 400 mg loading dose, then 200 mg p.o. qd. (Itraconazole has the highest corneal penetration of the available oral antifungal agents.)

    c. Miconazole or clotrimazole, 0.1% to 1.0% (1 to 10 mg/ml) drops, q 1 h. (Clotrimazole may be especially effective in Aspergillus infections.)

A corneal transplant may be necessary for a progressive fungal infection in a patient receiving maximal medical therapy. A corneal transplant or patch graft may also be required in an impending or complete corneal perforation.

❖ **Note** *Natamycin is the only commercially available topical antifungal; all others must be made from i.v. solutions with proper approval and sterile techniques. Other medications such as ketoconazole, fluconazole, nystatin, and flucytosine have been used either topically or systemically in recalcitrant fungal infections.*

Follow-up

Daily, as per Section 4.12, Infectious Corneal Infiltrate/Ulcer. The response to treatment is slower than in a bacterial infection. Lack of progression is a favorable sign.

4.14 ACANTHAMOEBA

Corneal infection with acanthamoeba should be considered in any patient with a history of soft contact lens wear, poor contact lens hygiene (e.g., using nonsterile homemade saline solutions to clean lenses, infrequent disinfection), and/or swimming or hot-tub use while wearing contact lenses. Heat disinfection and hydrogen peroxide systems with at least 2 hours contact time are effective in killing acanthamoeba cysts and trophozoites, whereas thimerosal, sorbic acid, EDTA, and quaternary ammonium compounds are mostly ineffective against acanthamoeba.

Symptoms

Severe ocular pain, redness, and photophobia over a period of several weeks.

Critical Signs

Early   Less corneal and anterior segment inflammation than would be expected for the degree of pain the patient is experiencing, epithelial and subepithelial infiltrates (sometimes along corneal nerves, producing a radial keratitis), pseudodendrites on the epithelium.

Late   A corneal stromal infiltrate in the shape of a ring.

❖ **Note** *Cultures for bacteria are negative, and the condition generally does not improve with antibiotic or antiviral medications.*

Other Signs

Eyelid swelling, conjunctival injection (especially circumcorneal), cells and flare in the anterior chamber. Generally little discharge or corneal vascularization. Corneal ulceration may occur later in the course.

Differential Diagnosis

- Herpes simplex keratitis (The patient often has a history of previous attacks in the same eye; typical branching corneal dendrites are common; the condition is much less painful than acanthamoeba; and multinucleated giant cells may be seen on Giemsa stain. See Section 4.15, Herpes Simplex Virus.)
- Fungal ulcer (Hyphae may be seen on histologic staining; fungi should grow on Sabouraud's dextrose agar. See Section 4.13, Fungal Keratitis.)
- Bacterial (e.g., *Pseudomonas* species) ulcer. (Much more acute course, over hours to days; should grow on bacterial culture and respond to fortified antibiotic drops. See Section 4.12, Infectious Corneal Infiltrate/Ulcer.)

Workup

See Section 4.12 for a general workup. The following are obtained when acanthamoeba is suspected:

1. Corneal scrapings for Giemsa, periodic acid-Schiff (PAS), and Gram's stains (Giemsa and PAS stains may show typical cysts).
2. Calcofluor white stain if available (requires a fluorescent microscope).
3. Culture on nonnutrient agar with *E. coli* overlay.

4. Consider a corneal biopsy if the stains and cultures are negative and the condition is not improving on the current regimen.
5. Consider cultures and smears of contact lens and case.

Treatment
The treatment of acanthamoeba is controversial and sometimes ineffective. The following are modes of therapy that have been found to be successful in many cases.

One or more of the following are generally used in combination, usually in the hospital initially:

1. Polymyxin/neomycin/gramicidin (e.g., Neosporin) drops, q 0.5 to 2 h.
2. Propamidine isethionate, 0.1% (e.g., Brolene) drops, q 0.5 to 2 h.
3. Itraconazole, 400 mg p.o. ×1 loading dose, and then 200 mg p.o. qd.
4. Polyhexamethyl biguanide, 0.02% (PHMB) drops, q 1 h.

Additional therapy includes clotrimazole, 1% drops, miconazole, 1% drops, or paromomycin drops, q 2 h. Dibromopropamidine isethionate 0.15% (e.g., Brolene) ointment is also available.

All patients:

5. Discontinue contact lens wear.
6. Cycloplegic (e.g., atropine, 1%, t.i.d.).
7. Oral nonsteroidal antiinflammatory agent (e.g., naproxen, 250 to 500 mg, p.o. b.i.d.) for pain and for scleritis if present. Additional oral analgesics (e.g., acetaminophen, codeine, oxycodone) if needed.

A corneal transplant may be indicated for medical failures, but this procedure can be complicated by recurrent infection.

Follow-up
Every day in the hospital until the condition is consistently improving. Medication may then be tapered judiciously and the patient checked as an outpatient. Treatment is usually continued for 6 to 8 weeks after resolution of inflammation, which may take up to 18 months in some cases.

❖ **Notes**
1. *Brolene is available in England and may be obtained in the U.S. with Food and Drug Administration (FDA) approval. Clotrimazole is not currently available as an ophthalmic suspension, but it can be formulated in artificial tears from a powder (with FDA approval). This solution must be shaken before each use.*
2. *Polyhexamethyl biguanide is available in the U.K. as Cosmocil; it can be prepared in the U.S. from Baquacil, a swimming pool disinfectant, on research protocol.*

4.15 HERPES SIMPLEX VIRUS

Symptoms

Red eye, pain, photophobia, tearing, decreased vision, skin (e.g., eyelid) rash; history of previous episodes; usually unilateral.

Signs

Any or all of the following may be present.

EYELID/SKIN INVOLVEMENT

Clear vesicles on an erythematous base that progress to crusting.

CONJUNCTIVITIS

Conjunctival injection with follicles and a palpable preauricular node.

CORNEAL EPITHELIAL DISEASE

May be seen as superficial punctate keratitis (SPK), stellate keratitis, dendritic keratitis (a thin, linear, branching lesion with club-shaped terminal bulbs at the end of each branch), or a geographic ulcer (a large, amoeba-shaped corneal ulcer with a dendritic edge). The edges of herpetic lesions are mildly heaped up with swollen epithelial cells that stain well with rose bengal; the central ulceration stains well with fluorescein. Corneal sensitivity may be decreased. Scars may develop underneath the epithelial lesions.

NEUROTROPHIC ULCER

A sterile ulcer with smooth epithelial margins over an area of interpalpebral stromal disease that persists despite antiviral therapy. May be associated with stromal melting and perforation.

CORNEAL STROMAL DISEASE

A. Disciform keratitis: Disc-shaped stromal edema with an intact epithelium. A mild iritis with localized granulomatous keratic precipitates is typical, and increased intraocular pressure (IOP) may be present. No necrosis or corneal neovascularization is present.
B. Necrotizing interstitial keratitis: Multiple or diffuse whitish gray corneal stromal infiltrates with an epithelial defect often accompanied by stromal inflammation, thinning, and neovascularization. Concomitant iritis, hypopyon, or glaucoma may be present. Bacterial superinfection must be ruled out.

UVEITIS

An anterior-chamber reaction may develop as a result of severe corneal stromal involvement. Less commonly, anterior-chamber reaction can develop without active corneal disease.

RETINITIS

Rare. In neonates, it is usually associated with a severe systemic herpes simplex virus (HSV) infection and is often bilateral.

Differential Diagnosis
(Conditions that produce dendritic-appearing corneal lesions)

- Herpes zoster virus (HZV; frequently painful skin vesicles are found along a dermatomal distribution of the face, not crossing the midline. Pain may be present before vesicles appear. The pseudodendrites in this condition are raised mucous plaques, do not have true terminal bulbs, and do not stain well with fluorescein. See Section 4.16, Herpes Zoster Virus.)
- Recurrent corneal erosion (A healing erosion often has a dendritiform appearance. Patients often provide a history of a corneal abrasion in the involved eye or have underlying anterior basement membrane dystrophy. Pain frequently develops on awakening from sleep. See Section 4.6, Recurrent Corneal Erosion.)
- Contact lens–related pseudodendrites (No skin involvement. Epithelial irregularities do not typically branch, do not have terminal bulbs, and stain minimally. See Section 4.17, Contact Lens–Related Problems.)
- Acanthamoeba keratitis pseudodendrites (History of soft contact lens wear, pain out of proportion to inflammation, chronic course. See Section 4.14, Acanthamoeba.)

Workup
1. History: Previous episodes? History of corneal abrasion; contact lens wear; or previous nasal, oral, or genital sores? Recent topical or systemic steroids? Immune deficiency state?
2. External examination: Note the distribution of skin vesicles if present.
3. Slit-lamp examination with IOP measurement.
4. Check corneal sensation before topical anesthetic.
5. Most cases of herpes simplex are diagnosed clinically and require no confirmatory laboratory tests. However, if the diagnosis is in doubt, any of the following tests may be supportive of the diagnosis:
   a. Scrapings of a corneal or skin lesion (scrape the edge of a corneal ulcer or the base of a skin lesion) for Giemsa stain, which shows multinucleated giant cells. (A Papanicolaou stain will show intranuclear eosinophilic inclusion bodies). Enzyme-linked immunosorbent assay (ELISA) testing also is available.
   b. Viral culture: A sterile, cotton-tipped applicator is used to swab the cornea, conjunctiva, or skin after unroofing vesicles with a sterile needle and is then placed into the viral transport medium.

❖ **Note** *Smears and cultures for bacteria should be taken if a corneal ulceration suddenly worsens. See Section 4.12, Infectious Corneal Infiltrate/ Ulcer.*

Treatment

EYELID/SKIN INVOLVEMENT

1. Antibiotic ointment (e.g., erythromycin or bacitracin) b.i.d. to the skin lesions. Topical acyclovir ointment, t.i.d., is an option, although it has not been proven effective.
2. Warm soaks to skin lesions, t.i.d.
3. If the eyelid margin is involved, add trifluorothymidine, 1% drops (e.g., Viroptic), or vidarabine, 3% ointment (good for small children; e.g., Vira-A), 5 times per day to the eye.

These medications are continued for 7 to 14 days until resolution of the symptoms.

❖ **Note** *Oral acyclovir, 400 mg p.o., 5 times per day for 7 to 14 days, is given by some physicians to adults suspected of having primary herpetic disease (e.g., flulike illness, fever, lymphadenopathy. Contraindicated in pregnancy and renal disease.)*

CONJUNCTIVITIS

Trifluorothymidine, 1% drops (e.g., Viroptic), or vidarabine, 3% ointment (e.g., Vira-A) 5 times per day. Discontinue the antiviral agent when the conjunctivitis has resolved after 7 to 14 days.

CORNEAL EPITHELIAL DISEASE

1. Trifluorothymidine, 1% drops (e.g., Viroptic), 9 times per day or vidarabine, 3% ointment (e.g., Vira-A), 5 times per day.
2. Cycloplegic agent (e.g., scopolamine, 0.25% t.i.d.) if an anterior-chamber reaction is present.
3. Patients taking topical steroids should have them tapered in the presence of corneal epithelial disease.
4. Consider gentle debridement of the infected epithelium as an adjunct to the antiviral agents.
   Technique: After topical anesthesia (e.g., proparacaine), a sterile, cotton-tipped applicator or semisharp instrument is used carefully to peel off the lesions at the slit lamp. After debridement, antiviral treatment should be instituted as described earlier.

❖ **Note** *Avoid debridement in children, in the presence of deep stromal lesions, or when a lesion has been previously treated with topical steroids.*

In epithelial defects that do not resolve after several weeks, antiviral toxicity and/or a neurotrophic ulcer should be suspected. At that point, the antiviral agent should be discontinued, and a nonpreserved artificial-tear ointment (e.g., Refresh PM) or an antibiotic ointment (e.g., erythromycin) should be used 2 to 8 times per day for several days with careful follow-up.

❖ **Note** *Oral acyclovir does not prevent stromal keratitis or iritis in patients with HSV epithelial keratitis.*

NEUROTROPHIC ULCER

See Section 4.5, Neurotrophic Keratopathy.

CORNEAL STROMAL DISEASE

A. Disciform keratitis
   Mild Cycloplegic (e.g., scopolamine, 0.25%, t.i.d.) alone.
   Severe and/or central (i.e., vision is reduced)
   1. Cycloplegic (e.g., scopolamine, 0.25%, t.i.d.).
   2. Topical steroid (e.g., prednisolone acetate, 1%, q.i.d.).
   3. Antiviral drops for prophylaxis (e.g., trifluorothymidine, 1%, 3 to 4 times per day).
   4. Adjunctive medications sometimes required include antibiotic prophylaxis (e.g., erythromycin ointment qhs) in the presence of epithelial defects, and aqueous suppressants (e.g., timolol, 0.5%, b.i.d.) for increased IOP.

❖ **Notes**
   1. *Topical steroids are contraindicated in those with corneal epithelial disease.*
   2. *Rarely a systemic steroid (e.g., prednisone, 60 to 80 mg, p.o. once a day tapered rapidly) is given to patients with severe stromal disease accompanied by an epithelial defect.*
   3. *Oral antivirals (e.g. acyclovir, famciclovir, and valacyclovir) have not been shown to be beneficial in the treatment of stromal disease but may be beneficial in herpetic iritis. (See Section 13.1, Anterior Uveitis)*

B. Necrotizing interstitial keratitis, treated as severe disciform keratitis. A corneal transplant may be required if the cornea perforates.

❖ **Note** *The persistence of an ulcer in the presence of stromal inflammation commonly is due to the underlying inflammation (requiring cautious steroid therapy); however, it may be due to antiviral toxicity. When an ulcer deepens, a new infiltrate develops, or the anterior-chamber reaction increases, smears and cultures should be taken for bacteria and fungi. (See Section 4.12, Infectious Corneal Infiltrate/Ulcer.)*

Follow-up

1. Patients are reexamined in 2 to 5 days to evaluate the response to treatment and then every 1 to 7 days, depending on the clinical findings. The following clinical parameters are evaluated: the size of the epithelial defect and ulcer, the corneal thickness and the depth to which the cornea is involved, the anterior-chamber reaction, and the IOP (see Section 10.4, Inflammatory Open-Angle Glaucoma, for glaucoma management).

2. Antiviral medications for corneal dendrites and geographic ulcers should be continued 5 to 9 times per day for 7 to 14 days and then tapered over 1 week.

3. Topical steroids used for corneal stromal disease are tapered slowly (often over months to years). The initial concentration of the steroid (e.g., prednisolone acetate 1%) is eventually reduced (e.g., prednisolone acetate 0.125%). Prophylactic antiviral agents are used t.i.d. No antiviral coverage is needed when the steroid is given once a day or less.

4. A corneal transplant may eventually be necessary in stromal disease if inactive postherpetic scars significantly affect vision.

❖ **Note** *Topical antivirals can cause a local toxic or allergic reaction (usually a papillary or follicular conjunctivitis). If such a reaction should occur, the antiviral agent should be replaced with another antiviral agent, because cross-reactivity is rare.*

4.16 HERPES ZOSTER VIRUS (HZV)

Symptoms

Skin rash, skin discomfort, and paresthesias. Headache, fever, malaise, blurred vision, eye pain, and red eye (may precede the skin rash).

Critical Sign

Acute vesicular skin rash that follows a dermatome of the fifth cranial nerve and can progress to scarring. Characteristically, the rash appears on one side of the forehead and scalp, does not cross the midline, and involves the upper eyelid only. Hutchinson's sign (rash in distribution of nasociliary branch of ophthalmic division) may predict higher risk of ocular involvement.

Other Signs

Less commonly, the rash involves the lower eyelid and cheek on one side, and rarely, one side of the jaw. Conjunctivitis, corneal involvement [e.g., multiple small epithelial dendrites early, followed by larger pseudodendrites (raised mucous plaques), superficial punctate keratitis (SPK), immune stromal keratitis, neurotrophic keratitis], uveitis, iris atrophy, scleritis, retinitis, choroiditis, optic neuritis, cranial nerve palsy, and glaucoma can occur. Late postherpetic neuralgia also may occur.

❖ **Note** *Corneal disease may follow the acute skin rash by many months to years. Occasionally it can precede the skin rash.*

Differential Diagnosis

- Herpes simplex virus (HSV) (The rash does not follow a dermatome nor obey the midline. Patients are often young. Corneal dendrites of HSV have true terminal bulbs and stain well with fluorescein; pseudodendrites of HZV generally appear stuck on the epithelium, do not have true terminal bulbs, and stain poorly with fluorescein. See Section 4.15, Herpes Simplex Virus.)

Workup

1. History: Duration of rash and pain? Immunocompromised or risk factors for acquired immunodeficiency syndrome (AIDS)?
2. Complete ocular examination, including a slit-lamp evaluation with fluorescein staining, intraocular pressure (IOP) check, and dilated optic nerve and retinal examination.
3. Systemic evaluation:
   a. Patients younger than 40 years: Medical evaluation to determine whether the patient may be immunocompromised.
   b. Patients aged 40 to 60 years: None (unless immunodeficiency is suspected from the history).
   c. Patients older than 60 years: If systemic steroid therapy is to be instituted, obtain a steroid workup as required. (See Drug Glossary for systemic steroid workup.)

❖ **Note** *Immunocompromised patients should not receive systemic steroids.*

Treatment

See Section 14.1, Acquired Immunodeficiency Syndrome, for the treatment of herpes zoster in immunocompromised patients.

SKIN INVOLVEMENT

A. Adults with an acute moderate to severe skin rash for less than 72 hours in which active skin lesions are present.
   1. Oral antiviral agent* (e.g., acyclovir, 800 mg p.o., 5 times per day; famciclovir, 500 mg t.i.d.; or valacyclovir, 1,000 mg p.o., t.i.d.) for 7 to 10 days; if the condition is severe or the patient is

---

*See Drug Glossary for systemic antiviral drug precautions.

systemically ill, hospitalize and prescribe acyclovir 5-10 mg/kg i.v., q 8 h, for 5 to 10 days.
2. Bacitracin or erythromycin ointment to the skin lesions b.i.d.
3. Warm compresses to periocular skin t.i.d. (to keep it clean).
B. Adults with a skin rash of more than 3 days' duration or without active skin lesions
1. Warm compresses to periocular skin t.i.d.
2. Bacitracin ointment to skin lesions b.i.d.
C. Children: Treat as in (B) unless there is evidence of systemic spread. For systemic spread, hospitalize and prescribe acyclovir 500 mg/m^2/day in three divided doses for 7 days.* The hospital pharmacy should have a conversion chart for height, weight, and surface area in square meters. The patient is usually transferred to the pediatric service.

OCULAR INVOLVEMENT

A. Conjunctival involvement: Cool compresses and erythromycin ointment to the eye b.i.d.
B. Corneal pseudodendrites or SPK: Lubrication with preservative-free artificial tears (e.g., Refresh Plus or Theratears) q 1 to 2 h and ointment (e.g., Refresh PM) qhs. Topical steroids (e.g., prednisolone acetate, 1%, q.i.d.) are occasionally helpful.
C. Immune stromal keratitis: Topical steroid (e.g., prednisolone acetate, 1%, q 1 to 6 h), tapering over months to years.
D. Uveitis (with or without immune stromal keratitis): Topical steroid (e.g., prednisolone acetate, 1%) q 1 to 6 h, cycloplegic (e.g., cyclopentolate, 1% to 2%, t.i.d.), and erythromycin ointment qhs. (See Section 13.1, Anterior Uveitis)
E. Neurotrophic keratitis: Treat mild epithelial defects with erythromycin or preservative-free artificial tear ointment q.i.d. If corneal ulceration occurs, obtain appropriate smears and cultures to rule out infection (see Section 4.12, Infectious Corneal Infiltrate/Ulcer). If the ulcer is sterile, consider a tarsorrhaphy or conjunctival flap when there is no response to ointment and patching. (See Section 4.5, Neurotrophic Keratopathy)
F. Scleritis: Treat as any other scleritis (see Section 5.7, Scleritis).
G. Retinitis, choroiditis, optic neuritis, or cranial-nerve palsy: Acyclovir, 5 to 10 mg/kg i.v., q 8 h for 1 week, and prednisone, 60 mg p.o., for 3 days, then tapering over 1 week.* Consider neurologic consultation to rule out CNS involvement.
H. Increased IOP: May be caused by the uveitis or steroids. If uveitis is present, increase the frequency of the steroid administration for a few days. If IOP remains increased, substitute fluorometholone, 0.1% (e.g., FML), rimexolone, 1% (e.g., Vexol), or loteprednol, 0.5% (e.g.,

---

*See Drug Glossary for systemic antiviral drug precautions.

Lotemax) drops for prednisolone acetate, and attempt to taper the dose. Topical aqueous suppressants (e.g., timolol, 0.5%, b.i.d., brimonidine, 0.2%, t.i.d., and/or dorzolamide, 2%, t.i.d.) will additionally help reduce IOP. (See Sections 10.4, Inflammatory Open-Angle Glaucoma, and 10.5, Steroid-Response Glaucoma.)

❖ **Note** *Pain may be severe during the first 2 weeks, and analgesics (e.g., acetaminophen with or without codeine) may be required. An antidepressant (e.g., amitryptyline, 25 mg p.o., t.i.d.) may be beneficial, as depression frequently develops during the acute phase of HZV infection. Antidepressants also may help postherpetic neuralgia. Capsaicin, 0.025% (e.g., Zostrix), or doxepin (e.g., Zonalon) ointment 3 to 4 times per day may be applied to the skin (not around the eyes) for postherpetic neuralgia after the initial skin lesions heal. Management of postherpetic neuralgia should involve the patient's primary medical doctor.*

Follow-up
If ocular involvement is present, examine the patient every 1 to 7 days, depending on the severity. Patients without ocular involvement can be followed up every 1 to 4 weeks. After the acute episode resolves, check the patient every 3 to 6 months, because relapses may occur months to years later, particularly as steroids are tapered. Systemic steroid administration requires collaboration with the patient's medical doctor.

❖ **Note** *HZV is contagious for children and adults who have not had chicken pox: it can be spread by inhalation. Pregnant women who have not had chicken pox must be especially careful to avoid contact with a herpes zoster patient.*

4.17 CONTACT LENS–RELATED PROBLEMS

Symptoms
Pain, photophobia, foreign-body sensation, decreased vision, red eye, itching.

❖ **Note** *Any contact lens wearer with pain or redness should remove the lens immediately and have a thorough ophthalmic examination as soon as possible.*

Signs
See the distinguishing characteristics of each etiology.

Etiology

- Corneal infiltrate/ulcer (bacterial, fungal, acanthamoeba). (White corneal lesion that may stain with fluorescein. Must always be ruled out in contact lens patients with eye pain. See Infectious Corneal Infiltrate/Ulcer, Section 4.12; Acanthamoeba, Section 4.14; and Fungal Keratitis, Section 4.13.)
- Giant papillary conjunctivitis (Itching, mucus discharge, and lens intolerance in a patient with large superior tarsal conjunctival papillae. See Section 4.18, Contact Lens–Induced Giant Papillary Conjunctivitis.)
- Hypersensitivity/toxicity reactions to preservatives in solutions [Conjunctival injection and ocular irritation typically develop shortly after lens cleaning and insertion, but can be present chronically. A recent change from one type or brand of solution to another often is elicited in the history. Commonly occurs in patients using older preserved solutions (e.g., thimerosal or chlorhexidine as a component), also occasionally with newer "all-purpose" solutions. May be due to inadequate rinsing of lenses after enzyme use. Signs include superficial punctate keratitis (SPK), conjunctival injection, bulbar conjunctival follicles, and subepithelial or stromal corneal infiltrates.]
- Contact lens deposits (Multiple small deposits on the contact lens, leading to corneal and conjunctival irritation. The contact lens is often old and may not have been cleaned or enzyme-treated properly in the past.)
- Tight-lens syndrome [Symptoms may be severe and often develop within 1 or 2 days of being fit with the responsible contact lens (usually a soft lens). The lens does not move with blinking and appears "sucked-on" to the cornea (this can occur after rewearing a soft lens that has dried out and then rehydrated). An imprint in the conjunctiva is often observed after the lens is removed. Corneal edema (usually anterior "brawny" edema), SPK, anterior-chamber reaction, and sometimes a sterile hypopyon may develop.]
- Corneal warpage [Seen predominantly in long-term polymethylmethacrylate (PMMA) hard contact lens wearers. Initially, the vision becomes blurred with glasses but remains good with contact lenses. Gradually, blurred vision and sometimes discomfort develop with contact lenses. There may or may not be SPK. Keratometry and computerized corneal topography reveal distorted mires.]
- Corneal neovascularization [Patients are often asymptomatic until the visual axis is involved. Superficial corneal neovascularization for 1 to 2 mm is common and generally not concerning in aphakic contact lens wearers (with the exception of post–corneal transplant patients, who are at a greater risk for graft rejection). Phakic and corneal transplant patients are generally treated.]
- Corneal epithelial changes (Range from epithelial thickening to pseudodendritic changes. Not infectious in origin, but rather a toxic/traumatic reaction to the contact lens.)

- Inadequate/incomplete blinking (Can lead to chronic inflammation and staining at the 3- and 9-o'clock positions.)
- Pseudosuperior limbic keratoconjunctivitis [Hyperemia and fluorescein staining of the superior bulbar conjunctiva, particularly at the limbus. Subepithelial infiltrates, haze, and irregularity may be found on the superior cornea. This may represent a hypersensitivity or toxicity reaction to a solution or contact lens–related product (especially thimerosal). Unlike superior limbic keratoconjunctivitis unassociated with contact lenses, there are no corneal filaments, papillary reaction, nor an association with thyroid disease.]
- Displaced contact lens (Most commonly the lens has actually fallen out of the eye and been lost, but if still present in the eye is usually found in the superior fornix. May require double-eversion of the upper eyelid to remove. Fluorescein will stain a soft lens to aid location.)
- Others [Contact lens inside out, corneal abrasion (see Section 3.2, Corneal Abrasion), poor lens fit, damaged contact lens, change in refractive error.]

Workup

1. History: What is the main complaint (severe pain, mild discomfort, itching)? What kind of contact lens does the patient wear (soft, hard, gas-permeable, daily-wear, extended-wear, or disposable)? How old are the lenses? For how many hours/days/weeks straight are the lenses worn? Does the patient sleep in lenses? How are the lenses cleaned and disinfected? Are enzyme tablets used? Are the products preservative-free? Any recent changes in contact lens habits or solutions?
2. In noninfectious conditions, while the contact lens is still in the eye, evaluate its fit and examine its surface for deposits and defects at the slit lamp.
3. Ocular examination, including slit-lamp examination with the contact lens in (if not too uncomfortable) to check fit. Then remove lens and examine the eye with fluorescein. Evert the upper eyelids of both eyes and inspect the superior tarsal conjunctiva for papillae.
4. Smears and cultures are taken when a corneal ulcer is suspected (see Infectious Corneal Infiltrate/Ulcer, Section 4.12; Acanthamoeba, Section 4.14; and Fungal Keratitis, Section 4.13).
5. The contact lenses and lens case are cultured, if possible, when an infectious corneal process is suspected.

Treatment

A. When the diagnosis of infection cannot be ruled out:
  1. Discontinue contact lens wear.
  2. Antibiotic treatment regimen varies with diagnosis as follows:
     - *Possible corneal ulcer* (corneal infiltrate, epithelial defect, anterior-chamber reaction, pain):

  a. Obtain appropriate smears and cultures.
  b. Start intensive topical antibiotics, either fortified or a fluoro-quinolone, and a cycloplegic (see Section 4.12, Infectious Corneal Infiltrate/Ulcer)
  • *Small subepithelial infiltrates, corneal abrasion, or diffuse SPK*
  a. Topical antibiotic (e.g., ofloxacin, or ciprofloxacin) drops 6 to 8 times per day and a cycloplegic.
  b. Can also add tobramycin or ciprofloxacin ointment qhs. Beware of toxicity with long-term use (especially tobramycin).
  3. Never pressure patch a contact lens wearer.
B. When a specific contact lens problem is suspected, it may be treated as follows:
  • Giant papillary conjunctivitis (see Contact Lens–Induced Giant Papillary Conjunctivitis, Section 4.18).
  • Hypersensitivity/toxicity reaction
    1. Discontinue contact lens wear.
    2. Preservative-free artificial tears (e.g., Refresh Plus or Theratears drops 4 to 6 times per day).
    3. New contact lenses and preservative-free solutions are used on resolution of the condition, and appropriate lens hygiene is explained.*
  • Contact lens deposits
    1. Discontinue contact lens wear.
    2. Replace with a new contact lens once the symptoms resolve. Consider changing the brand of contact lens, or to a planned replacement or disposable lens.
    3. Teach proper contact lens care, stressing weekly enzyme treatments for lenses replaced less frequently than every 2 weeks.
  • Tight-lens syndrome
    1. Discontinue contact lens wear.
    2. Consider a topical cycloplegic (e.g., scopolamine, 0.25%, t.i.d., or atropine, 1%, t.i.d.) in the presence of anterior-chamber reaction.

---

*The following regimen for contact lens care is one we recommend.

1. Daily cleaning and disinfection with removal of lenses while sleeping for all lens types, including those approved for "extended wear."
2. Daily cleaning regimen:
   a. Preservative-free daily cleaner (e.g., Miraflow),
   b. Preservative-free saline (e.g., Unisol),
   c. Disinfectant—preferably hydrogen peroxide type with a minimum 4-hour exposure time.
3. Weekly treatment with enzyme tablets (not necessary in disposable lenses replaced every 2 weeks or less).

3. Patients should be refit with a flatter contact lens after the symptoms and signs resolve.
4. If a soft lens has dried out, discard and refit.

❖ **Note** *Patients do not need to be cultured for their hypopyon when this syndrome is highly suspected.*

- Corneal warpage
  1. Discontinue contact lens wear (it is explained to patients that vision may be poor for the following 2 to 4 weeks).
  2. A gas-permeable hard contact lens should be fit when the refraction and keratometric readings have returned to normal (obtain the original keratometric readings).
- Corneal neovascularization
  1. Discontinue contact lens wear.
  2. Consider a topical steroid (e.g., prednisolone acetate, 1%, q.i.d.) for extensive neovascularization.
  3. Refit carefully with a highly oxygen transmissible daily-wear contact lens that moves adequately over the cornea.
- Corneal epithelial changes
  1. Discontinue contact lens wear.
  2. Consider a new contact lens when the epithelial changes resolve, which may take weeks or months.
  3. Use preservative-free solutions.
- Inadequate/incomplete blinking: Frequently apply preservative-free artificial tears (e.g., Refresh Plus or Theratears).
- Pseudosuperior limbic keratoconjunctivitis: Treated as described for hypersensitivity/toxicity reactions. When a large subepithelial opacity extends toward the visual axis, topical steroids may be added cautiously (e.g., prednisolone acetate, 1%, q 6 h), but they are often ineffective.
- Displaced lens: Inspect lens carefully for damage. If undamaged, clean and disinfect lens, then recheck fit when symptoms have resolved. If damaged, discard and refit.

Follow-up
- When a corneal infection cannot be ruled out, patients are reevaluated the following day. Treatment is maintained until the condition clears.
- In noninfectious conditions, patients are reevaluated in 1 to 4 weeks, depending on the clinical situation. Contact lens wear is resumed when the condition resolves. Patients using topical steroids should be followed up more closely and their intraocular pressure (IOP) monitored.

4.18 CONTACT LENS–INDUCED GIANT PAPILLARY CONJUNCTIVITIS

Symptoms

Itching, mucus discharge, decreased lens-wearing time, increased lens awareness, excessive lens movement.

Critical Sign

Giant papillae on the superior tarsal conjunctiva. (NOTE: The upper eyelid must be everted to make the diagnosis.)

Other Signs

Contact lens coatings, high-riding lens, ptosis, mild conjunctival injection.

Workup

1. History: Details of contact lens use, including age of lenses and cleaning and enzyme-treatment regimen.
2. Slit-lamp examination: Evert the upper eyelids and examine for large papillae.

Treatment

1. Start a topical mast cell stabilizer, either lodoxamide (e.g., Alomide) q.i.d., olopatadine (e.g., Patanol) b.i.d., or cromolyn sodium (e.g., Crolom or Opticrom) q.i.d.
2. Modify contact lens regimen as follows:
   - MILD TO MODERATE GIANT PAPILLARY CONJUNCTIVITIS (GPC)
     a. Replace the contact lens if it is older than 4 to 6 months or if it has numerous deposits. Refit with a new brand of soft contact lens (consider planned replacement or daily disposable lenses) or with a rigid gas-permeable (RGP) contact lens.
     b. Reduce contact lens wearing time (switch extended-wear contact lens patients to daily wear).
     c. Have the patient clean the lenses more thoroughly, preferably by using preservative-free solutions (e.g., Miraflow daily cleaner) and preservative-free saline (e.g., Unisol).
     d. Increase enzyme use (use at least every week).
   - SEVERE GPC
     a. Suspend contact lens wear.
     b. Restart with a new contact lens when the condition clears (usually 1 to 4 months), preferably with daily disposable soft or RGP lenses.
     c. Careful lens hygiene as explained earlier.

Follow-up
In 2 to 4 weeks. Mast cell stabilizers are continued or tapered slowly, depending on the clinical response.

❖ **Note** *GPC also can result from an exposed suture or ocular prosthesis. Exposed sutures are removed. Prostheses should be cleaned and polished. A coating (e.g., Biocoat) can be placed on the prosthesis to reduce GPC. Otherwise, these entities are treated as described earlier.*

4.19 INTERSTITIAL KERATITIS

Acute symptomatic interstitial keratitis (IK) most commonly occurs within the first or second decade of life. Signs of old IK often persist throughout life.

Acute Phase Symptoms
Pain, tearing, photophobia, red eye.

Critical Signs
Corneal stromal blood vessels and edema.

Other Signs
Anterior-chamber cells and flare, fine keratic precipitates on the corneal endothelium, conjunctival injection.

Signs of Old Disease
Deep corneal haze or scarring, often corneal stromal blood vessels containing minimal or no blood (ghost vessels), corneal stromal thinning.

Etiology
More common Congenital syphilis (usually affects both eyes within 1 year of each other).
Less common Acquired syphilis (unilateral, often sectorial), tuberculosis (TB) (unilateral, often sectorial), Cogan's syndrome [vertigo, tinnitus, hearing loss, negative syphilis serologies (FTA-ABS), often associated with systemic vasculitis, typically polyarteritis nodosa], leprosy, herpes simplex virus (HSV), and Lyme disease.

Workup
For active IK and old, previously untreated IK:

1. History: Venereal disease in the mother during pregnancy or in the patient? Difficulty hearing or tinnitus?

2. External examination: Look for saddle-nose deformity, Hutchinson's teeth, frontal bossing, or other signs of congenital syphilis; hypopigmented or anesthetic skin lesions and thickened skin folds, loss of the temporal eyebrow, and loss of eyelashes, as in leprosy.
3. Slit-lamp examination: Note whether the corneal nerves are segmentally thickened like beads on a string and whether iris nodules are present (leprosy); look for patchy hyperemia of the iris with fleshy, pink nodules (syphilis). Check intraocular pressure (IOP).
4. Dilated fundus examination: Look for the classic salt-and-pepper chorioretinitis or optic atrophy of syphilis.
5. VDRL or rapid plasma reagin (RPR), FTA-ABS, or microhemagglutination–*Treponema pallidum* (MHA-TP).
6. Purified protein derivative (PPD) with anergy panel.
7. Chest radiograph if negative FTA-ABS (or MHA-TP) or positive PPD.
8. Consider erythrocyte sedimentation rate (ESR), anti-nuclear antibody (ANA), rheumatoid factor, Lyme titer.

Treatment
  A. Acute disease
    1. Topical cycloplegic (e.g., atropine, 1%, t.i.d.).
    2. Topical steroid (e.g., prednisolone acetate, 1%, q 1 to 6 h, depending on the degree of inflammation).
    3. Treat any underlying disease.
  B. Old inactive disease: Corneal transplant surgery may improve vision when it has been impaired by central corneal scarring and no amblyopia is present.
  C. Acute or old, inactive disease
    • If FTA-ABS is positive and
      a. the patient has not been treated for syphilis in the past (or is unsure about treatment), or
      b. there are signs of active syphilitic disease (e.g., active chorioretinitis or papillitis), or
      c. the VDRL or RPR titer is positive and has not declined the expected amount after treatment
    then treatment for syphilis is indicated (see Congenital Syphilis, Section 14.3, or Acquired Syphilis, Section 14.2).
    • If PPD is positive (see Appendix 12) and
      a. the patient is younger than 35 years and has not been treated for TB in the past, or
      b. there is evidence of active systemic TB (e.g., positive finding on chest x-ray)
    then refer the patient to a medical internist for treatment of TB.
    • If Cogan's syndrome is present, then refer the patient to an ear, nose, and throat specialist and consider rheumatologic follow-up.

Follow-up
- A. Acute disease: Every 3 to 7 days initially, and then every 2 to 4 weeks. The frequency of steroid administration is slowly reduced as the inflammation subsides. IOP is monitored closely and reduced with medication when it is thought to be high enough to cause optic nerve damage (e.g., >30 mm Hg in a patient with a healthy optic nerve). (See Inflammatory Open-Angle Glaucoma, Section 10.4.)
- B. Old inactive disease: Routine follow-up every year unless treatment is required for underlying etiology.

4.20 PERIPHERAL CORNEAL THINNING

Symptoms

Pain, photophobia; may be asymptomatic.

Critical Sign

Corneal thinning (seen best with a narrow slit of light from the slit lamp), may have a sterile infiltrate or ulcer.

Etiology
- Collagen–vascular disease [(e.g., rheumatoid arthritis, Wegener's granulomatosis, relapsing polychondritis, polyarteritis nodosa, systemic lupus erythematosus, others). Peripheral, unilateral or bilateral, corneal thinning/ulcers, possibly with inflammatory infiltrates. May progress circumferentially to involve the entire peripheral cornea. Perforation may occur. This may be the first manifestation of systemic disease.]
- Terrien's marginal degeneration [Often asymptomatic, usually bilateral, slowly progressive thinning of the peripheral cornea, sparing the limbus, typically superiorly, most often in men. The anterior chamber is quiet, and the eye is typically not injected. A yellow line (lipid) may appear, with a fine pannus over the thinned areas of involvement. The ulceration may slowly spread circumferentially. Irregular and against-the-rule astigmatism is often present. The epithelium usually remains intact, but perforation may occur with minor trauma.]
- Mooren's ulcer (Unilateral or bilateral, idiopathic, painful corneal thinning and ulceration with inflammation, initially involving a focal area of peripheral cornea nasally or temporally without an adjacent perilimbal lucid zone, but later extending circumferentially or centrally. An epithelial defect, stromal thinning, and a leading undermined edge are present. Limbal blood vessels may grow into the ulcer, and perforation

can occur. This diagnosis can be made only after other etiologies are ruled out. Mooren's-like ulcer has been associated with systemic hepatitis C virus infection.)

- Pellucid marginal degeneration [Painless, bilateral corneal thinning of the inferior peripheral cornea (usually from the 4- to 8-o'clock portions). There is no anterior-chamber reaction, conjunctival injection, lipid deposition, or vascularization. The epithelium is intact. Corneal protrusion may be seen above the area of thinning. The thinning may slowly progress.]
- Furrow degeneration (Painless corneal thinning just peripheral to an arcus senilis, typically in the elderly. There is no vascular infiltration nor ocular inflammation, and perforation is rare. Usually nonprogressive and does not require treatment.)
- Dellen (Painless oval corneal thinning resulting from corneal drying and stromal dehydration adjacent to an abnormal conjunctival or corneal elevation. The epithelium is usually intact. See Section 4.21, Dellen.)
- Staphylococcal hypersensitivity (marginal keratitis). (Mildly painful peripheral, white corneal infiltrate separated from the limbus by a zone of clear cornea. Often multiple, bilateral infiltrates that may stain with fluorescein, may be mildly thinned, and are typically associated with blepharitis. See Section 4.22, Staphylococcal Hypersensitivity.)
- Dry-eye syndrome [Peripheral corneal ulcers may result from severe cases of dry eye. Patients may demonstrate a poor tear lake, decreased tear break-up time, superficial punctate keratitis (SPK) inferiorly or centrally, and corneal filaments. May be associated with a collagen–vascular disease. See Section 4.2, Dry-Eye Syndrome.]
- Exposure/neurotrophic keratopathy (Typically, a sterile oval ulcer develops inferiorly on the cornea without signs of significant inflammation. An eyelid abnormality, a fifth- or seventh-cranial-nerve defect, or proptosis is common. The ulcer may become superinfected. See Sections 4.4, Exposure Keratopathy, and 4.5, Neurotrophic Keratopathy.)
- Sclerokeratitis (Corneal ulceration is associated with severe ocular pain radiating to the temple and/or jaw due to accompanying scleritis. The sclera develops a blue hue, scleral vessels are engorged, and scleral edema with or without nodules is present. An underlying collagen–vascular disease, especially Wegener's granulomatosis, must be ruled out. See Section 5.7, Scleritis.)
- Vernal keratoconjunctivitis (Superior, shallow shield-shaped sterile corneal ulcer accompanied by giant papillae on the superior tarsal conjunctiva and/or limbal papillae. The conjunctivitis is usually bilateral, often occurs in children, and recurs during the summer months, but it can occur anytime in warm climates. See Section 5.1, Acute Conjunctivitis.)
- Ocular rosacea (Typically affects the inferior cornea in middle-aged patients. Erythema and telangiectasias of the eyelid margins, nose,

forehead, and cheeks are characteristic, and can progress to rhino-phyma. See Section 5.8, Ocular Rosacea.)
- Others (Cataract surgery, inflammatory bowel disease, and leukemia can rarely cause peripheral corneal thinning/ulceration.)

Differential Diagnosis
- Infectious infiltrate or ulcer (A dense, gray–white stromal infiltrate or ulcer that stains with fluorescein. The conjunctiva is injected, and an anterior-chamber reaction is usually present. Often lesions are treated as infectious until cultures are noted to be negative. See Section 4.12, Infectious Corneal Infiltrate/Ulcer.)

Workup
1. History: Contact lens wearer or previous herpes simplex keratitis (HSK) (infectious)? Known collagen–vascular disease or inflammatory bowel disease? Other systemic symptoms? Seasonal conjunctivitis with itching (vernal)?
2. External examination: Old facial scars of herpes zoster? Eyelid-closure problem causing exposure? Blue tinge to the sclera? Rosacea facies?
3. Slit-lamp examination: Look for infiltrate, corneal ulcer, hypopyon, uveitis, scleritis, old herpetic scarring, poor tear lake, SPK, blepharitis, or giant papillae on the superior tarsal conjunctiva or limbal papillae. Measure intraocular pressure (IOP).
4. Schirmer's test (see Section 4.2, Dry-Eye Syndrome).
5. Dilated fundus examination: Look for cotton-wool spots consistent with collagen–vascular disease or evidence of posterior scleritis (e.g., vitritis, subretinal fluid, chorioretinal folds, exudative retinal detachment).
6. Corneal scrapings and cultures when infection is suspected (see Infectious Corneal Infiltrate/Ulcer, Section 4.12).
7. Serum anti-nuclear antibody, rheumatoid factor, erythrocyte sedimentation rate, and complete blood count (CBC) with differential to rule out collagen–vascular disease and leukemia, if suspected. Serum anti-neutrophilic cytoplasmic antibody (ANCA) levels can be obtained if Wegener's granulomatosis is suspected.
8. Scleritis workup, when present (see Section 5.7, Scleritis).
9. Refer to an internist (or rheumatologist) when collagen–vascular disease or leukemia is suspected.

Treatment
The treatment of dellen, staphylococcal hypersensitivity, dry-eye syndrome, exposure and neurotrophic keratopathies, scleritis, vernal conjunctivitis, and ocular rosacea are discussed elsewhere in this book. See appropriate sections.

A. Corneal thinning due to collagen–vascular disease: Management is usually coordinated with a rheumatologist or internist.
   1. Antibiotic ointment (e.g., erythromycin ointment) and a pressure patch qhs.
   2. Ocular lubricants while awake (e.g., Refresh plus or Theratears q 1 h or Refresh PM ointment q 2 h).
   3. Cycloplegic drops (e.g., atropine, 1%) when an anterior-chamber reaction and/or pain are present.
   4. Systemic steroids (e.g., prednisone, 60 to 100 mg p.o., once per day; the dosage is adjusted according to the response) and an H_2-blocker (e.g., ranitidine, 150 mg p.o., b.i.d.) are used for significant and progressive corneal thinning, but not for perforation.
   5. An immunosuppressive agent such as cyclophosphamide is often required, especially for Wegener's granulomatosis. This should be done in cooperation with the patient's medical physician.
   6. Excision of adjacent inflamed conjunctiva is occasionally helpful when the condition progresses despite treatment.
   7. Punctal occlusion if dry eye syndrome also is present.
   8. Consider cyanoacrylate tissue adhesive or corneal transplant surgery for an impending or actual corneal perforation. A conjunctival flap can also be used for an impending corneal perforation.
   9. Patients with significant corneal thinning should wear their glasses [or protective glasses (e.g., polycarbonate lens)] during the day and an eye shield at night.

❖ **Note** *Topical steroids are generally not used when significant corneal thinning is present because of the risk of perforation due to inhibition of a proper healing response. Topical steroids should be gradually tapered if the patient is already taking them. Corneal thinning due to relapsing polychondritis, however, seems to improve with topical steroids (e.g., prednisolone acetate, 1%, q 1 to 2 h).*

B. Terrien's marginal degeneration: Correct astigmatism with glasses or contact lenses if possible. Protective eyewear (e.g., polycarbonate lens) during the day and an eye shield at night should be worn to prevent traumatic perforation if significant thinning is present. Lamellar grafts can be used if thinning is extreme.
C. Mooren's ulcer: Underlying systemic diseases must be ruled out before this diagnosis can be made. A step-wise approach to treatment is taken, by using any or all of the following therapeutic modalities. If the epithelial defect over the ulcer is not healing within a few days of initiating treatment, more aggressive therapy is pursued. Some cases are resistant to all forms of treatment.

1. Topical antibiotic drops [e.g., trimethoprim/polymyxin (e.g., Polytrim) q.i.d.] to prevent secondary bacterial infection.
2. Cycloplegic (e.g., atropine, 1%, t.i.d.).
3. Glasses during the day and an eye shield at night because of the risk of perforation with minor trauma.
4. Topical steroid (e.g., prednisolone acetate, 1%, q 1–6 h).
5. Systemic steroid (e.g., prednisone, 60 to 100 mg p.o., once per day) and an H_2-blocker (e.g., ranitidine, 150 mg p.o., b.i.d.) if unresponsive to topical alone.
6. Consider conjunctival excision, a conjunctival flap, or cryotherapy if the ulceration progresses.
7. Immunosuppressive agents (e.g., cyclophosphamide, methotrexate) for severe disease, after consultation with a medical physician familiar with these agents (e.g., hematologist/oncologist) to assist in monitoring for systemic toxicity. Topical cyclosporin A also may be beneficial.
8. Systemic interferon treatment has been shown to be effective in hepatitis C–related Mooren's ulcer.
9. Cyanoacrylate tissue adhesive or corneal surgery for actual or imminent corneal perforation.
D. Pellucid marginal degeneration: See Keratoconus, Section 4.23.
E. Furrow degeneration: No treatment is required.

❖ **Note** *If systemic steroid therapy is to be instituted, obtain a steroid workup (see Drug Glossary) as indicated, and involve the patient's primary medical physician.*

Follow-up

Patients with severe disease are examined daily in the hospital or as outpatients if compliant; those with milder conditions are checked less frequently. Watch carefully for signs of superinfection (e.g., increased pain, stromal infiltration, anterior-chamber cells and flare, conjunctival injection), increased IOP, and progressive corneal thinning. Treatment is maintained until the epithelial defect over the ulcer heals and is then gradually tapered. As long as an epithelial defect is present, there is a risk of progressive thinning and perforation.

4.21 DELLEN

Symptoms

Usually asymptomatic; irritation, foreign-body sensation.

Critical Sign

Corneal thinning, usually at the limbus, often in the shape of an ellipse, accompanied by an adjacent focal conjunctival or corneal elevation.

Other Signs

Fluorescein pooling in the area, but minimal staining. No infiltrate, no anterior-chamber reaction, often no hyperemia.

Etiology

Poor spread of the tear film over a focal area of cornea (with resultant stromal dehydration) due to an adjacent surface elevation (e.g., chemosis, conjunctival hemorrhage, filtering bleb from glaucoma surgery, pterygium, tumor, after muscle surgery).

Differential Diagnosis

See Peripheral Corneal Thinning, Section 4.20.

Workup

1. History: Previous eye surgery?
2. Slit-lamp examination with fluorescein staining. Look for an adjacent area of elevation.

Treatment

1. Lubricating or antibiotic ointment (e.g., Refresh PM, erythromycin ointment) and a pressure patch for 24 hours.
2. Lubricating ointment qhs after removal of the pressure patch. Maintain the ointment until the adjacent elevation is eliminated.
3. If the cause cannot be removed (e.g., filtering bleb), lubricating ointment should be applied nightly, and artificial-tear drops (e.g., Refresh Plus or Theratears) used 4 to 8 times per day, over the long term. (Most conjunctival elevations will regress with patching.)

Follow-up

Unless there is severe thinning, reexamination can be performed in 1 to 7 days, at which time the cornea can be expected to be of normal thickness. If it is not, full-time patching and lubrication should again be instituted.

4.22 STAPHYLOCOCCAL HYPERSENSITIVITY

Symptoms

Acute photophobia, mild pain, red eye, chronic eyelid crusting and itching; history of recurrent acute episodes.

Critical Signs

Usually multiple, often bilateral, peripheral corneal stromal infiltrates with a clear space between the infiltrates and the limbus, and minimal-to-no staining with fluorescein. The anterior chamber is usually quiet, and only a sector of the conjunctiva is typically injected.

Other Signs

Blepharitis, inferior superficial punctate keratitis (SPK), phlyctenule (a wedge-shaped, raised, sterile infiltrate near the limbus), peripheral scarring, and corneal neovascularization in the contralateral eye.

Etiology

Staphylococcal blepharitis (Infiltrates are a noninfectious reaction of the host's antibodies to the staphylococcal antigens.)

❖ **Note** *Patients with ocular rosacea (e.g., telangiectasias of the eyelids, nose, cheeks, and forehead that may progress to rhinophyma) are especially susceptible to this condition.*

Differential Diagnosis

- Infectious corneal infiltrates (A dense, white–gray stromal infiltrate, often central, painful, and associated with a marked anterior-chamber reaction. Not usually multiple and recurrent. See Section 4.12, Infectious Corneal Infiltrate/Ulcer.)
- Other causes of marginal thinning/infiltrates. (See Section 4.20, Peripheral Corneal Thinning)

Workup

1. History: Recurrent episodes? Contact lens wearer (a risk of infection)?
2. Slit-lamp examination with fluorescein staining and intraocular pressure (IOP) check.
3. If an infectious infiltrate is suspected, then corneal scrapings for culture and smears should be obtained. See Section 4.12, Infectious Corneal Infiltrate/Ulcer.

Treatment

MILD

Warm compresses, eyelid hygiene, and erythromycin or bacitracin ointment qhs (see Blepharitis/Meibomianitis, Section 5.10).

MODERATE-TO-SEVERE

Treat as described described earlier, but add a topical steroid (e.g., prednisolone acetate, 0.125%, q.i.d.) or a combination antibiotic/steroid (e.g., dexamethasone/tobramycin, q.i.d.). Maintain until the symptoms improve, and then slowly taper.

If recurrent episodes are not prevented by eyelid hygiene, consider systemic tetracycline (250 mg p.o., q.i.d., for 1 month, and then b.i.d. for 1 month, and then once per day) or doxycycline (100 mg p.o., b.i.d., for 1 month, and then once per day for 1 month, and then 50 to 100 mg daily, titrated as necessary) until the ocular disease is controlled for several months. These medications have an antiinflammatory effect on the sebaceous glands in addition to their antimicrobial action. Low-dose antibiotics may have to be maintained indefinitely.

❖ **Note** *Tetracycline and doxycycline are contraindicated in children younger than 8 years, pregnant women, and breast-feeding mothers. Erythromycin in the same dose as tetracycline can be substituted, but may not be as effective.*

Follow-up
In 2 to 7 days, depending on the clinical picture. IOP is monitored while patients are taking topical steroids.

4.23 KERATOCONUS

Symptoms
Progressive decreased vision, usually beginning in adolescence and continuing into middle age. Acute corneal hydrops can cause a sudden decrease in vision, pain, red eye, photophobia, and profuse tearing.

Critical Signs
Slowly progressive irregular astigmatism resulting from paracentral thinning and bulging of the cornea (maximal thinning near the apex of the protrusion), vertical tension lines in the posterior cornea (Vogt's stria), an irregular corneal retinoscopic reflex, and egg-shaped mires on keratometry. Inferior steepening is seen on corneal topographic evaluation. Usually bilateral but often asymmetric.

Other Signs
Fleischer's ring (epithelial iron deposits at the base of the cone), bulging of the lower eyelid when looking downward (Munson's sign), superficial corneal scarring. Corneal hydrops (sudden development of corneal edema) results from a rupture in Descemet's membrane.

Associations
Keratoconus is associated with Down's syndrome, atopic disease, and mitral valve prolapse. It may be related to chronic eye rubbing.

Differential Diagnosis
- Pellucid marginal degeneration (Corneal thinning in the inferior periphery. The cornea protrudes superior to the band of thinning.)
- Keratoglobus (Rare. Uniform circularly thinned cornea with maximal thinning in the midperiphery of the cornea. The cornea protrudes central to the area of maximal thinning.)

Treatment for these two conditions is the same as for keratoconus, except corneal transplants are technically more difficult and have a higher failure rate.

Workup
1. History: Duration and rate of decreased vision? Frequent change in eyeglass prescriptions? History of eye rubbing? Medical problems? Allergies?
2. Slit-lamp examination. (Note: Fleischer's ring is sometimes best seen with the blue light of the slit lamp.)
3. Retinoscopy and refraction. Look for irregular astigmatism and a waterdrop or scissors red reflex.
4. Computed corneal topography (can show central and inferior steepening) and keratometry (irregular mires and steepening).

Treatment
1. Patients are instructed not to rub their eyes.
2. Correct refractive errors with glasses (for mild cases) or rigid gas permeable (RGP) contact lenses (successful in most cases).
3. Corneal transplant surgery is usually indicated when contact lenses cannot be tolerated or no longer produce satisfactory vision.
4. Thermokeratoplasty, epikeratophakia, and lamellar keratoplasty are rarely used.

CORNEAL HYDROPS

1. Cycloplegic agent (e.g., scopolamine, 0.25%), sodium chloride 5% ointment, and occasionally a pressure patch.
2. Patients are instructed to remove the pressure patch in 24 to 48 hours, and start sodium chloride, 5% ointment, b.i.d., until resolved (usually several weeks to months).
3. Glasses or a shield should be worn by patients at risk for trauma or who cannot be relied on to avoid vigorous eye rubbing.

❖ **Note** *Acute hydrops is not an indication for an emergency corneal transplant, except in the extremely rare incidence of corneal perforation (reported cases are associated with minor trauma or topical steroid use).*

Follow-up
Every 3 to 12 months, depending on the progression of symptoms. After an episode of hydrops, examine the patient every 1 to 4 weeks until resolved (which can take several months).

4.24 CORNEAL DYSTROPHIES

Bilateral, inherited, progressive corneal disorders showing no signs of inflammation or corneal vascularization and without associated systemic disease.

Anterior Corneal Dystrophies
- Anterior basement membrane dystrophy (map–dot–fingerprint dystrophy)
  Diffuse gray patches (maps), large or tiny cysts (dots), or fine refractile lines (fingerprints) in the corneal epithelium best seen with retroillumination or a broad slit-lamp beam angled from the side; spontaneous corneal epithelial defects (erosions) and associated pain and photophobia may develop, particularly on opening the eyes after sleep. May also cause decreased vision. See Recurrent Corneal Erosion (Section 4.6) for treatment.
- Meesmann's dystrophy
  Rare, autosomal dominant, epithelial dystrophy that is seen in the first years of life but is usually asymptomatic until middle age. Retroillumination shows discrete, tiny epithelial vesicles diffusely involving the cornea but concentrated in the palpebral fissure. Although treatment is usually not required, bandage soft contact lenses, a superficial keratectomy, or a lamellar corneal transplant may be beneficial if significant photophobia is present or visual acuity is severely affected.
- Reis–Bucklers' Dystrophy
  Autosomal dominant, progressive dystrophy that appears early in life. Subepithelial, gray reticular opacities are seen primarily in the central cornea. Painful episodes from recurrent erosions are relatively common and require treatment. Corneal transplant surgery may be necessary to improve vision, but the dystrophy often recurs in the graft. Superficial lamellar keratectomy or excimer laser phototherapeutic keratectomy (PTK) may be adequate treatment in some cases.

Corneal Stromal Dystrophies
Patients with reduced vision from these conditions usually benefit from a corneal transplant or PTK.

- Lattice dystrophy
  Refractile branching lines, white subepithelial dots, and scarring of the corneal stroma centrally, best seen with retroillumination. Recurrent erosions are common (see Section 4.6, Recurrent Corneal Erosion).

The corneal periphery is clear. Autosomal dominant. Tends to recur after PTK or corneal transplantation over years.

- Granular dystrophy
  White, anterior stromal deposits in the central cornea, separated by discrete clear intervening spaces. The corneal periphery is spared. Appears in the first decade of life but rarely becomes symptomatic before middle age. Erosions uncommon. Autosomal dominant. Also may recur after PTK or corneal transplant.
- Macular dystrophy
  Gray–white stromal opacities with ill-defined edges extending from limbus to limbus with cloudy intervening spaces. Can involve full thickness of the stroma, more superficial centrally and deeper peripherally. Causes decreased vision more commonly than recurrent erosions. Autosomal recessive. Tends not to recur after corneal transplant.
- Central crystalline dystrophy of Schnyder
  Fine, yellow–white anterior stromal crystals located in the central cornea. Later develop full-thickness central haze and a dense arcus senilis. Can be associated with hyperlipidemia and hypercholesterolemia. Autosomal dominant. Workup includes fasting serum cholesterol and triglyceride levels. Rarely compromises vision enough to require transplantation.

Corneal Endothelial Dystrophies
- Fuchs' Dystrophy
  See Section 4.25, Fuchs' Endothelial Dystrophy.
- Posterior polymorphous dystrophy
  Changes at the level of Descemet's membrane, including vesicles arranged in a linear or grouped pattern, gray haze, or broad bands with irregular, scalloped edges. Iris abnormalities, including iridocorneal adhesions and a decentered pupil, may be present and are occasionally associated with corneal edema. Glaucoma may occur. Autosomal dominant with marked variability. See Developmental Anterior Segment and Lens Anomalies, (Section 9.11), for differential diagnosis.
- Congenital hereditary endothelial dystrophy (CHED)
  Bilateral corneal edema with normal corneal diameter, normal intraocular pressure (IOP), and no cornea guttata. See Congenital Glaucoma, (Section 9.10), for differential diagnosis. Some patients may benefit from a corneal transplant.
  Two distinct types distinguished by clinical presentation and genetics:
  a. *Autosomal recessive* Present at birth, nonprogressive, nystagmus present. Pain or photophobia uncommon.
  b. *Autosomal dominant* Is first seen during childhood, slowly progressive, no nystagmus. Pain, tearing, and photophobia are common.

4.25 FUCHS' ENDOTHELIAL DYSTROPHY

Symptoms

Glare and blurred vision, especially on awakening, that may progress to severe pain. Symptoms rarely develop before age 50 years. May be autosomal dominant.

Critical Signs

Cornea guttata and corneal stromal edema. Bilateral, but may be asymmetric.

❖ **Note** *Central cornea guttata without stromal edema is called endothelial dystrophy, which may progress to Fuchs' dystrophy.*

Other Signs

Fine pigment dusting on the endothelium, central epithelial edema and bullae, folds in Descemet's membrane, subepithelial scar tissue.

Differential Diagnosis

- Aphakic or pseudophakic bullous keratopathy (History of cataract surgery, unilateral. See Section 4.28, Aphakic Bullous Keratopathy.)
- Congenital hereditary endothelial dystrophy (Bilateral corneal edema at birth. See Section 4.24, Corneal Dystrophies.)
- Posterior polymorphous dystrophy (Autosomal dominant, seen early in life. Corneal endothelium shows either grouped vesicles, geographic-shaped gray lesions, or broad bands. Occasionally associated with corneal edema. Iridocorneal adhesions and pupillary abnormalities may be present. See Section 4.24, Corneal Dystrophies.)
- Iridocorneal endothelial (ICE) syndrome ("Beaten metal" corneal endothelial appearance, with corneal edema, increased intraocular pressure (IOP), possible iris thinning, and pupil distortion. Typically unilateral, in young to middle-aged adults. See Section 10.14, Iridocorneal Endothelial Syndrome.)

Workup

1. History: Previous cataract surgery?
2. Slit-lamp examination: Cornea guttata are often best seen with retroillumination. Fluorescein staining may demonstrate ruptured bullae.
3. Measure IOP.
4. Consider corneal pachymetry to determine the central corneal thickness.

Treatment

1. Topical sodium chloride, 5% drops, q.i.d. and ointment qhs.
2. May gently blow warm air from a hair dryer at arm's length toward the eyes for 5 to 10 minutes every morning to dehydrate the cornea.
3. Reduce the IOP with antiglaucoma medications if >20 to 22 mm Hg (e.g., timolol or levobunolol, 0.25% to 0.5%, b.i.d.), if no systemic contraindications.
4. Ruptured corneal bullae are painful and should be treated as a corneal abrasion (see Section 3.2, Corneal Abrasion).
5. Corneal transplant surgery is usually indicated when visual acuity decreases or the disease becomes advanced and painful.

Follow-up

Every 3 to 12 months to check IOP and assess corneal edema. The condition progresses very slowly, and visual acuity typically remains good until epithelial edema develops.

4.26 WILSON'S DISEASE (HEPATOLENTICULAR DEGENERATION)

Symptoms

Typically, no ocular complaints. Patients experience symptoms of cirrhosis, renal disease, or neurologic dysfunction (motor, but not sensory dysfunction). Patient is usually younger than 40 years at the onset of clinical manifestations. Autosomal recessive.

Critical Signs

In 95% of patients, a greenish brown (sometimes red) band is found in the corneal periphery, 1 to 3 mm in width, at the level of Descemet's membrane (deep in the cornea). It first appears superiorly, but eventually forms a ring (Kayser–Fleischer ring) that involves the entire corneal periphery. The ring usually extends to the limbus, without interspersed clear cornea. Serum and urine copper levels are increased, and the serum ceruloplasmin level is low.

Other Ocular Signs

Anterior and posterior subcapsular copper deposition, producing "sunflower" cataract.

Differential Diagnosis

- Other rare causes of a Kayser–Fleischer-like ring (Primary biliary cirrhosis, chronic active hepatitis, progressive intrahepatic cholestasis, and rarely, multiple myeloma. Normal serum ceruloplasmin levels, no neurologic symptoms.)
- Arcus senilis (Corneal stromal lipid deposition, first seen inferiorly and superiorly before it extends around the corneal periphery. Appears white, typically with a clear zone of cornea separating the edge of the arcus from the limbus. In patients younger than 40 years, a lipid profile with lipoprotein electrophoresis and serum cholesterol should be obtained to rule out hyperlipidemia, hyperlipoproteinemia, and hypercholesterolemia.)
- Chalcosis (Caused by copper-containing intraocular foreign body. Usually history of penetrating ocular trauma. Copper deposits in basement membranes, including Descemet's membrane. Also causes retinal toxicity. Severe inflammation if more than 85% copper.)

Workup

1. Slit-lamp examination: Narrow the beam of light to a thin slit and determine the level at which the deposition is located.
2. Gonioscopy if the Kayser–Fleischer ring is not evident on slit-lamp examination (pigment may be noted in peripheral Descemet's membrane before it is apparent on slit-lamp examination).
3. Serum copper and ceruloplasmin levels.
4. Urine copper level.
5. Serum protein electrophoresis when ceruloplasmin levels are normal.
6. Referral to an internist and a neurologist.

Treatment

Systemic therapy (e.g., D-penicillamine) is instituted by an internist. The ocular manifestations usually require no treatment.

Follow-up

- In conjunction with an internist and a neurologist who manage systemic therapy and monitor blood cell counts.
- Successful treatment should lead to reabsorption of the corneal copper deposition and clearing of the Kayser–Fleischer ring (although residual corneal changes may remain) and can be used as a guide for monitoring treatment. There are no ocular complications of a Kayser–Fleischer ring.

4.27 CORNEAL GRAFT REJECTION

Symptoms

Decreased vision, mild pain, redness, and photophobia in an eye that has undergone a prior corneal transplant, usually several weeks to years previously.

Critical Signs

Any of the following suggest corneal graft rejection: New keratic precipitates (KP) or a fine line of white blood cells on the corneal endothelium (endothelial rejection line), stromal edema or cellular infiltration, subepithelial infiltrates, epithelial edema, an irregularly elevated epithelial line (epithelial rejection line).

Other Signs

Conjunctival injection (particularly circumcorneal injection), anterior-chamber cells and flare, neovascularization growing up to or extending onto the graft (typically the rejection starts near a blood vessel adjacent to the graft wound). Tearing may occur, but discharge is not present.

Differential Diagnosis

- Suture abscess or corneal infection [May have a corneal infiltrate, hypopyon, or a purulent discharge. Remove the suture (by pulling the contaminated portion through the shortest track possible) and obtain smears and cultures, including a culture of the suture. Steroid frequency is usually reduced slowly rather than increased. Patients are treated with intensive topical fluoroquinolone or fortified antibiotics and monitored closely, sometimes in the hospital. See Section 4.12, Infectious Corneal Infiltrate/Ulcer.]
- Uveitis (May produce anterior-chamber cells and flare with KP. Often, a previous history of uveitis is obtained. It is best to treat uveitis as if it were a graft rejection.)
- Increased intraocular pressure (IOP) (A markedly increased IOP may produce epithelial corneal edema, but few-to-no other signs of graft rejection are present, and the edema often clears after the IOP is reduced.)
- Other causes of graft failure [Corneal endothelial decompensation in the graft, recurrent disease in the graft (e.g., herpes keratitis, corneal dystrophy)].

Workup
1. History: Time since the corneal transplant? Current eye medications? Recent change in topical steroid regimen? Previous ocular disease leading to the corneal transplant (e.g., herpes simplex virus)?
2. Slit-lamp examination, looking for the critical signs listed above. Look carefully for endothelial rejection line, KP, and subepithelial infiltrates.

Treatment
1. Topical steroids (e.g., prednisolone acetate, 1%, q 1 h while awake and dexamethasone, 0.1%, ointment at night) if significant endothelial rejection is present. If only subepithelial infiltrates, KP, or an epithelial rejection is present, prednisolone acetate, 1%, q.i.d., or twice the current level of topical steroids, whichever is more, should be prescribed.
2. Cycloplegic agent (e.g., scopolamine, 0.25%, 2 to 3 times per day).
3. Consider systemic steroids (e.g., prednisone, 40 to 80 mg p.o., once per day) or rarely subconjunctival steroids (e.g., betamethasone, 3 mg in 0.5 ml) to be used in addition when the graft rejection does not respond to topical steroids alone or for recurrent rejection.
4. Control IOP if increased (see Inflammatory Open-Angle Glaucoma, Section 10.4).
5. For multiple rejection episodes or severe rejection, consider hospitalization and single-pulse dose of methylprednisolone, 500 mg i.v., along with prednisolone acetate, 1%, q 1 h topically.

Follow-up
Treatment must be instituted immediately to maximize the likelihood of graft survival. Examine the patient every 3 to 7 days. Once improvement is noted, the steroids are tapered very slowly and may need to be maintained at low doses for months to years. IOP must be checked regularly in patients taking topical steroids.

4.28 APHAKIC BULLOUS KERATOPATHY/ PSEUDOPHAKIC BULLOUS KERATOPATHY

Symptoms
Decreased vision, pain, tearing, photophobia, red eye; history of cataract surgery in the involved eye.

Critical Sign
Corneal edema in an eye in which the natural lens has been removed.

Other Signs

Corneal bullae, corneal neovascularization, preexisting corneal endothelial guttata. Cystoid macular edema (CME) may be present.

Etiology

Often results from a combination of the following factors: corneal endothelial damage, intraocular inflammation, vitreous or subluxed intraocular lens touching (or intermittently touching) the cornea.

Workup

1. Slit-lamp examination: Stain the cornea with fluorescein to check for denuded epithelium, check the position of the intraocular lens if present, determine whether vitreous is touching the corneal endothelium, and evaluate the eye for inflammation. Evaluate the contralateral eye for corneal endothelial dystrophy.
2. Check intraocular pressure (IOP).
3. Dilated fundus examination: Look for CME and/or vitreous inflammation.
4. Consider a fluorescein angiogram to help detect CME.

Treatment

1. Topical sodium chloride, 5% drops, q.i.d. and ointment qhs if epithelial edema is present.
2. Reduce IOP with antiglaucoma medications if increased (e.g., >20 mm Hg). Avoid epinephrine derivatives and latanoprost (e.g., Xalatan) if possible because of the risk of CME. (See Primary Open-Angle Glaucoma, Section 10.1.)
3. Ruptured epithelial bullae (producing corneal epithelial defects) may be treated with an antibiotic ointment (e.g., erythromycin), a cycloplegic (e.g., scopolamine, 0.25%), and pressure patching for 24 to 48 hours. Alternatively, the antibiotic ointment can be used frequently (e.g., q 2 h) without patching. A bandage soft contact lens or anterior stromal puncture can be used for recurrent ruptured epithelial bullae (see Section 4.6, Recurrent Corneal Erosion).
4. Corneal transplant surgery (possibly including intraocular lens repositioning, replacement, or removal) is indicated when vision fails or the disease becomes advanced and painful. Conjunctival flap surgery may be indicated for a painful eye with poor visual potential.
5. See Section 12.14, Cystoid Macular Edema, for treatment of CME.

❖ **Note** *Although both CME and corneal disease may contribute to decreased vision, the precise role of each is often difficult to determine.*

Follow-up

In 24 to 48 hours until the epithelial defect heals. Otherwise, every 1 to 6 months, depending on the symptoms.

4.29 REFRACTIVE SURGERY COMPLICATIONS

The basic principle of corneal refractive surgery is to induce a change in curvature of the cornea to correct a preexisting refractive error.

A. Complications of Surface Photorefractive Keratectomy (PRK)

In surface PRK, the surgeon removes the corneal epithelium and partially ablates the corneal stroma by using an argon–fluoride excimer laser (193 nm, ultraviolet) to correct a refractive error.

Symptoms

Early (1 to 14 days) Decreasing visual acuity, increased pain. Note: There is a normal element of pain caused by an induced epithelial defect at surgery, which usually takes a few days to heal.

Later (2 weeks to several months) Decreasing visual acuity, severe glare, monocular diplopia.

Signs

Corneal infiltrate, central corneal scar.

Etiology

Early

- Dislocated bandage soft contact lens (See Section 4.17, Contact Lens–Related Problems)
- Nonhealing epithelial defect (See Section 3.2, Corneal Abrasion)
- Corneal ulcer (See Section 4.12, Infectious Corneal Infiltrate/Ulcer)
- Medication allergy (See Section 5.1, Acute Conjunctivitis)

Later

- Corneal haze (scarring) noted in anterior corneal stroma
- Irregular astigmatism (central island, decentered ablation)
- Regression or progression of refractive error
- Steroid-induced glaucoma (See Section 10.5, Steroid-Response Glaucoma)

Workup
1. Complete ophthalmic examination, including intraocular pressure (IOP).
2. Refraction if change in refractive error suspected. Refraction with hard contact lens may correct irregular astigmatism.
3. Corneal topography if irregular astigmatism suspected.

Treatment and Follow-up
1. Epithelial defect. (See Section 3.2, Corneal Abrasion)
2. Corneal infiltrate. (See Section 4.12, Infectious Corneal Infiltrate/Ulcer)
3. Corneal haze. Increase steroid drop frequency. Follow-up 1 to 2 weeks.
4. Refractive error or irregular astigmatism. Appropriate refraction. Consider PRK enhancement. If irregular astigmatism, may need repeated PRK or hard contact lens.
5. Steroid-induced glaucoma. (See Section 10.5, Steroid-Response Glaucoma)

B. Complications of Laser In Situ Keratomileusis (LASIK)

In LASIK, the surgeon creates a hinged partial-thickness corneal flap by using a microkeratome, and then ablates the underlying stroma by using an excimer laser to correct refractive error. The corneal flap is repositioned over the corneal stroma without sutures.

Symptoms
Early   (1 to 14 days) Decreasing visual acuity, increased pain.
Later   (2 weeks to several months) Decreasing visual acuity, severe glare, monocular diplopia.

Signs
Severe conjunctival injection, corneal infiltrate, large fluorescein-staining epithelial defect, dislocated corneal flap, central corneal scar.

Etiology
Early
- Flap dislocation or lost corneal flap
- Large epithelial defect
- Diffuse interstitial lamellar keratitis
  Also known as Sands of the Sahara because of its appearance of multiple fine inflammatory infiltrates in the flap interface. Usually occurs within 5 days of surgery.
- Corneal ulcer/infection in flap interface (See Section 4.12, Infectious Corneal Infiltrate/Ulcer)

- Medication allergy (See Section 5.1, Acute Conjunctivitis)

Later
- Epithelial ingrowth into flap interface
- Corneal haze (scarring). Less common than in PRK
- Irregular astigmatism (decentered ablation, central island, flap irregularity)
- Regression or progression of refractive error

Workup
1. Complete slit-lamp examination, including IOP measurement, fluorescein staining.
2. Refraction if irregular astigmatism or change in refractive error suspected. Refraction with hard contact lens.
3. Corneal topography if irregular astigmatism suspected.

Treatment and Follow-up
1. Flap dislocation. Requires urgent surgical repositioning.
2. Lost corneal flap. Treat as epithelial defect (See Section 3.2, Corneal Abrasion).
3. Epithelial defect. (See Section 3.2)
4. Diffuse interstitial lamellar keratitis. Aggressive treatment with topical steroids (e.g., prednisolone acetate, 1%, hourly).
5. Corneal infiltrate. (See Section 4.12, Infectious Corneal Infiltrate/Ulcer)
6. Epithelial ingrowth. Observation if not affecting vision and very peripheral. Surgical debridement if dense, approaching visual axis, or affecting vision.
7. Corneal haze. Increase steroid drop frequency. Follow-up 1 to 2 weeks.
8. Refractive error or irregular astigmatism. Appropriate refraction. Consider repositioning flap or LASIK enhancement. If irregular astigmatism, may need LASIK enhancement or hard contact lens.

C. Complications of Radial Keratotomy

In radial keratotomy (RK), the surgeon makes partial-thickness, spokelike cuts in the peripheral cornea by using a diamond blade (often 90% to 95% depth), which results in a flattening of the central cornea and correction of myopia. Astigmatic keratotomy (AK) is a similar procedure in which arcuate or tangential incisions are made to correct astigmatism.

Symptoms
Early   (1 to 14 days) Decreasing visual acuity, increased pain.
Later   (2 weeks to years) Decreasing visual acuity, severe glare, monocular diplopia.

❖ **Note** *Because the corneal integrity is weakened with RK, patients are at higher risk for a ruptured globe with trauma.*

Signs

Corneal infiltrate, large fluorescein-staining epithelial defect, rupture at RK incision site after trauma, anterior-chamber reaction.

Etiology

Early

- Large epithelial defect (See Section 3.2, Corneal Abrasion)
- Corneal ulcer/infection in RK incision (See Section 4.12, Infectious Corneal Infiltrate/Ulcer)
- Medication allergy (See Section 5.1, Acute Conjunctivitis)
- Endophthalmitis: rare (See Section 13.10, Postoperative Endophthalmitis)

Later

- RK incisions approaching the visual axis causing glare and starbursts
- Irregular astigmatism
- Regression or progression of refractive error
- Ruptured globe at RK incision site after trauma (See Section 3.14, Ruptured Globe and Penetrating Ocular Injury)

Workup

1. Complete slit-lamp examination, including IOP measurement, fluorescein staining.
2. Refraction if irregular astigmatism or change in refractive error suspected. Refraction with hard contact lens.
3. Corneal topography if irregular astigmatism suspected.

Treatment and Follow-up

1. Corneal infiltrate. (See Section 4.12, Infectious Corneal Infiltrate/Ulcer)
2. Epithelial defect. (See Section 3.2, Corneal Abrasion)
3. Endophthalmitis. (See Section 13.10, Postoperative Endophthalmitis)
4. Refractive error or irregular astigmatism. Appropriate refraction. Consider enhancement of RK incisions or AK. If irregular astigmatism, may require a hard contact lens.
5. Ruptured globe at RK incision. Requires surgical repair. (See Section 3.14, Ruptured Globe and Penetrating Ocular Injury)

CONJUNCTIVA/SCLERA/ EXTERNAL DISEASE

5.1 ACUTE CONJUNCTIVITIS

Symptoms

"Red eye" (conjunctival hyperemia), discharge, eyelids sticking (worse in morning), foreign-body sensation, *less than 4-week* duration of symptoms (otherwise, see Chronic Conjunctivitis, Section 5.2) See Fig. 5-1.

Gonococcal Conjunctivitis (GC)

Critical Sign
  Severe purulent discharge, hyperacute onset (within 12 to 24 hours).

Other Signs
  Conjunctival papillae, marked chemosis, preauricular adenopathy, eyelid swelling.

❖ **Note** *Neonatal conjunctivitis is not seen with follicular response (see Section 9.8, Ophthalmia Neonatorum).*

Workup
  1. Examine the entire cornea for peripheral ulcers (especially superiorly) because of the risk for rapid perforation.
  2. Conjunctival scrapings for immediate Gram's stain and for routine culture and sensitivities [e.g., blood agar, chocolate agar (37°C, 10% CO_2)].

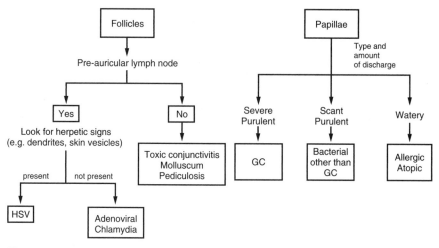

Figure 5-1

Treatment

Initiated if the Gram's stain shows gram-negative intracellular diplococci or there is a clinically high suspicion of GC.

1. Ceftriaxone, 1 g i.m., in a single dose. If corneal involvement exists, or cannot be excluded because of chemosis and eyelid swelling, then hospitalize the patient and treat with ceftriaxone, 1 g i.v., q 12 to 24 h. The duration of treatment depends on the clinical response. In penicillin-allergic patients, may consider ciprofloxacin, 500 mg p.o., single dose, or ofloxacin, 400 mg p.o., single dose, and consider consulting infectious disease specialist (fluoroquinolones are contraindicated in pregnant adults and children).
2. Topical bacitracin ointment q.i.d. or ciprofloxacin drops q 2 h. Topical ofloxacin, ciprofloxacin, gentamicin, or tobramycin q 1 h for corneal involvement.
3. Eye irrigation with saline q.i.d. until the discharge is eliminated.
4. Treat for possible coinfection with chlamydia (e.g., tetracycline or erythromycin, 250 to 500 mg p.o., q.i.d., doxycycline, 100 mg p.o., b.i.d., or clarithromycin, 250 to 500 mg p.o., b.i.d., for 3 to 6 weeks).

Follow-up

Daily, until consistent improvement is noted, and then examine every 2 to 3 days until the condition resolves. The patient and sexual partners should be evaluated by their medical doctors for other sexually transmitted diseases.

Viral Conjunctivitis (Usually Adenoviral)

Symptoms

Itching, burning, foreign-body sensation, and a history of a recent upper respiratory tract infection or contact with someone with red eye is common. It generally starts in one eye, and a few days later, involves the contralateral eye.

Critical Sign

Inferior palpebral conjunctival follicles.

Other Signs

Watery mucous discharge, red and edematous eyelids, palpable preauricular node, pinpoint subconjunctival hemorrhages, membrane/pseudomembrane. Subepithelial infiltrates (SEIs) may develop 1 to 2 weeks after the onset of the conjunctivitis.

Treatment

1. Artificial tears (e.g., Refresh Tears) 4 to 8 times per day for 1 to 3 weeks.
2. Cool compresses several times per day for 1 to 2 weeks.
3. Vasoconstrictor/antihistamine (e.g., naphazoline/pheniramine) q.i.d., if itching is severe.
4. If a membrane/pseudomembrane is present, it is gently peeled.
5. If a membrane/pseudomembrane is present or SEIs reduce vision, use topical steroids (e.g., fluorometholone or prednisolone acetate, 0.125%, q.i.d.). Steroid treatment is maintained for 1 week and then slowly tapered. SEIs may recur during or after tapering.
6. Viral conjunctivitis is very contagious, usually for 10 to 12 days from the day of onset. Patients should avoid touching their eyes, shaking hands with other people, sharing towels, etc. Restrict patients with significant exposure to others as long as the eyes are red and weeping.
7. Frequent handwashing.

Follow-up

In 1 to 2 weeks, but sooner if the condition worsens significantly. Viral conjunctivitis typically gets worse for the first 4 to 7 days after onset and may not resolve for 2 to 3 weeks.

Variants (treated the same as preceding)

- Pharyngoconjunctival fever—As earlier, but associated with pharyngitis and fever; usually in children.
- Acute hemorrhagic conjunctivitis—As earlier, but associated with a large subconjunctival hemorrhage. Associated with enterovirus and lasts 1 to 2 weeks. Tends to occur in tropical regions.

Herpes Simplex Virus Conjunctivitis

Patients may have a known history of ocular herpes simplex.

Symptoms
Foreign body sensation, pain, burning (rarely itching).

Critical Signs
Unilateral (sometimes recurrent) follicular conjunctival reaction; occasionally, concurrent herpetic skin vesicles along the eyelid margin or periocular skin; a palpable preauricular node.

Treatment
If the cornea or skin is involved, see Herpes Simplex Virus, Section 4.15.

1. Antiviral therapy [e.g., trifluorothymidine, 1% drops, 5 times per day, or vidarabine, 3% ointment, 5 times per day].
2. Cool compresses several times per day.

Follow-up
Every 2 to 5 days initially, to monitor for corneal involvement, and then every 1 to 2 weeks until resolved. Usually better in 1 week.

Allergic Conjunctivitis (e.g., hayfever)

Symptoms
Itching, watery discharge, and a history of allergies is typical.

Critical Signs
Chemosis, red and edematous eyelids, conjunctival papillae, preauricular node not palpable.

Treatment
1. Eliminate the inciting agent.
2. Cool compresses several times per day.
3. Topical drops, depending on the severity.
   a. Mild: Artificial tears (e.g., Refresh Tears or Theratears) 4 to 8 times per day.
   b. Moderate: Vasoconstrictor/antihistamine q.i.d. (e.g., naphazoline/pheniramine). Be aware of rebound vasodilation after prolonged use. Ketorolac 0.5% or levocabastine four times per day or olopatadine 2 to 3 times per day may help relieve itching.
   c. Severe: Mild topical steroid (e.g., fluorometholone, 0.1% q.i.d., for 1 to 2 weeks).

4. Oral antihistamine (e.g., diphenhydramine, 25 mg p.o., 3 to 4 times per day) in moderate-to-severe cases can be very helpful.

Follow-up

In 2 weeks. If topical steroids are being used, then patients should be followed up weekly, and the steroids slowly tapered.

Vernal/Atopic Conjunctivitis

Symptoms

Itching, thick ropy discharge, seasonal (spring/summer) recurrences, history of atopy. Usually seen in young patients, especially boys.

Critical Signs

Large conjunctival papillae seen under the upper eyelid or along the limbus (limbal vernal).

Other Signs

Superior corneal "shield" ulcer (a well-delineated sterile gray–white infiltrate), limbal or palpebral raised white dots (Horner–Trantas' dots) of degenerated eosinophils, superficial punctate keratopathy.

Treatment

- Treat as for allergic except add topical cromolyn sodium, 4%, q.i.d., lodoxamide, 0.1%, q.i.d., or olopatadine, 0.1%, b.i.d., for 2 to 3 weeks, before the season starts.
- If a shield ulcer is present add,
  1. Topical steroid (e.g., fluorometholone or prednisolone acetate, 1%, or dexamethasone, 0.1% ointment) 4 to 6 times per day.
  2. Topical antibiotic (e.g., erythromycin ointment q.i.d.).
  3. Cycloplegic agent (e.g., scopolamine, 0.25%, t.i.d.).
  4. Cromolyn sodium, 4%, q.i.d., lodoxamide, 0.1% (e.g., Alomide), q.i.d., or olopatadine, 0.1% (e.g., Patanol), b.i.d., if not already using.
  5. Cool compresses q.i.d.
- If atopic conjunctivitis is associated with atopic dermatitis of eyelids, may use topical steroid ointment such as fluorometholone, 0.1%, q.i.d.

Follow-up

Every 1 to 3 days in the presence of a shield ulcer; otherwise, every few weeks. Topical medications are tapered slowly as improvement is noted. Cromolyn sodium, lodoxamide, or olopatadine is maintained for the duration of the season and often reinitiated a few weeks before the next spring.

Patients on topical steroids should be monitored regularly to check intraocular pressure.

Bacterial Conjunctivitis (Other Than Gonococcal)

Symptoms

Redness, foreign body sensation, itching is much less prominent.

Critical Sign

Purulent discharge of mild to moderate degree.

Other Signs

Conjunctival papillae, chemosis, typically without preauricular adenopathy.

Workup

Conjunctival swab for routine cultures and sensitivities (blood and chocolate agars) and Gram's stain if severe.

Etiology

Common organisms are *Staphylococcus aureus* (often associated with blepharitis, phlyctenules, and marginal sterile infiltrates), *S. epidermidis, Streptococcus pneumoniae,* and *Haemophilus influenzae* (especially in children).

❖ **Note** *If suspect GC, then see Gonococcal Conjunctivitis.*

Treatment

1. In general, use topical antibiotic therapy [e.g., trimethoprim/polymyxin (e.g., Polytrim) q.i.d., ofloxacin or ciprofloxacin drops q.i.d., or bacitracin ointment q.i.d.] for 5 to 7 days.
2. *Haemophilus influenzae* conjunctivitis should be treated with oral amoxicillin/clavulanate (20 to 40 mg/kg/day in three divided doses) because of occasional nonocular involvement (i.e., otitis media, pneumonia, and meningitis).

❖ **Note** *Routine use of antibiotics for viral or allergic conjunctivitis is discouraged.*

Follow-up

Every 2 days initially, then every 3 to 5 days until resolved. Antibiotic therapy is adjusted according to culture and sensitivity results if the condition does not respond.

Pediculosis (Lice, Crabs)

Typically develops from contact with pubic lice (usually sexually transmitted). May be unilateral or bilateral.

Symptoms

Itching, minimal injection.

Critical Sign

Adult lice, nits, and blood-tinged debris on the eyelids and eyelashes.

Other Signs

Conjunctival follicles.

Treatment

1. Mechanical removal of lice and eggs with jeweler's forceps.
2. Any bland ophthalmic ointment (e.g., erythromycin or bacitracin) to the eyelids t.i.d. for 10 days to smother the lice and nits. Physostigmine, 0.25% (e.g., Eserine) ointment to the eyelids, two applications 1 week apart may be used instead, but this therapy has ocular side effects.
3. Antilice (e.g., Kwell, Nix, Rid) lotion and shampoo as directed to *non*ocular areas for patient and close contacts.
4. Thoroughly wash and dry all clothes and linens.

For chlamydial, toxic, and molluscum contagiosum–related conjunctivitis, see Section 5.2, Chronic Conjunctivitis.

Also see related sections: Ophthalmia Neonatorum (Section 9.8), Stevens–Johnson Syndrome (Section 14.9), and Ocular Cicatricial Pemphigoid (Section 5.9).

❖ **Note** *Many systemic diseases can cause a nonspecific conjunctivitis (e.g., measles, mumps, influenza). The underlying disease should be managed appropriately; the eyes are treated with artificial tear drops 4 to 8 times per day.*

5.2 CHRONIC CONJUNCTIVITIS

Symptoms

Discharge, eyelids sticking (worse in morning), "red eye" (conjunctival hyperemia), foreign body sensation, duration *greater than 4 weeks* (otherwise see Acute Conjunctivitis, Section 5.1).

Differential Diagnosis
- Parinaud's Oculoglandular Conjunctivitis (Section 5.3)
- Silent dacryocystitis (See Section 6.8, Dacryocystitis)
- Verruca vulgaris papilloma
- Contact lens related (See Section 4.17, Contact Lens–Related Problems)

Chlamydial Inclusion Conjunctivitis

Sexually transmitted, typically found in young adults. A history of vaginitis, cervicitis, or urethritis may be present.

Signs

Inferior tarsal conjunctival follicles, superior corneal pannus, palpable preauricular node (PAN), and/or tiny, gray–white peripheral subepithelial infiltrates. A stringy, mucous discharge is typical.

Workup
1. History: Determine duration of red eye, any prior treatment, concomitant vaginitis, cervicitis, or urethritis. Sexual contacts with chlamydia?
2. Slit-lamp examination.
3. In adults, direct chlamydial immunofluorescence test and/or chlamydial culture of conjunctiva.

❖ **Note** *Topical fluorescein can interfere with immunofluorescence tests.*

4. Consider conjunctival scraping for Giemsa stain: shows basophilic intracytoplasmic inclusion bodies in epithelial cells, polymorphonuclear leukocytes, and lymphocytes in newborns.

Treatment
1. Tetracycline, 250 to 500 mg p.o., q.i.d., doxycycline, 100 mg p.o., b.i.d., erythromycin, 250 to 500 mg p.o., q.i.d., or clarithromycin, 250 to 500 mg p.o., b.i.d., for 3 to 6 weeks is given to the patient and sexual partners.*
2. Erythromycin, tetracycline, or sulfacetamide ointment 2 to 3 times per day for 2 to 3 weeks.

Follow-up

In 1 to 3 weeks, depending on the severity. The patient and sexual partners should be evaluated by their medical doctors for other sexually transmitted

---

*The tetracyclines are contraindicated in children younger than 8 years, pregnant women, and breast-feeding mothers.

diseases and should be treated to prevent reinfection (though they may be asymptomatic).

Trachoma

Principally occurs in developing countries in areas of poor sanitation and crowded conditions.

Signs
MacCallan Classification

Stage 1 Superior tarsal immature follicles, mild superior superficial punctate keratitis (SPK) and pannus, often preceded by purulent discharge and tender PAN.

Stage 2 Florid superior tarsal follicular reaction (IIa) and/or papillary hypertrophy (IIb) associated with superior corneal subepithelial infiltrates, pannus, and limbal follicles.

Stage 3 Follicles and scarring of superior tarsal conjunctiva.

Stage 4 No follicles, extensive conjunctival scarring.

Late complications Severe dry eyes, trichiasis, entropion, keratitis, corneal scarring, superficial fibrovascular pannus, Herbert's pits (scarred limbal follicles), corneal bacterial superinfection, and ulceration.

World Health Organization (WHO) Classification

TF (Trachomatous inflammation: follicular) More than five follicles on the upper tarsus.

TI (Trachomatous inflammation: intense) Inflammation with thickening obscuring more than 50% of the tarsal vessels.

TS (Trachomatous scarring) Cicatrization of tarsal conjunctiva with fibrous white bands.

TT (Trachomatous trichiasis) Trichiasis of at least one eyelash.

CO (Corneal opacity) Corneal opacity involving at least part of the pupillary margin.

Workup
1. History of exposure to areas in which it is endemic (i.e., North Africa, Middle East, India, Southeast Asia, rarely in United States).
2. Examination and diagnostic studies as noted for chlamydial inclusion conjunctivitis, described previously.

Treatment
1. Tetracycline or erythromycin, 250 to 500 mg p.o., q.i.d., doxycycline, 100 mg b.i.d.,* or clarithromycin, 250 to 500 mg p.o., b.i.d., for 3 to 6 weeks.

---

*The tetracyclines are contraindicated in children younger than 8 years, pregnant women, and breast-feeding mothers.

2. Tetracycline, erythromycin, or sulfacetamide ointment 2 to 4 times per day for 3 to 4 weeks.

Follow-up

Every 2 to 3 weeks initially, then as needed. Although the previously described treatment is usually curative, reinfection is common if hygienic conditions do not improve.

Molluscum Contagiosum

Critical Sign

Dome-shaped, usually multiple, umbilicated, shiny nodules on the eyelid or eyelid margin.

Other Signs

Follicular conjunctival response from toxic viral products, corneal pannus. If many lesions are present, consider the possibility of human immunodeficiency virus (HIV).

Treatment

Removal of lesions by simple excision, incision and curettage, or cryosurgery.

Follow-up

Every 2 to 4 weeks until the conjunctivitis resolves.

Toxic Conjunctivitis (Eye Drops)

Signs

Inferior papillary reaction, especially with aminoglycosides, antivirals, and preservatives. With long-term use, usually >1 month, a follicular response may be seen with atropine, miotics, epinephrine agents, antibiotics, and antivirals. Inferior superficial punctate keratitis (SPK) and scant discharge may be noted.

Treatment

Discontinuing the offending eye drop is usually sufficient. Artificial tears without preservatives (e.g., Refresh Plus or Theratears) 4 to 8 times per day may help as well.

Follow-up

In 1 to 2 weeks, as needed.

5.3 PARINAUD'S OCULOGLANDULAR CONJUNCTIVITIS

Symptoms
Red eye, mucopurulent discharge, foreign-body sensation.

Critical Signs
Granulomatous nodule(s) on the palpebral conjunctiva, visibly swollen preauricular or submandibular lymph node on the same side.

Other Signs
Fever, rash, follicular conjunctivitis.

Etiology
- Cat-scratch disease from *Bartonella henselae* (most common cause). (Often a history of being scratched or licked by a kitten within 2 weeks before the onset of symptoms.)
- Tularemia (History of contact with rabbits, other small wild animals, or ticks. Patients have severe headache, fever, and other systemic manifestations.)
- Tuberculosis and other mycobacteria
- Rare causes: syphilis, leukemia, lymphoma, mumps, mononucleosis, fungi, sarcoidosis, and others.

Workup
Initiated when etiology is not known (e.g., no recent cat scratch).

1. Conjunctival biopsy with scrapings for Gram's, Giemsa, and acid-fast stains.
2. Conjunctival cultures on blood, Lowenstein–Jensen, Sabouraud's, and thioglycolate media.
3. Complete blood count, rapid plasma reagin (RPR), fluorescent treponemal antibody, absorbed (FTA-ABS), and, if the patient is febrile, blood cultures.
4. Chest x-ray, purified protein derivative (PPD), and anergy panel.
5. If tularemia is suspected, serologic titers are necessary.
6. If diagnosis of cat-scratch disease is uncertain, cat-scratch serology and cat-scratch skin test (Hanger–Rose) may be performed.

Treatment
1. Warm compresses for tender lymph nodes.
2. Antipyretics prn.

3. Specifically:

Cat-scratch disease   The disease generally resolves spontaneously in 6 weeks. Consider tetracycline, 250 mg q.i.d., trimethoprim/sulfamethoxazole DS, p.o., b.i.d., or ciprofloxacin, 250 mg p.o., b.i.d., for 4 weeks plus a topical antibiotic (e.g., bacitracin/polymyxin B ointment or gentamicin drops, q.i.d.) for 4 weeks. The cat does not need to be removed.

Tularemia   Streptomycin, 1 g i.m., b.i.d., for 7 days and gentamicin drops q 2 h for 1 week and then 5 times per day until resolved. Refer to a medical internist for systemic management.

Tuberculosis   Refer to an internist for antituberculosis medication.

Syphilis   Systemic penicillin (dose depends on the stage of the syphilis) and topical tetracycline ointment. See Section 14.2.

Follow-up

Repeat the ocular examination in 1 to 2 weeks. Conjunctival granulomas and lymphadenopathy may take 4 to 6 weeks to resolve for cat-scratch disease.

5.4 SUBCONJUNCTIVAL HEMORRHAGE

Symptoms

Red eye, may have mild irritation, usually asymptomatic.

Critical Sign

Blood underneath the conjunctiva, often in a sector of the eye. The entire view of the sclera may be obstructed by blood.

Etiology

- Valsalva (e.g., coughing or straining)
- Traumatic (May be isolated or associated with a retrobulbar hemorrhage or ruptured globe.)
- Hypertension
- Bleeding disorder
- Idiopathic

Differential Diagnosis

- Kaposi's sarcoma [Red or purple lesion beneath the conjunctiva, usually elevated slightly. These patients should be evaluated for acquired immunodeficiency syndrome (AIDS).]

- Other conjunctival neoplasms (e.g., lymphoma) with secondary hemorrhage.

Workup
1. History: Bleeding or clotting problems? Medications (e.g., aspirin, Coumadin)? Eye rubbing, trauma, heavy lifting or Valsalva? Recurrent subconjunctival hemorrhage? Acute or chronic cough?
2. Ocular examination: Rule out a conjunctival lesion and check intraocular pressure (IOP). In traumatic cases, rule out a ruptured globe (abnormally deep anterior chamber, significant subconjunctival edema, hyphema, vitreous hemorrhage, and/or limitation of extraocular motility) and a retrobulbar hemorrhage (associated with proptosis, increased IOP, and occasionally, conjunctival swelling).
3. Check blood pressure.
4. If the patient has recurrent subconjunctival hemorrhages or a history of bleeding problems, a bleeding time, prothrombin time, partial thromboplastin time, and complete blood count (to evaluate for leukemia) with platelets and protein C and S should be obtained with a consultation to an internist considered.

Treatment
None required. Artificial tear drops (e.g., Refresh Tears) q.i.d. can be given if mild ocular irritation is present. In addition, elective use of aspirin products and nonsteroidal antiinflammatory drugs (NSAIDs) should be discouraged.

Follow-up
This condition usually clears spontaneously within 1 to 2 weeks. Patients are told to return if the blood does not fully resolve or if they suffer a recurrence. Referral to an internist or family physician should be made as indicated for hypertension or a bleeding diathesis.

5.5 SUPERIOR LIMBIC KERATOCONJUNCTIVITIS (SLK)

Symptoms
Red eye, burning, foreign-body sensation, pain, tearing, mild photophobia, frequent blinking. The course may be chronic with exacerbations and remissions.

Critical Sign
Thickening and inflammation of the superior bulbar conjunctiva, especially at the limbus.

Other Signs
Fine papillae on the superior palpebral conjunctiva; fine punctate fluorescein staining on the superior cornea, limbus, and conjunctiva; superior corneal micropannus and filaments. Usually bilateral.

Workup
1. History: Recurrent episodes?
2. Slit-lamp examination with fluorescein staining, particularly of the superior cornea and adjacent conjunctiva. The upper eyelid often must be lifted by the examiner to see the superior limbal area, and then should be everted to visualize the tarsus. Sometimes the localized hyperemia of the superior bulbar conjunctiva is best appreciated by direct inspection without a slit lamp by raising the eyelids of the patient while they are in downgaze.
3. Thyroid function tests (T_3, T_4, TSH), because 50% of patients have associated dysthyroid disease.

Treatment

MILD

1. Aggressive lubrication: artificial tears (e.g., Refresh Plus or Theratears) 4 to 8 times per day and artificial-tear ointment (e.g., Refresh PM) qhs.
2. May consider punctal occlusion.
3. Treat any concurrent blepharitis.

MODERATE TO SEVERE (IN ADDITION TO ABOVE)

1. Silver nitrate 0.5 to 1.0% **solution** (from wax ampules) applied on a cotton-tipped applicator for 10 to 20 seconds to the superior tarsal and superior bulbar conjunctiva after topical anesthesia (e.g., proparacaine). Then irrigation and antibiotic ointment (e.g., erythromycin) qhs for 1 week.

❖ **Note** *Do* not *use silver nitrate cautery sticks, which cause severe ocular burns.*

2. If significant amounts of mucus or filaments are present, then acetylcysteine, 10% drops (e.g., Mucomyst), 3 to 5 times per day are usually added.
3. If two to three separate silver nitrate solution applications are unsuccessful, then consider cautery, or surgical resection or recession of the superior bulbar conjunctiva.

Follow-up

Every week or two during an exacerbation. If signs and symptoms persist, a reapplication of silver nitrate solution, as described previously, may be performed at the weekly follow-up visit.

5.6 EPISCLERITIS

Symptoms

Acute onset of redness and mild pain in one or both eyes, typically in young adults; a history of recurrent episodes is common. No discharge.

Critical Signs

Sectoral (and less commonly, diffuse) redness of one or both eyes, mostly due to engorgement of the episcleral vessels. These vessels are large and run in a radial direction beneath the conjunctiva.

Other Signs

Mild to moderate tenderness over the area of episcleral injection or a nodule that can be moved slightly over the underlying sclera may be seen. Associated anterior uveitis and corneal involvement are rare. Vision is normal.

Etiology

- Idiopathic (Most common.)
- Collagen–vascular disease (e.g., rheumatoid arthritis, polyarteritis nodosa, systemic lupus erythematosus, Wegener's granulomatosis)
- Gout (Serum uric acid increased.)
- Infectious [Herpes zoster virus (scars from an old facial rash may be present), herpes simplex virus, Lyme disease, syphilis (fluorescent treponemal antibody, absorbed [FTA-ABS] positive), hepatitis B].
- Others (e.g., inflammatory bowel disease, rosacea, atopy, and thyroid disease)

Differential Diagnosis

- Scleritis [Pain is deep, severe, and often radiates to the ipsilateral side of the head or face. The sclera may have a bluish hue when observed in natural light. Scleral (and deep episcleral) vessels, as well as conjunctival and superficial episcleral vessels, are injected. The scleral vessels do not blanch on application of topical phenylephrine, 2.5%. Corneal involvement may be present. See Section 5.7, Scleritis.]

- Iritis (Cells and flare are present in the anterior chamber. May be present with scleritis.)
- Conjunctivitis (Characterized by a discharge, and inferior tarsal conjunctival follicles or papillae. See Sections 5.1, Acute Conjunctivitis, and 5.2, Chronic Conjunctivitis.)

Workup
1. History: Assess for a history of rash, arthritis, venereal disease, recent viral illness, other medical problems.
2. External examination in natural light: Look for the bluish hue of scleritis.
3. Slit-lamp examination: Anesthetize (e.g., topical proparacaine) and move the conjunctiva with a cotton-tipped applicator to determine the depth of the injected blood vessels. Evaluate for any corneal or anterior-chamber involvement. Check intraocular pressure (IOP).
4. Place a drop of phenylephrine, 2.5%, in the affected eye and reexamine the vascular pattern 10 to 15 minutes later. Episcleral vessels should blanch.
5. If the history suggests an underlying etiology, the appropriate laboratory tests should be obtained [e.g., anti-nuclear antibody (ANA), rheumatoid factor, erythrocyte sedimentation rate (ESR), serum uric acid level, rapid plasma reagin (RPR), FTA-ABS, anti-neutrophil cytoplasmic antibody (ANCA)].

Treatment
- If mild, treat with artificial tears (e.g., Refresh Tears), q.i.d.
- If moderate to severe, a mild topical steroid (e.g., fluorometholone) q.i.d. often relieves the discomfort. Rarely, more potent or frequent topical steroid application is necessary.
- In cases in which topical steroids do not provide relief, oral non-steroidal antiinflammatory drugs (NSAIDs) may help (e.g., ibuprofen, 200 to 600 mg p.o., 3 to 4 times per day, or aspirin, 325 to 650 mg p.o., 3 to 4 times per day, with food and/or antacids). Some prefer oral NSAIDs to topical steroids as initial therapy.

Follow-up
Patients treated with artificial tears need not be seen for several weeks for their episcleritis unless it worsens or discomfort continues. Patients taking topical steroids are checked weekly (including an IOP check) until their symptoms have resolved. The frequency of steroid administration is then tapered. Patients are informed that episcleritis may recur in the same or contralateral eye.

5.7 SCLERITIS

Symptoms

Severe and boring eye pain (most prominent feature), which may radiate to the forehead, brow, or jaw and may awaken the patient at night. Usually, gradual onset with red eye and insidious decrease in vision. Recurrent episodes are common. Scleromalacia perforans may have minimal symptoms.

Critical Signs

Inflammation of scleral, episcleral, and conjunctival vessels (scleral vessels are large, deep vessels that cannot be moved with a cotton swab and do not blanch with topical phenylephrine)—can be sectoral or diffuse. The sclera has a characteristic bluish hue (best seen in natural light by gross inspection) and may be thin or edematous.

Other Signs

Scleral nodules, corneal changes (peripheral keratitis, limbal guttering, and/or keratolysis), glaucoma, subretinal granuloma, uveitis, exudative retinal detachment (RD), cataract, proptosis (posterior scleritis), or rapid-onset hyperopia (posterior scleritis).

❖ **Note** *The patient should be examined in all directions of gaze in daylight or with adequate room illumination without a slit lamp.*

Classification

Diffuse anterior scleritis:
• Widespread inflammation of the anterior segment.

Nodular anterior scleritis:
• Immovable inflamed nodule(s).

Necrotizing anterior scleritis with inflammation:
• Extreme pain.
• The sclera becomes transparent (choroidal pigment visible) because of necrosis.
• High level of association with a systemic inflammatory disease.

Necrotizing anterior scleritis without inflammation (scleromalacia perforans):
• Almost complete lack of symptoms.
• Mainly seen in patients with long-standing rheumatoid arthritis (RA).

Posterior scleritis:
- May start posteriorly or be an extension of anterior scleritis.
- May simulate an amelanotic choroidal mass.
- Exudative RD, disc swelling, retinal hemorrhage, choroidal folds, choroidal detachment.
- Restricted extraocular movements.
- Proptosis, pain, tenderness.
- Usually unrelated to systemic disease.

Etiology

Fifty percent of patients with scleritis have an associated systemic disease.

More common   Connective tissue disease (e.g., RA, Wegener's granulomatosis, relapsing polychondritis, systemic lupus erythematosus, Reiter's syndrome, polyarteritis nodosa, ankylosing spondylitis), herpes zoster ophthalmicus, syphilis, after ocular surgery, gout.

Less common   Tuberculosis (TB), other bacteria (*Pseudomonas* species), Lyme disease, sarcoidosis, hypertension, foreign body, parasite.

Differential Diagnosis

- Episcleritis (Sclera not involved. Blood vessels blanch with topical phenylephrine. More acute onset than scleritis. Tend to be younger in age and with very mild symptoms if any. See Section 5.6, Episcleritis.)

Workup

1. History: Previous episodes? Medical problems?
2. Examine the sclera in all directions of gaze by gross inspection in natural light or adequate room light.
3. Slit-lamp examination with a red-free filter (green light) to determine whether avascular areas of the sclera exist. Check for corneal or anterior-chamber involvement.
4. Dilated fundus examination to rule out posterior involvement.
5. Complete physical examination (especially joints, skin, cardiovascular and respiratory systems, often performed by an internist or rheumatologist).
6. Complete blood count, erythrocyte sedimentation rate (ESR), uric acid, rapid plasma reagin (RPR), fluorescent treponemal antibody, absorbed (FTA-ABS), rheumatoid factor, anti-nuclear antibody (ANA), fasting blood sugar, angiotensin-converting enzyme (ACE), CH 50, C3, C4, and serum anti-neutrophilic cytoplasmic antibody (ANCA).
7. Other tests if clinical suspicion warrants additional workup: PPD with anergy panel, chest radiograph, radiograph of sacroiliac joints, B-scan ultrasonography to detect posterior scleritis, and magnetic resonance imaging (MRI) or computed tomography (CT) scan if indicated.

Treatment

1. *Diffuse and nodular scleritis: One or more of the following may be required. Concurrent antacid or H_2-blocker* (e.g., ranitidine, 150 mg p.o., b.i.d.) is advisable.
   a. Nonsteroidal antiinflammatory drugs (NSAIDs) (e.g., ibuprofen, 400 to 600 mg p.o., q.i.d., or indomethacin, 25 mg p.o., t.i.d., diflunisal, 500 mg, b.i.d., flurbiprofen, 100 mg, t.i.d., naproxen, 250 to 500 mg, b.i.d., and others). If there is failure to improve while taking one NSAID after 1 to 3 weeks, another one or two others should be tried. If still no improvement, consider systemic steroids.
   b. Systemic steroids: prednisone, 60 to 100 mg p.o., once per day for one week, followed by a taper to 20 mg per day over next 2 to 3 weeks, followed by a slower taper. The addition of an NSAID often facilitates the tapering of the steroid. If steroids are unsuccessful, consider immunosuppressive therapy. See Drug Glossary before prescribing systemic steroids.
   c. Immunosuppressive therapy (e.g., cyclophosphamide, methotrexate, cyclosporine, azathioprine): If one drug is ineffective or not tolerated, another should be tried, up to two to three different drugs. Systemic steroids may be used in conjunction. Immunosuppressive therapy is given with an internist or rheumatologist. The role of topical cyclosporine 2% drops is unclear.
2. Necrotizing scleritis:
   a. Systemic steroid and immunosuppressive therapies are used as in 1b and 1c.
   b. For scleromalacia perforans, abundant lubrication is also important.
   c. Scleral (or Tutoplast) patch grafting may be necessary, if there is significant risk of perforation.
3. Posterior scleritis: Therapy is controversial and may include systemic aspirin, NSAIDs, steroids, or immunosuppressive therapy as above.
4. Infectious etiologies: Treat with appropriate topical and systemic antimicrobial. If a foreign body is present, surgical removal is indicated.
5. Glasses or eye shield should be worn at all times if there is significant thinning and a risk of perforation.

❖ **Notes**

1. *Topical steroids are not effective in scleritis.*
2. *Subconjunctival steroids are generally contraindicated, especially in necrotizing scleritis, and may lead to scleral thinning and perforation.*

Follow-up

Depends on the severity of the symptoms and the degree of corneal thinning. Decreased pain is a sign of response to treatment, even if inflammation appears unchanged.

5.8 OCULAR ROSACEA

Symptoms

Bilateral chronic ocular irritation, redness, burning, and foreign-body sensation. Patients are typically middle-aged adults, but it can be found in children.

Critical Signs

Telangiectasias, pustules, papules, and/or erythema of the cheeks, forehead, and nose. The findings may be subtle and are often best seen in natural light. Superficial or deep corneal vascularization, particularly in the inferior cornea, is sometimes seen, and it may extend into a stromal infiltrate.

Other Signs

Rhinophyma of the nose occurs in the late stages of the disease. Blepharitis (telangiectasias of the eyelid margin with inflammation) and chalazia are common. Conjunctival injection, superficial punctate keratitis (SPK), phlyctenules, perilimbal infiltrates of staphylococcal hypersensitivity, iritis, or even corneal perforation may occur.

Differential Diagnosis

- Herpes simplex keratitis (Usually unilateral. Stromal keratitis with neovascularization may appear similar. The typical facial lesions of rosacea are absent. See Section 4.15, Herpes Simplex Virus.)
- See Superficial Punctate Keratitis, Section 4.1, for additional differential diagnoses.

Workup

1. External examination: Look at the face for the characteristic skin findings and inspect the eyelids for chalazia.
2. Slit-lamp examination: Look for telangiectasias of the eyelid margins, conjunctival injection, and corneal scarring and vascularization, especially inferiorly.

Treatment

1. Tetracycline, 250 mg p.o., q.i.d., or doxycycline, 100 mg p.o., b.i.d., for 2 to 6 weeks; taper the dose slowly once relief of symptoms is obtained. Some patients are maintained on low-dose tetracycline (e.g., 250 mg q day) indefinitely if active disease recurs when the patient is off medication. Erythromycin, in the same dose as tetracycline, may be substituted if tetracycline or doxycycline cannot be used (e.g., in a pregnant woman, nursing mother, or child younger than 8 years).

❖ **Note** *Patients diagnosed with ocular rosacea who are asymptomatic and who do not demonstrate progressively worsening eye disease need not be treated with oral antibiotics.*

2. Warm compresses and eyelid hygiene for blepharitis or meibomianitis (see Section 5.10, Blepharitis/Meibomianitis). Treat dry eyes if present (see Section 4.2, Dry-Eye Syndrome).
3. Treat chalazia as needed (see Section 6.1, Chalazion/Hordeolum).
4. Corneal perforations may be treated with cyanoacrylate tissue adhesive if small, whereas larger perforations may require surgical correction. (Tetracycline is usually administered in the preoperative and postoperative periods.)
5. If infiltrates stain with fluorescein, smears, cultures, and antibiotic treatment may be necessary for possible infectious corneal ulcer (see Section 4.12, Infectious Corneal Infiltrates/Ulcer).

Follow-up
Variable; depends on the severity of disease. Patients without corneal involvement are seen weeks to months later. Those with corneal disease are examined more often.

❖ **Note** *Tetracycline and doxycycline should not be given to pregnant women, nursing women, or children younger than 8 years. Patients should be told to take the tetracycline on an empty stomach and be warned of susceptibility to sunburn while taking tetracycline and doxycycline.*

5.9 OCULAR CICATRICIAL PEMPHIGOID

Symptoms
Insidious onset of redness, foreign-body sensation, tearing, and photophobia. Bilateral involvement. The course is characterized by remissions and exacerbations. Usually occurs in patients older than 55 years.

Critical Signs
Inferior symblepharon (linear folds of conjunctiva connecting the palpebral conjunctiva of the lower eyelid to the inferior bulbar conjunctiva), foreshortening and tightness of the lower fornix.

Other Signs
Secondary bacterial conjunctivitis, superficial punctate keratitis (SPK), corneal ulcer. Later, poor tear film, resulting in severe dry-eye syndrome, entropion, trichiasis, corneal opacification with pannus and keratinization,

obliteration of the fornices with eventual limitation of ocular motility, and ankyloblepharon can occur. Open-angle glaucoma also may be present.

Systemic Signs

Mucous membrane (nose, oral cavity, pharynx, larynx, esophagus, anus, vagina, urethra) vesicles, scarring and/or strictures; ruptured or formed bullae; denuded epithelium. In the mouth, a desquamative gingivitis is common. Vesicles and bullae also may be noted on the skin, sometimes with erythematous plaques or scars near affected mucous membranes.

Differential Diagnosis

- Stevens–Johnson syndrome (erythema multiforme major). [Acute onset, usually with fever and malaise. Similar ocular involvement as ocular pemphigoid. The lips are typically swollen and crusted, and target lesions of the skin (red centers surrounded by a pale zone) are often found. Often precipitated by drugs (e.g., sulfa, penicillin, other antibiotics, Dilantin) or infections (e.g., herpes and mycoplasma). See Section 14.9, Stevens–Johnson Syndrome.]
- Membranous conjunctivitis with scarring (Usually adenovirus or β-hemolytic streptococcus. Symblepharon can follow any severe membranous/pseudomembranous conjunctivitis.)
- Severe chemical burn. See Section 3.1, Chemical Burn.
- Chronic topical medicine [e.g., glaucoma medications (especially epinephrine and pilocarpine), antiviral agents].
- Others (e.g., atopic keratoconjunctivitis, radiation treatment, squamous cell carcinoma).

Workup

1. History: Long-term topical medications? Acute onset of severe systemic illness in the past? Recent systemic medications?
2. Skin and mucous membrane (especially the mouth) examination.
3. Slit-lamp examination: Especially examine for inferior symblepharon. (Pull down the lower eyelid and have the patient look up.) Check intraocular pressure (IOP).
4. Gram's stain and culture of the cornea or conjunctiva if secondary bacterial infection is suspected.
5. Consider a conjunctival biopsy for immunofluorescence studies.
6. Dermatology; ear, nose, and throat; gastrointestinal; and pulmonary consults if needed.

Treatment

(Often needs to be coordinated with an internist, rheumatologist, and/or dermatologist.)

1. Artificial tears (e.g., Refresh Plus or Theratears drops) 4 to 10 times per day. Can add an artificial tear ointment (e.g., Refresh PM) 2 to 4 times per day and qhs.

2. Treat blepharitis vigorously with eyelid hygiene, warm compresses, and antibiotic ointment (e.g., bacitracin, t.i.d.). Oral tetracycline can be used if eyelid disease is severe. See Blepharitis/Meibomianitis, Section 5.10.
3. Goggles or glasses with sides to provide a moist environment for the eyes.
4. Punctal occlusion if puncta are not already closed by scarring.
5. Topical steroids (e.g., prednisolone acetate, 1%, q.i.d.) may rarely help in suppressing acute exacerbations, but be cautious of corneal melting.
6. Systemic steroids (e.g., prednisone, 60 mg p.o., once per day) may additionally help in suppressing acute exacerbations.
7. Dapsone is often used for progressive disease. Starting dose is 25 mg p.o., for 3 to 7 days, increase by 25 mg every 4 to 7 days until the desired result is achieved (usually 100 to 150 mg p.o., q.d.). Dapsone is maintained for several months and tapered slowly.

❖ **Note** *Dapsone can cause a dose-related hemolysis; therefore, complete blood count and glucose-6-phosphate dehydrogenase (G-6-PD) must be checked before administration. Dapsone should be avoided in patients with G-6-PD deficiency. A complete blood count with reticulocyte count is obtained weekly as the dose is increased, every 3 to 4 weeks until blood counts are stable, and then every few months.*

8. Immunosuppressive agents (e.g., cyclophosphamide, methotrexate, or azathioprine) may be used for progressive disease.
9. Consider surgical correction of entropion and cryotherapy or electrolysis of trichiasis. (May be necessary, but carries a risk of further scarring and of provoking an acute exacerbation.)
10. Mucous membrane grafts (e.g., buccal) can be used to reconstruct the fornices if needed.
11. Consider a keratoprosthesis in an end-stage eye with apparently good macular and optic nerve function.

Follow-up
Every 1 to 2 weeks during acute exacerbations, and every 1 to 3 months during remissions.

5.10 BLEPHARITIS/MEIBOMIANITIS

Symptoms
Itching, burning, mild pain, foreign-body sensation, tearing, crusting around the eyes on awakening.

Critical Sign

Crusty, red, thickened eyelid margins with prominent blood vessels (blepharitis) and/or inspissated oil glands at the eyelid margins (meibomianitis).

Other Signs

Conjunctival injection, swollen eyelids, mild mucous discharge, superficial punctate keratitis (SPK); acne rosacea may be present. Corneal infiltrates and phlyctenules may be present.

Treatment

See Section 5.8 in the presence of acne rosacea.

1. Scrub the eyelid margins with mild shampoo (e.g., Johnson's baby shampoo) twice a day on a cotton-tipped applicator or a wash cloth.
2. Warm compresses for 10 to 15 minutes, b.i.d. to q.i.d.
3. If associated with dry eyes, then use artificial tears (e.g., Refresh Plus or Theratears) 4 to 8 times per day.
4. If moderately severe, then add erythromycin or bacitracin ointment to the eyelids qhs.
5. Recurrent meibomianitis can be treated with tetracycline, 250 mg p.o., q.i.d., or doxycycline, 100 mg p.o., b.i.d., for 1 to 2 weeks, and then taper slowly.

❖ **Note** *Tetracycline and doxycycline should not be used in pregnant women, nursing mothers, or children younger than 8 years. Erythromycin, 250 mg p.o., q.i.d., can be used instead.*

Follow-up

Follow up in 3 to 4 weeks as needed. Eyelid scrubs and warm compresses may be reduced to once per day as the condition improves. They often need to be maintained indefinitely.

❖ **Note** *Rarely, intractable, unilateral, or asymmetric blepharitis is the only manifestation of sebaceous cell carcinoma of the eyelid.*

5.11 CONTACT DERMATITIS

Symptoms

Sudden onset of a periorbital rash or eyelid swelling, mild watery discharge.

Critical Signs

Periorbital edema, erythema, vesicles, lichenification of the skin. Conjunctival chemosis out of proportion to injection and papillary response.

Other Signs

Watery discharge; crusting of the skin may develop when secondary infection arises.

Etiology

Most commonly, eye drops and cosmetics, including nail polish.

Treatment

1. Avoid the offending agent(s).
2. Cool compresses 4 to 6 times per day.
3. Preservative-free artificial tears (e.g., Refresh Plus or Theratears) 4 to 8 times per day and topical antihistamines (e.g., levocabastine q.i.d.).
4. Consider a mild steroid cream (e.g., dexamethasone cream, 0.05%) applied to the periocular area 2 to 3 times per day for 4 to 5 days for skin involvement.
5. Consider an oral antihistamine [e.g., diphenhydramine (e.g., Benadryl) 25 to 50 mg p.o., 3 to 4 times per day] for several days.

Follow-up

Reexamine within 1 week.

EYELID

6.1 CHALAZION/HORDEOLUM

Symptoms

Eyelid lump, swelling, pain, tenderness, erythema.

Critical Signs

Visible or palpable, well-defined subcutaneous nodule within the eyelid (in some cases, a nodule cannot be identified).

Other Signs

Blocked meibomian orifice, eyelid swelling and erythema, localized eyelid tenderness. There may be associated blepharitis or acne rosacea.

Differential Diagnosis

- Preseptal cellulitis (Eyelid erythema, edema, and warmth. Often there is a periorbital skin abrasion, laceration, or site of infection. Patients may be febrile. See Section 6.10, Preseptal Cellulitis.)
- Sebaceous gland carcinoma (Should be suspected in recurrent chalazion, thickening of both the upper and lower eyelids, chronic unilateral blepharitis, or a chalazion associated with loss of the eyelashes. It usually develops in older patients. A biopsy with frozen sections can establish the diagnosis. A special request must be made for lipid stains on frozen sections. See Section 6.11, Malignant Tumors of the Eyelid.)
- Pyogenic granuloma [Deep red, pedunculated lesion that may be associated with a chalazion/hordeolum or may develop after trauma or surgery to the conjunctiva or skin. It may be excised or treated with a topical antibiotic–steroid combination (e.g., sulfacetamide/pred-

nisolone acetate q.i.d. for 1 to 2 weeks). Intraocular pressure (IOP) must be monitored if topical steroids are used.]

Workup
1. History: Previous ocular surgery or trauma?
2. Palpate the involved eyelid, feeling for a nodule.
3. Slit-lamp examination: Evaluate the meibomian glands and evert the involved eyelid (this may allow better visualization of the nodule).

Treatment
1. Warm compresses for 15 to 20 minutes q.i.d. with light massage over the lesion.
2. Consider a topical antibiotic (e.g., bacitracin or erythromycin ointment b.i.d.).
3. If the chalazion does not disappear after 3 to 4 weeks of appropriate medical therapy and the patient wishes to have it removed, incision and curettage are performed. Occasionally an injection of steroid (e.g., 0.2 to 1.0 ml of triamcinolone, 40 mg/ml) into the lesion is performed instead of minor surgery, especially if the chalazion is near the lacrimal apparatus. The total dosage depends on the size of the lesion.

❖ **Note** *A steroid injection can lead to permanent depigmentation and/or atrophy of the skin at the injection site.*

Follow-up
Patients are not seen after instituting medical therapy unless the lesion persists beyond 3 to 4 weeks. Patients who have incision and curettage are usually reexamined in 1 week or as needed.

6.2 ECTROPION

Symptoms
Tearing, eye or eyelid irritation; may be asymptomatic.

Critical Sign
Outward turning of the eyelid margin.

Other Signs
Superficial punctate keratitis (SPK; from corneal exposure); conjunctival injection, thickening, and eventual keratinization (from chronic conjunctival drying).

Etiology
- Involutional (Aging.)
- Paralytic (Seventh-nerve palsy.)
- Cicatricial (Due to chemical burn, surgery, eyelid laceration scar, skin diseases, and others.)
- Mechanical (Due to herniated orbital fat, eyelid tumor, and others.)
- Allergic (Contact dermatitis.)
- Congenital (Facial dysmorphic syndromes or isolated abnormality.)

Workup
1. History: Previous surgery, trauma, chemical burn, or seventh-nerve palsy?
2. External examination: Check orbicularis oculi function, look for an eyelid tumor, eyelid scarring, herniated orbital fat, and other causes.
3. Slit-lamp examination: Check for SPK due to exposure and evaluate conjunctival integrity.

Treatment
1. Treat exposure keratopathy with lubricating agents (see Section 4.4, Exposure Keratopathy).
2. Treat an inflamed, exposed eyelid margin with warm compresses and antibiotic ointment (e.g., bacitracin or erythromycin t.i.d.).
3. Taping the eyelids into position with adhesive tape may be a temporizing measure.
4. Definitive treatment usually requires surgery. Surgery is delayed for 3 to 6 months in patients with a seventh-nerve palsy, as the ectropion may resolve spontaneously (see Section 11.8, Isolated Seventh-Nerve Palsy).

Follow-up
Patients with signs of corneal or conjunctival drying are examined in 1 to 2 weeks to evaluate the efficacy of therapy. Otherwise, follow-up is not urgent.

6.3 ENTROPION

Symptoms
Ocular irritation, foreign-body sensation, tearing, red eye.

Critical Sign
Inward turning of the eyelid margin.

Other Signs

Superficial punctate keratitis (SPK) (from eyelashes contacting the globe), conjunctival injection.

Etiology

- Involutional (Aging.)
- Cicatricial (Due to conjunctival scarring in ocular cicatricial pemphigoid, Stevens–Johnson syndrome, chemical burns, trauma, trachoma, and others.)
- Spastic (Due to surgical trauma, ocular irritation, or blepharospasm.)
- Congenital

Workup

1. History: Previous surgery, trauma, chemical burn, severe eye disease?
2. Slit-lamp examination: Check for SPK, conjunctival and eyelid scarring.

Treatment

See Section 6.6, Blepharospasm, if blepharospasm is present.

1. Antibiotic ointment (e.g., erythromycin or bacitracin t.i.d.) for SPK.
2. Everting the eyelid margin away from the globe and taping it in place with adhesive tape may be a temporizing measure.
3. Surgery is often required for permanent correction (spastic entropion may respond to the previously described measures and not require surgery).

Follow-up

If the cornea is relatively healthy, the condition does not require urgent attention. If the cornea is significantly damaged, aggressive treatment is indicated (see Superficial Punctate Keratitis, Section 4.1).

6.4 TRICHIASIS

Symptoms

Ocular irritation, foreign-body sensation, tearing, red eye.

Critical Sign

Misdirected eyelashes rubbing against the globe.

Other Signs

Superficial punctate keratitis (SPK), conjunctival injection.

Etiology

- Idiopathic
- Chronic blepharitis (Thickened, crusted, erythematous, or inflamed eyelid margin with mild discharge and telangiectatic blood vessels. See Section 5.10, Blepharitis/Meibomianitis.)
- Cicatricial (Due to eyelid scarring from trauma, surgery, ocular cicatricial pemphigoid, trachoma, others.)

Differential Diagnosis

All of the following can cause lashes to contact the globe.

- Entropion (Inward turning of the entire eyelid margin, including lashes. See Section 6.3, Entropion.)
- Epiblepharon (Congenital, sometimes familial, condition in which an extra lower eyelid skin fold redirects lashes into a vertical position, where they may contact the globe.)
- Distichiasis [Aberrant second row of lashes emanates from Meibomian gland openings. Either congenital (rare) or acquired in the setting of chronic inflammation (more common).]

Workup

1. History: Recurrent episodes? Severe systemic illness in the past? Previous trauma?
2. Slit-lamp examination with fluorescein staining: Evert the eyelids and inspect the palpebral conjunctiva.

Treatment

1. Epilation: remove the misdirected lashes.
   a. A few misdirected lashes: Remove them at the slit lamp with fine forceps. Recurrence is common, and cooperative patients may be instructed to epilate themselves carefully at home.
   b. Diffuse, severe, or recurrent trichiasis: Can attempt to epilate as described; however, definitive therapy generally requires electrolysis, cryotherapy, or surgery.
2. Treat SPK with antibiotic ointment (e.g., erythromycin or bacitracin t.i.d.) for several days.
3. Treat any underlying blepharitis (See Section 5.10, Blepharitis/Meibomianitis).

Follow-up

As needed, dictated by symptoms.

6.5 FLOPPY EYELID SYNDROME

Symptoms

Chronically red, irritated eye, often worst on awakening from sleep, and a mild mucus discharge. Patients are typically obese, often with associated sleep apnea syndrome.

Critical Signs

Upper eyelid is easily everted, without an accessory finger or cotton-tipped applicator exerting counterpressure.

Other Signs

Soft and rubbery superior tarsal plate, superior tarsal papillary conjunctivitis, Superficial punctate keratitis (SPK), upper-eyelash ptosis. May have associated keratoconus.

❖ **Note** *The symptoms are thought to result from spontaneous eversion of the upper eyelid during sleep, allowing the superior palpebral conjunctiva to rub against a pillow or sheets.*

Differential Diagnosis

All of the following may produce superior tarsal papillary conjunctivitis, but in none of them are the eyelids easily everted as described previously.

- Vernal conjunctivitis (Seasonal, itching, ropy discharge, giant papillary reaction. See Section 5.2, Chronic Conjunctivitis.)
- Giant papillary conjunctivitis (Often related to contact lens wear or an exposed suture. See Section 4.18, Contact Lens–Induced Giant Papillary Conjunctivitis.)
- Superior limbic keratoconjunctivitis (Hyperemia and thickening of the superior bulbar conjunctiva, often with filaments and corneal pannus. See Section 5.5, Superior Limbic Keratoconjunctivitis.)
- Toxic keratoconjunctivitis (Papillae and/or follicles are usually more abundant on the inferior tarsal conjunctiva in a patient using eyedrops. See Section 5.2, Chronic Conjunctivitis.)

Workup

1. Pull the skin of the upper eyelid toward the patient's forehead, and watch to see if the eyelid spontaneously everts or is abnormally lax.
2. Slit-lamp examination of the cornea and conjunctiva with fluorescein staining.

Treatment
1. Topical antibiotics or lubricants for any mild corneal or conjunctival abnormality [e.g., erythromycin ointment 2 to 3 times per day for SPK, and then artificial-tear ointment (e.g., Refresh PM) qhs when corneal pathology resolves].
2. The eyelids are taped closed during sleep and/or an eye shield is worn to protect the eyelid from rubbing against the pillow or bed. Patients are asked to refrain from sleeping face down.
3. An eyelid-tightening surgical procedure is often required.

Follow-up
1. Every 2 to 7 days initially, and then every few weeks to months as the condition stabilizes.
2. Refer to an internist or pulmonologist for evaluation and management of possible sleep apnea syndrome.

6.6 BLEPHAROSPASM

Symptoms
Uncontrolled blinking, twitching, or closure of the eyelids; decreased vision; always bilateral.

Critical Signs
Episodic involuntary contractions of the orbicularis oculi muscles.

Other Signs
Disappears during sleep, may have uncontrollable orofacial, head, and neck movements.

Etiology
- Idiopathic
- Ocular irritation (e.g., corneal or conjunctival foreign body, trichiasis, blepharitis, dry eye).

Differential Diagnosis
- Hemifacial spasm [Unilateral contractures involve the entire side of the face, does not disappear during sleep; damage to the seventh nerve at the level of the brainstem is the most common etiology. Magnetic resonance imaging (MRI) of the cerebellopontine angle should be obtained to rule out tumor. Treatment options include observation, bot-

ulism toxin injections, or neurosurgical decompression of the seventh cranial nerve (Janetta procedure).]

- Tourette's syndrome (Multiple compulsive muscle spasms associated with utterances of bizarre sounds or vile words.)
- Tic douloureux (trigeminal neuralgia) (Acute episodes of pain in the distribution of the fifth cranial nerve, often causing a wince or tic.)
- Tardive dyskinesia (Orofacial dyskinesia, often with restlessness and dystonic movements of the trunk and limbs, typically from long-term use of antipsychotic medications.)
- Eyelid myokymia (Eyelid twitches, often brought on by stress and caffeine.)

Workup

1. History: Unilateral or bilateral? Are the eyelids alone involved, or are the facial and limb muscles also involved? Medications?
2. Slit-lamp examination: Search for a local ocular disorder.
3. Neuroophthalmic examination to rule out other accompanying abnormalities.
4. Computed tomography (CT) scan (axial and coronal views) and/or magnetic resonance imaging (MRI) of the posterior fossa in atypical cases.

Treatment

1. Treat any underlying eye disorder causing ocular irritation (e.g., treat dry eye/blepharitis with eyelid hygiene and artificial tears 4 to 6 times per day; See the appropriate section.)
2. Consider botulinum toxin injections into the orbicularis muscles around the eyelids if the blepharospasm is severe (usually lasts 3 to 4 months).
3. If the spasm is not relieved with botulinum toxin injections, consider surgical excision of the orbicularis muscle from the upper eyelids and brow.

Follow-up

Not an urgent condition, but with severe blepharospasm, patients can be functionally blind.

6.7 CANALICULITIS

Symptoms

Tearing or discharge, red eye, mild tenderness over the nasal aspect of the lower or upper eyelid.

Critical Signs

Erythematous pouting of the punctum, erythema of the skin surrounding the punctum. Mucopurulent discharge or concretions may be expressed from the punctum when pressure is applied over the nasal corner of the lower eyelid (the lacrimal sac area).

Other Signs

Recurrent conjunctivitis confined to the nasal aspect of the eye, gritty sensation on probing of the canaliculus.

Etiology

- *Actinomyces israelii* (streptothrix) (Most common. Gram-positive rod with fine, branching filaments seen on Gram's stain.)
- Other bacteria (e.g., *Fusobacterium* and *Nocardia* species)
- Fungal (e.g., *Candida, Fusarium,* and *Aspergillus* species)
- Viral (e.g., herpes simplex and varicella-zoster)

Differential Diagnosis

- Dacryocystitis (Much more swelling, tenderness, and pain than canaliculitis. Swelling of the skin is more prominent than pouting of the punctum. See Section 6.8, Dacryocystitis.)
- Nasolacrimal duct obstruction (Tearing, minimal-to-no erythema or tenderness around the punctum. See Section 9.9, Congenital Nasolacrimal Duct Obstruction.)
- Conjunctivitis (Conjunctival follicles and/or papillae, discharge. No pouting punctum nor punctal discharge. See Sections 5.1, Acute Conjunctivitis, and 5.2, Chronic Conjunctivitis.)

Workup

1. Apply gentle pressure over the lacrimal sac with a cotton-tipped swab and roll it toward the punctum; observe for a punctal discharge.
2. Smears and cultures of the material expressed from the punctum: Gram's stain, Giemsa stain, and a KOH smear if available (1 drop of KOH, 10% to 20%, is placed on a slide, the discharge is added to the drop with a spatula, and a coverslip is placed over the mixture before microscopic examination); consider thioglycolate and Sabouraud's cultures.

Treatment

1. Remove obstructing concretions. Can try expressing the concretions through the punctum at the slit lamp, but a surgical canaliculotomy (with marsupialization of the canaliculus) is usually required to remove them all.

2. After removing the concretions, irrigate the canaliculus with penicillin G solution, 100,000 units/ml, or iodine, 1% solution. The patient is irrigated while in the upright position so the solution drains out of the nose and not into the nasopharynx.

3. If a fungus is found on smears and cultures, nystatin, 1:20,000 drops, t.i.d., and nystatin, 1:20,000 solution, irrigation several times per week may be effective.

   If evidence of herpes virus is found on smears, treat with trifluorothymidine, 1% drops (e.g., Viroptic) 5 times per day for several weeks. Silicone intubation is sometimes required in viral canaliculitis, along with appropriate antiviral therapy.

4. Warm compresses to the punctal area q.i.d.

5. More extensive surgical treatment is occasionally required.

Follow-up

This is generally not an urgent condition.

6.8 DACRYOCYSTITIS
(INFLAMMATION OF THE LACRIMAL SAC)

Symptoms

Pain, redness, and swelling over the innermost aspect of the lower eyelid (over the lacrimal sac); tearing; discharge; fever; may be recurrent.

Critical Signs

Erythematous, tender swelling centered over the nasal aspect of the lower eyelid and extending around the periorbital area nasally. A mucoid or purulent discharge can be expressed from the punctum when pressure is applied over the lacrimal sac.

❖ **Note** *Swelling in dacryocystitis is below the medial canthal tendon. Suspect lacrimal sac tumor (rare) if mass is above the medial canthal tendon.*

Other Signs

Fistula formation (often emerging from the skin beneath the medial canthal tendon), a lacrimal sac cyst, or a mucocele can occur in chronic cases. Rarely orbital or facial cellulitis may develop as a complication.

Etiology

May be related to nasolacrimal duct obstruction, diverticulum of the lacrimal sac, dacryolith, nasal or sinus surgery, trauma, or lacrimal sac tumor (rare). Most common organisms found are staphylococci, strepto-cocci, and diphtheroids.

Differential Diagnosis
All of the following may produce inflammation of the periorbital area nasally.

- Facial cellulitis involving the medial canthus (Discharge cannot be expressed from the punctum by placing pressure over the lacrimal sac. The lacrimal drainage system is patent on irrigation and special lacrimal drainage system radiographic studies.)
- Acute ethmoid sinusitis (Pain, tenderness, and erythema over the nasal bone, just medial to the inner canthus. Frontal headache and nasal obstruction are common. Patients are often febrile.)
- Acute frontal sinusitis (Inflammation predominantly involves the upper eyelid. The forehead is tender on palpation.)

Workup
1. History: Previous episodes? Concomitant ear, nose, or throat infection?
2. External examination, including gentle compression of the lacrimal sac (nasal corner of the lower eyelid) with a cotton-tipped swab in an attempt to express discharge from the punctum. This should be performed bilaterally to uncover a subtle contralateral dacryocystitis.
3. Ocular examination: Specifically check extraocular motility and look for proptosis (Hertel exophthalmometry).
4. Obtain a Gram's stain and blood agar culture (and chocolate agar culture in children) of any discharge expressed from the punctum.
5. Consider a CT scan (axial and coronal views) of the orbit and paranasal sinuses in atypical or severe cases or those that do not respond to, or worsen with, appropriate antibiotics.

❖ **Note** *Do not attempt to probe or irrigate the lacrimal system during the acute stage of the infection.*

Treatment
1. Systemic antibiotics in the following regimen:
   Children:
   a. Afebrile, systemically well, mild case, and reliable parent: Amoxicillin/clavulanate (e.g., Augmentin), 20 to 40 mg/kg/day p.o., in three divided doses. Alternative treatment: cefaclor (e.g., Ceclor), 20 to 40 mg/kg/day p.o., in three divided doses.
   b. Febrile, acutely ill, moderate to severe case, or unreliable parent: Hospitalize and treat with cefuroxime, 50 to 100 mg/kg/day i.v., in three divided doses.

Adults:
   a. Afebrile, systemically well, mild case, and reliable patient:
      Cephalexin (e.g., Keflex), 500 mg p.o., q 6 h.
      Alternative treatment: Amoxicillin/clavulanate (e.g., Augmentin), 500 mg p.o., q 8 h.
   b. Febrile, acutely ill:
      Hospitalize and treat with cefazolin (e.g., Ancef), 1 g i.v., q 8 h.
      Alternative treatment: See Orbital Cellulitis, Section 7.4.

The antibiotic regimen is adjusted according to the clinical response and the culture and sensitivity results. The intravenous antibiotics can be changed to comparable oral antibiotics depending on the rate of improvement, but systemic antibiotic therapy should be continued for a full 10- to 14-day course.

2. Topical antibiotic drops [e.g., trimethoprim/polymyxin (e.g., Polytrim), q.i.d.].
3. Warm compresses and gentle massage to the inner canthal region q.i.d.
4. Pain medication (e.g., acetaminophen with or without codeine) prn.
5. Consider incision and drainage of a pointing abscess.
6. Consider surgical correction [e.g., dacryocystorhinostomy (DCR) with silicone intubation] once the acute episode has resolved, particularly with chronic dacryocystitis.

Follow-up

Daily. If the condition of an outpatient worsens, hospitalization and i.v. antibiotics are recommended.

6.9 ACUTE INFECTIOUS DACRYOADENITIS
(INFECTION OF THE LACRIMAL GLAND)

Symptoms

Unilateral pain, redness, and swelling over the outer one third of the upper eyelid, often with tearing or discharge. Typically occurs in children and young adults.

Critical Signs

Erythema, swelling, and tenderness over the outer one third of the upper eyelid; may be associated with hyperemia of the palpebral lobe of the lacrimal gland.

Other Signs

Ipsilateral preauricular lymphadenopathy, ipsilateral conjunctival chemosis temporally, fever, elevated white blood cell count (WBC).

Etiology

- Bacterial (e.g., *Staphylococcus aureus, Neisseria gonorrhoeae,* streptococci)
- Viral (e.g., mumps, infectious mononucleosis, influenza, herpes zoster)

Differential Diagnosis

- Chalazion (A palpable subcutaneous nodule or a blocked meibomian orifice may be present, afebrile, normal WBC. See Section 6.1, Chalazion/Hordeolum.)
- Adenoviral conjunctivitis (May produce eyelid swelling and erythema with preauricular lymphadenopathy and a discharge. Typically produces inferior tarsal conjunctival follicles, often bilateral. See Section 5.1, Acute Conjunctivitis.)
- Preseptal cellulitis [Erythema, edema, and warmth of the eyelid(s) and surrounding soft tissue. May have a periorbital skin laceration or site of infection. See Section 6.10, Preseptal Cellulitis.]
- Orbital cellulitis (Proptosis and limitation of ocular motility often accompany eyelid erythema and swelling. See Section 7.4, Orbital Cellulitis.)
- Inflammatory dacryoadenitis from orbital pseudotumor (No preauricular lymphadenopathy. May have concomitant proptosis, downward displacement of the globe, or limitation of ocular motility. Typically afebrile with a normal WBC. Does not respond to antibiotics, but improves dramatically with systemic steroids. See Section 7.3, Orbital Inflammatory Pseudotumor.)
- Malignant lacrimal gland tumor (Commonly produces displacement of the globe or proptosis, often palpable, evident on CT scan. See Section 7.7, Lacrimal Gland Mass.)

Workup

The following is performed when an acute infectious etiology is suspected. When the disease does not respond to medical therapy or another etiology is being considered, see Lacrimal Gland Mass, Section 7.7.

1. History: Acute or chronic? Fever? Discharge? Systemic infection or viral syndrome?
2. Palpate the eyelid and along the orbital rim for a mass.
3. Evaluate the resistance of each globe to retropulsion.
4. Look for proptosis (Hertel exophthalmometry).

5. Complete ocular examination, particularly extraocular motility assessment.
6. Smears and bacterial cultures of any discharge.
7. Examine the parotid glands (often, but not always, enlarged in mumps, sarcoidosis, tuberculosis, lymphoma, and syphilis.)
8. If the patient is febrile, a complete blood count with differential, and sometimes blood cultures are obtained.
9. CT scan of the orbit and brain (axial and coronal views) when proptosis or a motility restriction is present or a mass is suspected.

Treatment
  A. Bacterial or infectious (but unidentified) etiology
   If mild-to-moderate:
   Amoxicillin/clavulanate (e.g., Augmentin)
    Children: 20 to 40 mg/kg/day, p.o., in three divided doses.
    Adults: 250 to 500 mg, p.o., q 8 h.
   or
   Cephalexin (e.g., Keflex)
    Children: 25 to 50 mg/kg/day, p.o., in four divided doses.
    Adults: 250 to 500 mg, p.o., q 6 h.
   If moderate-to-severe, hospitalize and treat with:
   ticarcillin/clavulanate (e.g., Timentin)
    Children: 200 mg/kg/day, i.v., in four divided doses.
    Adults: 3.1 g i.v., q 4 to 6 h.
   or
   Cefazolin (e.g., Ancef)
    Children: 50 to 100 mg/kg/day, i.v., in three to four divided doses.
    Adults: 1 gm, i.v., q 8 h.
   The antibiotic regimen should be adjusted according to the clinical response and culture and sensitivity test results. Intravenous antibiotics can be changed to comparable oral antibiotics depending on the rate of improvement, but systemic antibiotics should be continued for a full 7- to 14-day course. If an abscess develops, incision and drainage are necessary.
  B. Viral (e.g., mumps, infectious mononucleosis)
   1. Cool compresses to the area of swelling and tenderness.
   2. Analgesic as needed (e.g., acetaminophen, 650 mg, p.o., q 4 h prn).

❖ **Note** *Do not give aspirin to children with a viral syndrome because of the risk of Reye's syndrome.*

Follow-up
  Daily. Watch for signs of orbital involvement (decreased motility or proptosis). Outpatients are admitted to the hospital for i.v. antibiotic therapy

and an orbital CT scan if the condition worsens. Patients who fail to respond to medical therapy are managed as are those with chronic dacryoadenitis (see Lacrimal Gland Mass, Section 7.7).

6.10 Preseptal Cellulitis

Symptoms
Tenderness and redness of the eyelid, mild fever, irritability.

Critical Signs
Eyelid erythema, edema, warmth, tenderness. No proptosis, no restriction of extraocular motility, no pain with eye movement (unlike orbital cellulitis). The patient may not be able to open the eye because of the eyelid edema.

Other Signs
Conjunctival chemosis, tightness of the eyelid skin, fluctuant lymphedema of the eyelids.

❖ **Note** *Preseptal cellulitis due to* Haemophilus influenzae *generally occurs in children younger than 5 years and is characterized by the presence of an excessive amount of upper- and lower-eyelid edema, which may extend into the cheeks. Classically, there is a distinctive red–purple discoloration of the involved area. The child may have malaise, ipsilateral otitis media, sinusitis, leukocytosis, or a bacteremia.*

Etiology
Puncture wound, laceration, retained foreign body from trauma, vascular extension, or extension from sinuses or another infectious site (e.g., dacryocystitis in children, chalazion). May be primarily infectious or inflammatory with secondary infectious potential.

Organisms
Staphylococcus aureus and streptococci most common, but *H. influenzae* should be considered in children. Suspect anaerobes if a foul-smelling discharge or necrosis is present or there is a history of an animal or human bite. Consider a viral cause if preseptal cellulitis is associated with a skin rash (e.g., herpes simplex or herpes zoster).

Differential Diagnosis

- Orbital cellulitis (Proptosis, pain with eye movement, restricted motility, decreased sensation along the first division of the trigeminal nerve, decreased vision, fever, or chemosis. See Section 7.4, Orbital Cellulitis.)
- Other orbital disorders (Proptosis, globe displacement, or restricted ocular motility. See Section 7.1, Orbital Disease.)
- Chalazion (Focal eyelid inflammation, palpable mass, pointing meibomian gland. See Section 6.1, Chalazion/Hordeolum.)
- Allergic eyelid swelling (Sudden onset, bright-red eyelid discoloration, prominent itching, absence of tenderness, positive history of contact allergies or new eye or skin medication. See Section 5.11, Contact Dermatitis.)
- Viral conjunctivitis with eyelid swelling (Conjunctival follicles, palpable preauricular lymph node, itching, tearing, eyelid sticking, or watery discharge. See Section 5.1, Acute Conjunctivitis.)
- Cavernous sinus thrombosis (Proptosis; paresis of the third, fourth, and sixth cranial nerves out of proportion with the eyelid swelling; decreased sensation of the first and second division of the trigeminal nerve; typically bilateral. See Section 11.9, Cavernous Sinus/Superior Orbital Fissure Syndrome.)
- Erysipelas (Rapidly advancing streptococcal cellulitis, often with a clear demarcation line, high fever, and chills.)
- Others (Insect bite, angioedema, trauma, maxillary osteomyelitis, and others.)

Workup

1. History: Pain with eye movements? Prior trauma or cancer?
2. Complete ocular examination: Look carefully for restriction of ocular motility or proptosis. An eyelid speculum or Desmarres eyelid retractor may facilitate the ocular examination if the eyelids are excessively swollen.
3. Check facial sensation in the distribution of first and second divisions of the trigeminal nerve.
4. Palpate the periorbital area and the head and neck lymph nodes for a mass.
5. Check vital signs.
6. Gram's stain and culture of any open wound or drainage.
7. CT scan of the brain and orbits (axial and coronal views) if there is a history of significant trauma or a concern about the possibility of an orbital or intraocular foreign body, orbital cellulitis, a subperiosteal abscess, cavernous sinus thrombosis, or cancer.
8. Consider obtaining a complete blood count with differential and blood cultures in severe cases or when a fever is present.

Treatment
1. Antibiotic therapy
   A. Mild preseptal cellulitis, older than 5 years, afebrile, reliable patient/parent:
      Amoxicillin/clavulanate (e.g., Augmentin)
      Children: 20 to 40 mg/kg/day, p.o., in three divided doses.
      Adults: 500 mg, p.o., q 8 h.

      or
      Cefaclor (e.g., Ceclor)
      Children: 20 to 40 mg/kg/day, p.o., in three divided doses; maximum dose, 1 g/day.
      Adults: 250 to 500 mg, p.o., q 8 h.

      If the patient is allergic to penicillin, then:
      Trimethoprim/sulfamethoxazole (e.g., Bactrim)
      Children: 8 to 12 mg/kg/day trimethoprim with 40 to 60 mg/kg/day sulfamethoxazole, p.o., in two divided doses.
      Adults: 160 to 320 mg trimethoprim with 800 to 1,600 mg sulfamethoxazole (one to two double strength tablets), p.o., b.i.d.

      or
      Erythromycin
      Children: 30 to 50 mg/kg/day, p.o., in three to four divided doses.
      Adults: 250 to 500 mg, p.o., q 6 h.

❖ **Note** *Oral antibiotics are maintained for 10 days.*

   B. Moderate-to-severe preseptal cellulitis, or any one of the following:
      • Patient appears toxic,
      • Patient may be noncompliant with outpatient treatment and follow-up.
      • Child 5 years of age or younger,
      • Infection with *H. influenzae* is suspected,
      • No noticeable improvement or worsening after a few days of oral antibiotics.

      Admit to the hospital for i.v. antibiotics as follows:
      Ceftriaxone
      Children: 100 mg/kg/day, i.v., in two divided doses.
      Adults: 1 to 2 g, i.v., q 12 h.

      and
      Vancomycin
      Neonates: 15 mg/kg load, then 10 mg/kg q 12 h.
      Children: 40 mg/kg/day, i.v., in three to four divided doses.
      Adults: 0.5 to 1 g, i.v., q 12 h.

❖ **Note** *Intravenous antibiotics can be changed to comparable oral antibiotics after significant improvement is observed. Systemic antibiotics are maintained for a complete 10- to 14-day course. See Orbital Cellulitis, Section 7.4, for alternative treatment.*

2. Warm compresses to the inflamed area, t.i.d., prn.
3. Polymyxin B/bacitracin ointment (e.g., Polysporin) to the eye, q.i.d., if secondary conjunctivitis is present.
4. Tetanus toxoid if needed (see Appendix 10).
5. Exploration and debridement of the lesion if a fluctuant mass or abscess is present. Incise over the mass or reopen a healing laceration with a scalpel, fully explore the wound, and Gram's stain and culture any drainage. Avoid the orbital septum if possible. A drain may need to be placed.

Follow-up

Daily until clear and consistent improvement is demonstrated, then every 2 to 7 days until the condition has totally resolved. If a preseptal cellulitis progresses despite antibiotic therapy, the patient is admitted to the hospital and a repeated (or initial) orbital CT scan is obtained. For patients taking oral antibiotics, i.v. antibiotic treatment is started (see Orbital Cellulitis, Section 7.4). Consultation with an infectious disease specialist may be helpful.

6.11 MALIGNANT TUMORS OF THE EYELID

Symptoms

Asymptomatic or mildly irritating eyelid lump.

Signs

Skin ulceration and inflammation with distortion of the normal eyelid anatomy are common findings in malignant lesions. Abnormal color, texture, or persistent bleeding suggest malignancy. Loss of eyelashes (madarosis) or whitening of eyelashes (poliosis) over the lesion may occur.

Etiology

- Basal cell carcinoma (Most common malignant eyelid tumor, usually occurs in middle-aged or elderly patients.) Presents as:
   1. Nodular: Indurated, firm mass, commonly with telangiectases over the tumor margins. Sometimes the center of the lesion is ulcerated.
   2. Morpheaform: Firm, flat, subcutaneous lesion with indistinct borders.

❖ **Note** *Basal cell carcinoma does not metastasize, but it may be highly locally invasive, particularly when it is present in the medial canthal region.*

- Squamous cell carcinoma (Variable presentation, often appearing similar to a basal cell carcinoma. Metastasis may occur but is uncommon. A premalignant lesion, actinic keratosis, may appear as a scaly erythematous flat lesion or as a cutaneous horn.)
- Sebaceous gland carcinoma (Usually occurs in middle-aged or elderly patients. Most arise from the meibomian glands. Must be considered in the presence of a recurrent "chalazion" or intractable "blepharitis," as it may simulate each of these conditions. Loss of eyelashes and destruction of the meibomian gland orifices in the region of the tumor may occur. The tumor may be multifocal, involving both the upper and lower eyelids. Metastasis or orbital extension can occur.)
- Others (Malignant melanoma; lymphoma; sweat gland carcinoma; metastasis, usually breast or lung; and others.)

Differential Diagnosis
(Benign eyelid masses)

- Seborrheic keratosis (Middle-aged or elderly patients. Brown–black well-circumscribed, crustlike lesion, usually elevated slightly and uninflamed. May be removed by shave biopsy if desired.)
- Hordeolum (stye) (Acute, erythematous, tender, well-circumscribed lesion, often associated with blepharitis. See Section 6.1, Chalazion/Hordeolum, for treatment.)
- Chalazion (A chronically obstructed meibomian gland. See Section 6.1 for treatment.)
- Keratoacanthoma [Appears similar to basal and squamous cell carcinomas, as it is elevated and possesses a central ulcer crater. These tumors, however, grow rapidly to a large size (1 to 2 cm) and then slowly shrink, often resolving spontaneously. Lesions that involve the eyelid or eyelash margin can be destructive and are surgically excised.]
- Cysts (e.g., epidermal inclusion, sudoriferous, sebaceous) (Well-circumscribed white or yellow lesions on the eyelid margin or underneath the skin. Ultrasound may help differentiate a cyst from a solid lesion. May be surgically excised.)
- Molluscum contagiosum (Frequently multiple small papules with umbilicated centers. Viral in origin, found mostly in younger patients, can be severe in patients with acquired immunodeficiency syndrome (AIDS). May produce a chronic follicular conjunctivitis. If treatment is desired, these lesions are usually surgically excised, but cryotherapy or other methods may also be used. See Section 5.2, Chronic Conjunctivitis.)

- Nevus (Light-to-dark-brown, sometimes amelanotic, well-circumscribed lesion, sometimes with hair arising from the surface. It does not grow in size.)
- Xanthelasma (Multiple, often bilateral, yellow plaques in the upper, and sometimes the lower, eyelids. Patients should have a serum cholesterol and lipid profile evaluation to rule out a cholesterol or lipid disorder. Diabetes also may be present. Surgical excision can be performed as desired for cosmesis.)
- Squamous papilloma [Soft, elevated (villous) or flat (sessile) benign skin-colored lesion. May enlarge slowly over time. Often spontaneously regress. Some squamous carcinomas can appear papillomatous; a biopsy/excision should be performed on suggestive lesions.]
- Actinic keratosis (Round, premalignant lesion with scaly surface. Found in sun-exposed areas of skin. Treated with excisional biopsy.)
- Others [Verrucae (viral warts related to human papillomavirus), benign tumors of hair follicles or sweat glands, inverted follicular keratosis, neurofibroma, neurilemoma, capillary hemangioma, cavernous hemangioma, pseudoepitheliomatous hyperplasia, necrobiotic xanthogranuloma nodules of multiple myeloma (yellow plaques or nodules often mistaken for xanthelasma).]

Workup
1. History: How long has the lesion been present? Rapid or slow growth? Previous malignant skin lesion?
2. External examination: Check the skin for additional lesions, palpate the preauricular and submaxillary nodes for metastasis.
3. Slit-lamp examination: Look for telangiectasias on nodular tumors, evaluate for loss of eyelashes in the region of the tumor, and inspect the meibomian orifices to determine whether they have been destroyed.
4. Photograph and/or draw the lesion and its location for documentation.
5. Perform a biopsy of the lesion: An incisional biopsy is most commonly performed when a malignancy is suspected, although an excisional biopsy with wide margins on all sides is preferable to detect malignant melanoma. Margins of potential malignant melanoma are sent for permanent section.
6. When a sebaceous gland carcinoma is suspected, the pathologist should be alerted, and frozen or nonfixed tissue must be obtained [for lipid stains (e.g., oil red-O)]. Patients confirmed to have this tumor are referred to a medical internist for a metastatic workup (typically metastatic to the lymph nodes, lung, brain, liver, and bone).

Treatment
- Basal cell carcinoma: Surgical excision with histologic evaluation of the tumor margins. Cryotherapy and radiation are used rarely. Patients

are informed about the etiologic role of the sun and are advised to avoid sunlight when possible and to use protective sunscreens.

- Squamous cell carcinoma: Same as for basal cell carcinoma. Radiation therapy is the second-best treatment after surgical excision. Patients are informed about the etiologic role of the sun.
- Sebaceous gland carcinoma: Surgical excision, taking wide margins of normal tissue on all sides. Frozen section evaluation of the margins is recommended.

Follow-up

After the initial follow-up period (every 1 to 4 weeks to ensure proper healing of the surgical site), patients are reevaluated every 6 to 12 months. Patients who have had one skin malignancy are at greater risk for additional malignancies.

ORBIT

7.1 ORBITAL DISEASE

This introductory section provides an overview to aid in distinguishing a variety of orbital diseases. Specific details on individual disease entities are covered in the remainder of the chapter.

Symptoms
Eyelid swelling, bulging eye(s), and double vision are common. Pain and decreased vision can occur.

Critical Signs
Proptosis and restriction of ocular motility, which can be confirmed by forced duction testing (see Appendix 5). There is often resistance on attempted retropulsion of the globe.

Other Signs
See the individual entities.

Etiology
One or more of the critical signs are usually present, but it is the specific characteristics listed that help to distinguish the individual entities. When specified, computed tomography (CT) scan is done with axial *and* coronal cuts through the orbits.

- Thyroid eye disease (Eyelid retraction and eyelid lag. Painless unless exposure keratopathy develops. Often bilateral. CT scan: Thickening of the extraocular muscles without involvement of the associated tendons.)

- Orbital inflammatory pseudotumor [Often painful. The patient is usually afebrile with a normal white blood cell count (WBC). CT scan: Extraocular muscles are commonly thickened, with involvement of the associated tendons. The sclera, orbital fat, or lacrimal gland may be involved. Acute disease usually responds dramatically to systemic steroids.]
- Orbital cellulitis (Patients are usually febrile and often have an elevated WBC. CT scan: Sinusitis, especially ethmoid sinusitis, is usually present.)
- Orbital tumors [A palpable mass may be present. The globe may be displaced away from the location of the tumor. CT or magnetic resonance imaging (MRI) scan: A mass lesion is evident.]
- Lacrimal gland tumors (Tumor is located in the outer one third of the upper eyelid. The globe is usually is displaced inferiorly and medially with ptosis of the involved eyelid. CT or MRI scan: A mass lesion is present in the lacrimal gland.)
- Trauma (e.g., intraorbital foreign body, retrobulbar hemorrhage; An intraorbital foreign body may not produce orbital signs for a long period. Retrobulbar hemorrhage can result in optic nerve compression. CT scan with or without orbital ultrasound is diagnostic.)
- Orbital vasculitis [e.g., Wegener's granulomatosis, polyarteritis nodosa; Systemic signs and symptoms of vasculitis (especially sinus, renal, pulmonary, and skin disease), fever, markedly increased erythrocyte sedimentation rate (ESR).]
- Mucormycosis (Orbital, nasal, and sinus disease in a diabetic, immuno-compromised, or debilitated patient. Rapidly progressive and potentially life threatening. See Cavernous Sinus/Superior Orbital Fissure Syndrome, Section 11.9.)
- Varix [A large dilated vein within the orbit that produces proptosis when it fills and dilates (e.g., during a Valsalva maneuver or with the head in a dependent position). When the vein is not engorged, the proptosis disappears, and enophthalmos may even be present. CT scan: Demonstrates the dilated vein if an enhanced scan is performed during a Valsalva maneuver. MRI with gadolinium may be done if CT scan is negative.]

Differential Diagnosis
- Arteriovenous fistula [e.g., carotid–cavernous fistula. May mimic orbital disease. It follows trauma or can occur spontaneously. A bruit is sometimes heard by the patient and may be detected if ocular auscultation is performed. Arterialized conjunctival vessels and chemosis may be present. CT scan: Enlarged superior ophthalmic vein (SOV), sometimes accompanied by enlarged extraocular muscles. Orbital color Doppler ultrasound: reversed, arterialized flow in SOV.]

- Cavernous sinus thrombosis (Orbital cellulitis signs, plus decreased sensation of the fifth cranial nerve, dilated and sluggish pupil, paresis of the third, fourth, and sixth cranial nerves out of proportion to the degree of orbital edema, decreasing level of consciousness, nausea, and vomiting. Usually bilateral with rapid progression.)
- Cranial nerve palsy (May produce mild proptosis with limitation of eye movement in specific directions. No resistance to retropulsion, negative forced duction testing. Orbital CT scan is normal.)
- Enlarged globe (e.g., myopia; May produce pseudoproptosis. Large, myopic eyes frequently have tilted discs and peripapillary crescents, and ultrasound reveals a long axial length.)
- Enophthalmos of the fellow eye (e.g., after an orbital floor fracture; May produce pseudoproptosis.)

Workup
1. History: Rapid or slow onset? Pain? Ocular bruit? Fever, chills, systemic symptoms? History of cancer, diabetes, pulmonary disease, or renal disease? Skin rash? Trauma?
2. External examination:
   a. Look from over the patient's forehead to examine for proptosis. Measure the amount with a Hertel exophthalmometer.*
   b. Look for displacement of the globe. Measure from the bridge of the nose with a ruler.
   c. Test for resistance to retropulsion. Have the patient close his or her eyes while gently pushing each globe back into the orbit with your thumb. Assess the resistance of each eye.)
   d. Feel along the orbital rim for a mass.
   e. Measure any ocular misalignment with prisms (see Appendix 2).
3. Ocular examination: Specifically check the pupils, visual fields, color vision (by using color plates), intraocular pressure (IOP), optic nerve, and peripheral retina.
4. Imaging studies: Orbital CT scan (axial and coronal views) and/or MRI with surface coil, depending on suspected etiology. Occasionally, orbital ultrasound with or without color Doppler imaging is useful if the diagnosis is uncertain or when a cystic or vascular lesion is identified. (See Chapter 16 for more information on ophthalmic imaging.)
5. Vital signs, particularly temperature.
6. Laboratory tests when appropriate: T_3, T_4, thyroid-stimulating hormone (TSH), complete blood count (CBC), ESR, anti-nuclear antibody (ANA), blood urea nitrogen (BUN), creatinine, fasting blood sugar, blood cultures, others.

---

*Normal upper limits for proptosis are approximately 22 mm in whites and 24 mm in blacks. There should be no more than a 2-mm difference between the two eyes.

7. Consider a forced duction test (see Appendix 5 for technique.)
8. Consider an excisional, incisional, or fine-needle biopsy, as dictated by the working diagnosis.

Additional workup, treatment, and follow-up vary according to the suspected diagnosis. See individual sections.

7.2 THYROID EYE DISEASE
(GRAVES' OPHTHALMOPATHY)

Ocular Symptoms
Prominent eyes, chemosis, eyelid swelling, double vision, foreign-body sensation, pain, photophobia, decreased vision in one or both eyes.

Critical Ocular Signs
Retraction of the eyelids, eyelid lag on downward gaze, and often, unilateral or bilateral proptosis. When extraocular muscles are involved, elevation and abduction are commonly restricted. There is resistance on forced duction testing. Orbital CT scan shows thickening of the involved extraocular muscles with sparing of the tendon.

❖ **Note** *Optic nerve compression caused by thickened extraocular muscles at the orbital apex can produce an afferent pupillary defect, reduced color vision, and visual-field and visual-acuity loss. The optic disc may be swollen. Optic nerve compression can develop in the presence of minimal exophthalmos. Involvement of more than one muscle with restriction of both elevation and horizontal eye movements is an indication that the patient is at risk for this complication.*

Other Ocular Signs
Reduced frequency of blinking (stare), injection of the blood vessels over the insertion sites of involved extraocular muscles, resistance to retropulsion, superficial punctate keratitis (SPK), or ulceration from exposure keratopathy.

Systemic Signs
Hyperthyroidism common [rapid pulse, hot and dry skin, diffusely enlarged thyroid gland (goiter), weight loss, muscle wasting with proximal muscle weakness, hand tremor, pretibial dermopathy or myxedema, and sometimes, cardiac arrhythmias]. Some patients are euthyroid, and some are hypothyroid taking replacement therapy. Concomitant myasthenia gravis with fluctuating double vision and ptosis is rarely present.

Differential Diagnosis

See Orbital Disease, Section 7.1, for conditions that produce proptosis. Two rare conditions that may produce eyelid retraction or eyelid lag are

- Third-nerve palsy with aberrant regeneration (The upper eyelid may elevate with downward gaze, simulating eyelid lag. Ocular motility may be limited, but forced duction testing and orbital CT scan are normal.)
- Parinaud's syndrome (Eyelid retraction and limitation of upward gaze may accompany mildly dilated pupils that react poorly to light, but react normally to convergence.)

Workup

See Orbital Disease, Section 7.1, for a general workup of proptosis of unknown etiology.

1. History: Duration of symptoms? Pain? Known thyroid disease or cancer?
2. Complete ocular examination to establish the diagnosis and to determine whether the patient is developing exposure keratopathy (slit-lamp examination with fluorescein staining) or optic nerve compression (pupillary assessment and evaluation of color vision by using color plates). Diplopia is measured with prisms (see Appendix 2) and proptosis is measured with a Hertel exophthalmometer. Check intraocular pressure (IOP).
3. CT scan of the orbit (axial and coronal views) is performed when the diagnosis is uncertain (e.g., proptosis is present without other signs of thyroid disease) or surgery is planned.
4. Forced duction testing as needed to establish the diagnosis (see Appendix 5).
5. Formal visual-field examination when signs or symptoms of optic nerve compression are present (e.g., Humphrey, Octopus, or Goldmann).
6. Thyroid-function tests (T_3, T_4, TSH).
7. Edrophonium chloride (e.g., Tensilon) test for suspected myasthenia gravis (see Section 11.10).

Treatment

1. Refer the patient to a medical internist or endocrinologist for management of systemic thyroid disease, if present.
2. Treat exposure keratopathy with artificial tears and lubricating ointment (e.g., Refresh Plus drops q 1 to 6 h and/or Refresh PM ointment qhs, t.i.d.) or by taping eyelids closed at night (see Section 4.4, Exposure Keratopathy).
3. Elevate the head of the bed at night if the patient is developing eyelid edema.

4. Orbital disease may need to be treated more aggressively when exposure keratopathy is worsening despite treatment (or is already severe), bothersome diplopia is present (particularly when looking straight ahead or reading), or optic nerve compression is developing.

The following recommendations are somewhat controversial:

1. Proptosis and corneal ulceration: Prednisone, 100 mg p.o., daily for 1 to 2 days followed by orbital decompression surgery.
2. Acute disturbing double vision with an inflamed eye: Prednisone, 60 to 100 mg p.o., daily, which may be tapered slowly as the condition improves. If no improvement occurs within 10 days, then quickly taper and discontinue the steroids. Orbital irradiation also may be considered as an alternative to steroid treatment. When thyroid disease is no longer active and orbital disease is stable, extraocular muscle surgery may be performed as needed.
3. Visual loss from optic neuropathy: Treat immediately. Options include prednisone, 100 mg p.o., daily, radiation therapy, and posterior orbital decompression surgery. Often prednisone is started immediately in preparation for radiation or surgical therapy. If the vision does not improve or continues to deteriorate after 2 to 7 days of systemic steroids, posterior orbital decompression surgery is recommended if it can be performed by a surgeon very familiar with the technique.
4. Orbital irradiation as a steroid-sparing modality has gained increasing acceptance, and its use continues to evolve. It is best performed according to strict protocols with carefully controlled dosage and shielding, under the supervision of a radiation oncologist familiar with the technique. Typically a total dose of 2,000 cGy is administered in 10 fractions over 2 weeks. Improvement in orbitopathy is often seen within 2 weeks after completion of treatment, but it may take several months to attain maximum benefit. It is unusual for radiation to succeed if steroids have failed.

❖ **Note** *See the Drug Glossary for systemic steroid workup.*

5. A step-wise approach is used for surgical treatment, starting with orbital decompression (if needed) followed by strabismus surgery (for diplopia, if present), followed by eyelid surgery. Alteration of this sequence leads to unpredictable results.

Follow-up

Optic nerve compression is the most urgent ocular complication of thyroid eye disease; it requires immediate attention. Patients with advanced exposure keratopathy and severe proptosis also require prompt attention. Patients with minimal-to-no exposure problems and mild-to-moderate

proptosis are reevaluated every 1 to 2 months. Patients who develop fluctuating diplopia and/or ptosis should be considered for an edrophonium
chloride (e.g., Tensilon) test to rule out myasthenia gravis.

7.3 ORBITAL INFLAMMATORY PSEUDOTUMOR
(NONSPECIFIC ORBITAL INFLAMMATORY DISEASE)

Symptoms
May be acute, recurrent, or chronic. Pain, prominent red eye, double
vision, or decreased vision are common in acute disease. Children may
have concomitant constitutional symptoms (including fever), which are
not typical in adults. Asymptomatic proptosis may develop in chronic
disease.

Critical Signs
Proptosis and/or restriction of ocular motility, usually unilateral. Orbital
CT scan shows a thickened posterior sclera (or a ring of scleral thickening
360 degrees around the globe), orbital fat or lacrimal gland involvement,
or thickening of extraocular muscles (including the tendons). Bone
destruction is very rare.

Other Signs
Eyelid erythema and edema, lacrimal gland enlargement or a palpable
orbital mass, decreased vision, uveitis, increased intraocular pressure
(IOP), hyperopic shift, optic nerve swelling or atrophy, decreased sensitivity of the first division of the trigeminal nerve, conjunctival chemosis, and
injection.

❖ **Note** *Bilateral pseudotumor in adults can occur, but should prompt a care-*
ful evaluation to rule out a systemic vasculitis (e.g., Wegener's granulo-
matosis, polyarteritis nodosa) and lymphoma. Bilateral pseudotumor is
more common in children than in adults.

Etiology
Idiopathic.

Differential Diagnosis
See Orbital Disease, Section 7.1.

Workup

See Section 7.1, for general orbital workup.

1. History: Previous episodes? Any other systemic symptoms or diseases? History of cancer?
2. Complete ocular examination, including ocular motility, exophthalmometry, IOP, and optic nerve evaluation.
3. Vital signs, particularly temperature.
4. Orbital CT scan (axial and coronal views).
5. Blood tests as needed (e.g., bilateral or atypical cases): ESR, CBC with differential, anti-nuclear antibody (ANA), blood urea nitrogen (BUN), creatinine (to rule out vasculitis), and fasting blood sugar (before instituting systemic steroids). Consider anti-neutrophilic cytoplasmic antibody (ANCA) if Wegener's granulomatosis is suspected.
6. Orbital biopsy (fine-needle aspiration or incisional biopsy) when the diagnosis is uncertain, the case is atypical, the patient has a history of cancer, or a patient with an acute case does not respond to systemic steroids within a few days.

Treatment

Prednisone, 80 to 100 mg p.o., daily, with an antiulcer medication (e.g., ranitidine, 150 mg p.o., b.i.d.). Low-dose radiation therapy may be used when the patient does not respond to systemic steroids, when disease recurs as steroids are tapered, or when steroids pose a significant risk to the patient, after the diagnosis is confirmed by biopsy.

❖ **Note** *See Drug Glossary for systemic steroid workup.*

Follow-up

Reevaluate in 3 to 5 days. Patients who respond to the systemic steroids are maintained at the initial dose for 1 to 2 weeks and then tapered off of them slowly, usually over several months. Patients who do not respond to the steroids usually undergo biopsy (unless the diagnosis is known for certain, in which case, radiation therapy is attempted). The IOP must be followed closely in patients being treated with steroids.

7.4 ORBITAL CELLULITIS

Symptoms

Red eye, pain, blurred vision, headache, double vision.

Critical Signs

Eyelid edema, erythema, warmth, tenderness. Conjunctival chemosis and injection, proptosis, and restricted ocular motility with pain on attempted eye movement are usually present.

Other Signs

Decreased vision, retinal venous congestion, optic disc edema, purulent discharge, decreased periorbital sensation, fever. CT scan usually shows a sinusitis (typically an ethmoid sinusitis).

Etiology

- Direct extension from a sinus infection (especially ethmoiditis), focal orbital infection (e.g., dacryoadenitis, dacryocystitis, panophthalmitis), orbital fracture, or dental infection.
- Complication of orbital trauma (e.g., blowout fracture or penetrating trauma). (NOTE: When a foreign body is retained, the cellulitis may develop months after injury.)
- Complication of eye surgery (especially orbital surgery) or paranasal sinus surgery.
- Vascular extension (e.g., seeding from a systemic bacteremia, or locally from facial cellulitis via venous anastomoses).

Organisms

Staphylococcus species, *Streptococcus* species, *Haemophilus influenzae* (especially in children), bacteroides, gram-negative rods (especially after trauma).

Differential Diagnosis

See Orbital Disease, Section 7.1.

Workup

See Section 7.1 for a nonspecific orbital workup.

1. History: Trauma? Ear, nose, throat, or systemic infection? Stiff neck or mental status changes? Diabetes or an immunosuppressive illness?
2. Complete ophthalmic examination: Look for an afferent pupillary defect, limitation of or pain with eye movements, proptosis, decreased skin sensation, or an optic nerve or fundus abnormality.
3. Check vital signs, mental status, and neck flexibility.
4. CT scan of the orbits and sinuses (axial and coronal views, with and without contrast, if possible) to confirm the diagnosis and to rule out a foreign body, orbital or subperiosteal abscess, and sinus disease.
5. CBC with differential.
6. Blood cultures.

7. Explore and debride wound, if present, and obtain a Gram's stain and culture of any drainage (e.g., blood and chocolate agars, Sabouraud's dextrose agar, thioglycolate broth.)

8. Obtain a lumbar puncture for suspected meningitis. Consider a neurology consult.

❖ **Note** *Mucormycosis, a life-threatening disease, must be considered in all diabetics and immunocompromised patients with orbital cellulitis. Immediate action may need to be taken. See Cavernous Sinus/Superior Orbital Fissure Syndrome, Section 11.9.*

Treatment

1. Admit the patient to the hospital.

2. Broad-spectrum i.v. antibiotics to cover gram-positive, gram-negative, and anaerobic organisms are required for at least 1 week or until the condition improves significantly. The specific recommendations frequently change. We presently prefer the following (or equivalent) drugs:

CHILDREN (AGE 13 YEARS OR YOUNGER)

> ceftriaxone, 100 mg/kg/day i.v., in two divided doses (maximum, 4 g/day)
> *plus*
> vancomycin, 40 mg/kg/day i.v, in two to three divided doses.

ADULTS

> ceftriaxone, 1 to 2 g i.v., q 12 h
> *plus*
> vancomycin, 1 g i.v., q 12 h;
> *or*
> ampicillin/sulbactam (e.g., Unasyn), 3 g i.v., q 6 h.

Consider adding metronidazole, 15 mg/kg i.v. load, and then 7.5 mg/kg i.v., q 6 h for adults with chronic orbital cellulitis or when an anaerobic infection is suspected.

If the patient is allergic to penicillin/cephalosporin:
vancomycin, 1 g i.v., q 12 h
or
clindamycin, 300 mg i.v., q 6 h
plus
gentamicin, 5.0 mg/kg i.v., q 24 h (in adults).

❖ **Note** *Antibiotic dosages may need to be reduced in the presence of renal insufficiency or failure. Peak and trough levels of vancomycin and gentamicin are usually monitored, and dosages are adjusted as needed. BUN and creatinine levels are monitored closely.*

3. Ear, nose, and throat consult for surgical drainage of the sinuses as needed, usually after the initial episode is treated.

4. Nasal decongestant spray (e.g., Afrin, b.i.d.) as needed.
5. Erythromycin ointment, q.i.d., for corneal exposure if there is severe proptosis.

Follow-up

Reevaluate every day in the hospital; may take 24 to 36 hours to show improvement.

1. Progress may be monitored by
   a. Temperature and WBC.
   b. Visual acuity.
   c. Ocular motility.
   d. Degree of proptosis and any displacement of the globe (significant displacement may indicate an abscess).

If any of these are worsening, then a CT scan of the orbit and brain should be repeated to look for an abscess. If an abscess is found, then surgical drainage may be required. Other conditions that must be considered when the patient is not improving are cavernous sinus thrombosis and meningitis.

2. Evaluate the cornea for signs of exposure.
3. Check intraocular pressure (IOP).
4. Examine the retina and optic nerve for signs of posterior compression (e.g., choroidal folds), inflammation, or exudative retinal detachment.
5. When orbital cellulitis is clearly and consistently improving, then the regimen can be changed to oral antibiotics (depending on the culture and sensitivity results) to complete a total 14-day course. We often use amoxicillin/clavulanate (e.g., Augmentin)
   20 to 40 mg/kg/day in three divided doses in children;
   250 to 500 mg, t.i.d., in adults
   or
   cefaclor (e.g., Ceclor)
   20 to 40 mg/kg/day in three divided doses in children;
   250 to 500 mg, t.i.d., in adults

The patient is examined every few days as an outpatient until the condition resolves.

7.5 ORBITAL TUMORS IN CHILDREN

Presentation

Proptosis and/or globe displacement. See the specific etiologies for additional presenting signs and imaging characteristics.

Etiology

- Dermoid and epidermoid cysts [Present from birth to young adulthood and progress slowly, unless the cyst ruptures. May develop in the orbit (especially superotemporally) or outside of the orbit in the temporal upper eyelid or brow. When external to the orbit, the cyst is usually a smooth, round, nontender mass. CT scan: Well-defined lesion that may mold the bone of the orbital walls. MRI with contrast: Well-defined mass, T_1-weighted image (T_1W): hypointense to orbital fat, contrast enhances capsule only, T_2-weighted image (T_2W): iso/hypointense to fat, can sometimes see fat/fluid level in lesion. Ultrasound (B-scan): Cystic lesion with good transmission of echoes.]
- Capillary hemangioma [Seen first from birth to early infancy, slow progression, usually in the superonasal orbit. May be observed through the eyelid as a bluish mass or be accompanied by a red hemangioma of the skin (strawberry nevus), which blanches with pressure. Proptosis may be exacerbated by crying. It can enlarge over the first year but spontaneously regresses over the following several years. CT scan: Irregular, contrast-enhancing, usually extraconal lesion. MRI with fat suppression: Fairly well-defined mass; T_1W, hypointense to fat, hyperintense to muscle; T_2W, hyperintense to fat and muscle.]
- Rhabdomyosarcoma (Average age of presentation is 7 years, but may occur from infancy to adulthood. Malignant and may metastasize. Rapid onset and progression. May have edema of the eyelids, a palpable superonasal eyelid or subconjunctival mass, or a history of nosebleeds. *Must be managed by urgent biopsy*. CT scan: Bone destruction is typical. The mass may be well circumscribed and is commonly in the superior orbit, especially nasally. MRI with contrast and fat suppression: Well-circumscribed mass; T_1W, hypointense to fat, hyperintense to muscle, enhances with contrast; T_2W, hyperintense to fat and muscle.)
- Lymphangioma [Usually seen in the first decade of life with a slowly progressive course, but may abruptly worsen if the tumor bleeds. Proptosis may be intermittent and exacerbated by upper respiratory infections. Concomitant conjunctival, eyelid, or oropharyngeal lymphangiomas may be noted (a conjunctival lesion appears as a multicystic mass). CT scan: Nonencapsulated, irregular mass. MRI with contrast and fat suppression: Cystic, possibly multiloculated, nonhomogeneous mass; T_1W, hypointense to fat, hyperintense to muscle, diffuse contrast enhancement; T_2W, markedly hyperintense to fat and muscle. Ultrasound (B-scan): Cystic spaces are often seen.]
- Optic nerve glioma (juvenile pilocytic astrocytoma) [Usually first seen at age 2 to 6 years and is slowly progressive. Decreased visual acuity and a relative afferent pupillary defect usually develop. Optic atrophy or optic nerve swelling may be present. May be associated with neurofibromatosis (in which case, it may be bilateral). CT scan: Fusiform enlargement

of the optic nerve. The optic canal or chiasm may be involved. MRI with contrast: tubular or fusiform mass; T_1W, hypointense to gray matter, variable contrast enhancement; T_2W, homogeneous hyperintensity.]
- Leukemia (granulocytic sarcoma) [Seen first in the first decade of life with rapidly evolving unilateral or bilateral proptosis and occasionally, swelling of the temporal fossa area due to a mass. Typically, these lesions precede blood or bone marrow signs of leukemia, usually acute myelogenous leukemia, by several months. CT scan: Irregular mass, sometimes with bony erosion. There may also be extension of the mass into the temporal fossa.]

❖ **Note** *Acute lymphoblastic leukemia also can produce unilateral or bilateral proptosis.*

- Metastatic neuroblastoma (Seen first in the first few years of life. Abrupt presentation with unilateral or bilateral proptosis, eyelid ecchymosis, and globe displacement. The child is usually systemically ill. The vast majority of patients have already been diagnosed with abdominal cancer. CT scan: Poorly defined mass with bony destruction, especially of the lateral orbital wall.)
- Plexiform neurofibroma (First seen in the first decade of life and is pathognomonic of neurofibromatosis. Ptosis, eyelid hypertrophy, S-shaped deformity of the upper eyelid, or pulsating proptosis may be present. Facial asymmetry and a palpable anterior orbital mass may also be evident. CT scan: Diffuse, irregular soft-tissue mass. A defect in the orbital roof may be seen. MRI: Well-circumscribed oval or fusiform mass; T_1W, isointense or slightly hyperintense to muscle; T_2W, hyperintense to fat and muscle. See Section 14.11.)
- Teratoma (Seen at birth with severe unilateral proptosis that may progress. Vision is often lost from increased intraocular pressure (IOP), optic nerve atrophy, and corneal exposure. The mass transilluminates. CT scan: Multiloculated soft-tissue mass and enlarged orbit; intracranial extension is possible.)

Differential Diagnosis
See Section 7.1, Orbital Disease.

Workup
1. History: Determine the age of onset and the rate of progression. Does the proptosis vary in degree (e.g., with crying)? Nosebleeds? Systemic illness?
2. External examination: Look for an anterior orbital mass, a skin hemangioma, or a temporal fossa lesion. Measure any proptosis (Hertel exophthalmometer) or globe displacement (measure from the bridge of the nose with a ruler). Abdominal examination to rule out mass or organomegaly.

3. Complete ocular examination, including visual acuity, pupillary assessment, color vision, intraocular pressure (IOP), refraction, and optic nerve evaluation.

4. CT scan (axial and coronal views) of the orbit and brain and/or orbital MRI (with gadolinium-DTPA contrast and fat suppression if indicated).

5. Orbital ultrasound with or without color Doppler imaging, if needed to define the lesion further.

6. In cases of acute onset and rapid progression, an emergency incisional biopsy for frozen, permanent, and electron-microscopic evaluation is indicated to rule out an aggressive malignancy (e.g., rhabdomyosarcoma).

7. Other tests as determined by the working diagnosis (usually performed in conjunction with a pediatric oncologist):

> *Rhabdomyosarcoma* Physical examination (look especially for enlarged lymph nodes), chest and bone radiographs, bone marrow aspiration, lumbar puncture, liver-function studies.
>
> *Leukemia* CBC with differential, bone marrow studies, others.
>
> *Neuroblastoma* Abdominal CT scan, urine for vanilyllmandelic acid (VMA).

❖ **Note:** *If clinical suspicion for rhabdomyosarcoma is high, emergency biopsy and initiation of therapy is indicated.*

Treatment

- Dermoid and epidermoid cysts: Complete surgical excision with the capsule intact. If the cyst ruptures, the contents can incite an acute inflammatory response.

- Capillary hemangioma: Observe if mild. A local steroid injection (e.g., betamethasone, 6 mg, and triamcinolone, 40 mg) may be given to shrink the lesion if necessary. Treatment is often indicated if strabismus, anisometropia, or amblyopia develop (see Amblyopia, Section 9.6).

- Rhabdomyosarcoma (managed by urgent referral to a pediatric oncologist in most cases): Local radiation therapy and systemic chemotherapy are given once the diagnosis is confirmed by biopsy.

- Lymphangioma: Surgical excision is performed for a significant cosmetic deformity, ocular dysfunction (e.g., strabismus and amblyopia), or compressive optic neuropathy from acute orbital hemorrhage. Incidence of hemorrhage into lesion is increased after surgery. May recur after excision.

- Optic nerve glioma: Controversial. Observation, surgery, and/or radiation are used variably on a case-by-case basis.

- Leukemia (managed by a pediatric oncologist in most cases): Systemic chemotherapy for the leukemia. Some physicians administer orbital

radiation therapy alone when systemic leukemia cannot be confirmed on bone marrow studies.
- Metastatic neuroblastoma (managed by a pediatric oncologist in most cases): Local radiation and systemic chemotherapy.
- Plexiform neurofibroma: Surgical excision is reserved for patients with significant symptoms or disfigurement.
- Teratoma: Surgical excision (sometimes with the help of a neurosurgeon). Aspiration of the cyst may facilitate complete removal of large lesions. Preservation of ocular function may be possible.

Follow-up

Tumors with rapid onset and progression require urgent attention to rule out malignancy. Tumors that progress more slowly may be managed less urgently.

7.6 ORBITAL TUMORS IN ADULTS

Symptoms

Prominent eye, double vision, pain, decreased vision; may be asymptomatic.

Critical signs

Proptosis, displacement of the globe away from the location of the tumor, orbital mass on CT scan.

Other Signs

A palpable mass, limitation of ocular motility, optic disc edema, or choroidal folds may be present. See the individual etiologies for more specific findings and imaging characteristics.

Etiology
- Metastatic [Most common orbital mass in adults. Usually occurs in middle-aged to elderly people with a rapid onset of orbital signs. Common primary sources include the breast (most common), lung, genitourinary tract (especially prostate), and gastrointestinal tract. Enophthalmos (not proptosis) may be seen with scirrhous breast carcinoma. CT scan: Poorly defined, diffuse tumor that may conform to the shape of the adjacent orbital structures; bone destruction may be seen. MRI with contrast: Diffuse, infiltrating, nonencapsulated mass; T_1W,

hypointense to fat, isointense to muscle, moderate to marked contrast enhancement; T_2W, hyperintense to fat and muscle.]

- Cavernous hemangioma [Most common benign orbital mass in adults. Typically occurs in young adulthood to middle age, with a slow onset of orbital signs. CT scan: Well-defined mass, usually within the muscle cone. MRI with contrast: Well-circumscribed homogeneous mass; T_1W, iso/hyperintense to muscle, diffuse contrast enhancement; T_2W, hyperintense to muscle and fat. Ultrasound (A-scan): High-amplitude internal echoes.]
- Mucocele (Often a frontal headache and a history of chronic sinusitis. Usually nasally or superonasally located. CT scan: A frontal or ethmoid sinus cyst usually seen extending through eroded bone into the orbit; affected sinuses may be opacified.)
- Lymphoid tumors (Usually occurs in middle-aged to elderly adults. Slow onset and progression. Typically develop superiorly in the anterior aspect of the orbit. May be accompanied by a subconjunctival, salmon-colored lesion. Less responsive to systemic steroids than orbital pseudotumor. Can occur without evidence of systemic lymphoma. CT scan: Irregular mass conforming to the shape of the orbital bones or globe, no bony erosion. MRI with contrast: Nonspecific irregular mass; T_1W, hypointense to fat, iso/hyperintense to muscle, moderate to marked contrast enhancement; T_2W, hyperintense to muscle.)
- Optic nerve sheath meningioma [Typically occurs in middle-aged women with painless, slowly progressive visual loss, often with mild proptosis. An afferent pupillary defect develops with visual loss. Ophthalmoscopy can reveal optic nerve swelling, optic atrophy, or abnormal collateral vessels around the disc (optociliary shunt vessels). Meningiomas arising intracranially can produce a temporal-fossa mass. CT scan with contrast: Tubular enlargement of the optic nerve, sometimes with a "railroad-track" appearance (a linear shadow is seen within the lesion). MRI with contrast and fat suppression: Variable-intensity lesion surrounding optic nerve; T_1W, marked contrast enhancement, difficult to differentiate from orbital fat unless fat suppression is used.]
- Localized neurofibroma [Occurs in young to middle-aged adults with slow development of orbital signs. Some have neurofibromatosis, but most do not. CT scan: Well-defined mass in the superior orbit (rarely inferiorly). MRI: Well-circumscribed, possibly heterogeneous mass; T_1W, iso/hyperintense to muscle; T_2W, hyperintense to fat and muscle.]
- Neurilemoma (benign schwannoma) (Progressive painless proptosis. Rarely associated with neurofibromatosis. CT scan: Well-circumscribed fusiform or ovoid mass, usually located in the superior orbit. MRI with contrast: Well-circumscribed mass; T_1W, iso/hyperintense to muscle, variable contrast enhancement; T_2W, variable intensity.)

- Fibrous histiocytoma [Occurs at any age. Cannot be distinguished from a hemangiopericytoma before biopsy. (See the following.) CT scan: Well-circumscribed mass anywhere in the orbit. MRI with contrast: Heterogeneous mass; T_1W, hypointense to fat, iso/hyperintense to muscle, irregular contrast enhancement; T_2W, hypointense areas similar to T_1W.]
- Hemangiopericytoma [Occurs at any age. Relatively slow development of signs. Usually superiorly located. CT scan: May appear well defined and indistinguishable from a cavernous hemangioma or fibrous histiocytoma. Sometimes extends through the orbital bones into the temporal fossa and cranial cavity. MRI: Well-circumscribed mass; T_1W, hypointense to fat, iso/hyperintense to muscle, moderate diffuse contrast enhancement; T_2W, variable. Ultrasound (A-scan): Low-to-medium internal reflectivity.]
- Others (Dermoid cyst, osteoma, hematocele, lymphangioma, extension of an ocular or periocular tumor, others.)

Differential Diagnosis
See Sections 7.1, Orbital Disease, and 7.7, Lacrimal Gland Mass.

Workup
1. History: Determine the age of onset and rate of progression. Headache or chronic sinusitis? History of cancer? Trauma (e.g., hematocele, orbital foreign body, ruptured dermoid)?
2. Complete ocular examination, particularly visual acuity, pupillary response, ocular motility, color vision and visual field of each eye, measurement of globe displacement (from the bridge of the nose with a ruler) and proptosis (Hertel exophthalmometer), intraocular pressure (IOP), and optic nerve evaluation.
3. CT scan (axial and coronal views) of the orbit and brain and/or orbital MRI with surface coil, depending on suspected etiology.
4. Orbital ultrasound with or without color Doppler imaging as needed to further define the lesion.
5. When a metastasis is suspected and primary tumor is unknown, the following should be performed:
   a. Fine-needle aspiration biopsy or incisional biopsy to confirm the diagnosis, with estrogen-receptor assay if breast carcinoma is suspected.
   b. Breast examination and palpation of axillary lymph nodes.
   c. Medical workup as directed by the biopsy result (e.g., chest radiograph, mammogram).
6. When a lymphoma is suspected, a medical consult is obtained, and a systemic workup is instituted (e.g., CBC with differential, serum protein electrophoresis, bone marrow biopsy, CT scan of the abdomen

and brain). If the workup is negative, an incisional biopsy is performed (often need nonfixed tissue for special studies, e.g. flow cytometry). If the workup is positive, the systemic lymphoma is treated, and the orbital lesion is observed for its response to treatment. Occasionally a fine-needle biopsy is performed to confirm the orbital diagnosis.

Treatment

- Metastatic disease: Systemic chemotherapy as required for the primary malignancy. Radiotherapy is often used paliatively for the orbital mass. Carcinoid tumors are occasionally resected.
- Cavernous hemangioma: Complete surgical excision is performed when there is compromised visual function or for cosmetic purposes. If the patient is asymptomatic, he or she can be followed every 6 to 12 months.
- Mucocele: Systemic antibiotics (e.g., vancomycin, 1 g i.v., q 12 h, and ceftazidime, 1 g i.v., q 8 h) followed by surgical drainage of the mucocele and exenteration of the involved sinus.
- Lymphoid tumors: Lymphoid hyperplasia and orbital lymphoma without systemic involvement are treated with local radiation therapy. Systemic lymphoma is treated with chemotherapy.
- Optic nerve sheath meningioma: Surgery is usually indicated when the tumor is growing and producing visual loss. Otherwise, the patient may be followed every 3 to 6 months with serial clinical examinations and imaging studies (CT scan or MRI) as needed.
- Localized neurofibroma: Surgical removal is performed for enlarging tumors that are producing symptoms.
- Neurilemoma: Same as for cavernous hemangioma (see previous).
- Fibrous histiocytoma: Complete surgical removal. Recurrences are generally more aggressive and more malignant, sometimes necessitating orbital exenteration.
- Hemangiopericytoma: Complete surgical excision (because there is a potential for malignant transformation and metastasis).

Follow-up

Variable. Referral for treatment is not an emergency, except when optic nerve compromise is present. Metastatic disease requires workup without much delay.

❖ **Note** *See also Lacrimal Gland Mass, Section 7.7, especially if the mass is in the outer one third of the upper eyelid, and Orbital Tumors in Children, Section 7.5.*

7.7 LACRIMAL GLAND MASS/ CHRONIC DACRYOADENITIS

Symptoms

Persistent or progressive swelling of the outer one third of the upper eyelid. Pain and/or double vision may or may not be present.

Critical Signs

Chronic eyelid swelling and erythema, predominantly in the outer one third of the upper eyelid, with or without proptosis and displacement of the globe inferiorly and medially.

Other Signs

A palpable mass may be present in the outer one third of the upper eyelid. Extraocular motility may be restricted.

Etiology

- Sarcoidosis [May be bilateral. May have concomitant lung, skin, or ocular disease. Lymphadenopathy, parotid gland enlargement, or seventh-nerve palsy may be present. More common in blacks. Serum angiotensin-converting enzyme (ACE) level may be increased.]
- Orbital inflammatory pseudotumor (Commonly, pain and swelling develop acutely, with or without limitation of ocular motility, displacement of the globe, or proptosis. CT scan may show stranding of orbital fat if not confined to lacrimal gland. A rapid response to systemic steroids is typical in acute cases.)
- Benign mixed epithelial tumor (pleomorphic adenoma) (Slowly progressive, painless proptosis or displacement of the globe in middle-aged adults. CT scan may show a well-circumscribed mass with pressure-induced remodeling and enlargement of the lacrimal gland fossa. No bony erosion occurs.)
- Dermoid (Typically a painless, subcutaneous mass that enlarges slowly and is found in a child. May rarely rupture, causing acute swelling and inflammation. Well-defined, extraconal mass noted on CT scan.)
- Lymphoid tumor (Slowly progressive proptosis and globe displacement in a middle-aged patient. May have a pink–white "salmon-patch" area of subconjunctival extension. CT scan shows an irregularly shaped lesion that conforms to the globe and lacrimal fossa. Bony erosion is not usually found.)
- Adenoid cystic carcinoma (Acute onset of pain and proptosis, which progress rapidly. Globe displacement, ptosis, and a motility disturbance

are common. This highly malignant lesion often exhibits perineural invasion. CT scan shows an irregular mass, often with bony erosion.)

- Malignant mixed epithelial tumor (pleomorphic adenocarcinoma) (Occurs primarily in elderly patients, acutely producing pain and progressing rapidly. Usually develops within a long-standing benign mixed epithelial tumor, or secondarily, as a recurrence of a previously resected benign mixed tumor. CT scan findings are similar to those for adenoid cystic carcinoma.)
- Lacrimal gland cyst (dacryops) (Usually an asymptomatic mass that may fluctuate in size. Typically occurs in a young adult or middle-aged patient.)
- Others (Tuberculosis, syphilis, leukemia, mumps, mucoepidermoid carcinoma, plasmacytoma, others.)

❖ **Note** *Primary neoplasms (except lymphoma) are almost always unilateral; inflammatory disease may be bilateral. Lymphoma is more commonly unilateral, but may be bilateral.*

Workup
1. History: Determine the duration of the abnormality and rate of progression. Associated pain, tenderness, double vision? Weakness, weight loss, fever, or other signs of systemic malignancy? Breathing difficulty, skin rash, or history of uveitis (sarcoidosis)? Any known medical problems? Prior lacrimal gland biopsy or surgery?
2. Complete ocular examination: Specifically look for keratic precipitates, iris nodules, posterior synechiae, and old retinal periphlebitis from sarcoidosis.
3. Orbital CT scan (axial and coronal views). MRI is rarely required.
4. Consider a chest radiograph (may diagnose sarcoidosis and rarely, tuberculosis).
5. Consider CBC with differential, ACE, rapid plasma reagin (RPR), fluorescent treponemal antibody, absorbed (FTA-ABS), and purified protein derivative (PPD) with anergy panel if clinical history suggests a specific etiology.
6. Systemic workup by an internist or hematologist/oncologist when a lymphoma is suspected (e.g., abdominal and head CT scan, bone marrow biopsy).
7. Lacrimal gland biopsy is indicated when a malignant tumor is suspected, or if the diagnosis is uncertain and a malignancy or inflammatory etiology is probable. (Biopsy may be unnecessary when a lymphoma is suspected clinically and is confirmed on systemic workup.)

❖ **Note** *Do not perform a biopsy on lesions thought to be benign mixed tumors or dermoids. Incomplete excision of a benign mixed tumor may lead to a* *recurrence with or without malignant transformation. Rupture of a dermoid cyst may lead to a severe inflammatory reaction. These two lesions must be completely excised without rupturing the capsule or pseudocapsule.*

Treatment
- Sarcoidosis: Systemic steroids (see Section 13.4, Sarcoidosis).
- Orbital inflammatory pseudotumor: Systemic steroids (see Section 7.3, Orbital Inflammatory Pseudotumor).
- Benign mixed epithelial tumor: Complete surgical removal.
- Dermoid cyst: Complete surgical removal.
- Lymphoid tumor:
  a. Confined to the orbit: Orbital irradiation.
  b. Systemic involvement: Chemotherapy (orbital irradiation is usually withheld until the response of the orbital lesion to chemotherapy can be evaluated).
- Adenoid cystic carcinoma: Consider orbital exenteration with irradiation. (Rarely chemotherapy is used.)
- Malignant mixed epithelial tumor: Same as for adenoid cystic carcinoma.
- Lacrimal gland cyst: Excise if symptomatic.

Follow-up
Depends on the specific cause.

OCULAR TUMORS

8.1 CONJUNCTIVAL TUMORS

The following are the most common and important conjunctival tumors. Phlyctenulosis and pterygium/pingueculum are discussed in Sections 4.9 and 4.10, respectively.

Amelanotic Lesions

Limbal Dermoid

Congenital benign tumor, usually located in the inferotemporal quadrant of the limbus; it may involve the cornea. Lesions are white, solid, fairly well circumscribed, elevated, and may have hair arising from their surface. They may enlarge, particularly at puberty. They may be associated with eyelid colobomas, preauricular skin tags, and vertebral abnormalities (Goldenhar's syndrome). Surgical removal may be performed for cosmetic purposes or if they are affecting the visual axis, although a white corneal scar may persist postoperatively.

❖ **Note** *The cornea or sclera underlying a dermoid may be very thin or even absent, and penetration of the eye can occur with surgical resection.*

Dermolipoma

Congenital benign tumor, usually occurring under the bulbar conjunctiva in the temporalmost aspect of the eye. It appears as a yellow–white solid tumor, and may have hair arising from its surface. Surgical removal is usually avoided if possible because of the frequent extension of this tumor into the orbit, involving some of the orbital structures. Partial resection of the anterior portion can usually be done without difficulty if necessary.

Pyogenic Granuloma

Benign, deep-red, pedunculated mass. It typically develops at a site of prior surgery, trauma, or chalazion. It may respond to topical steroids; use of a topical steroid–antibiotic combination (e.g., prednisolone acetate–tobramycin, q.i.d., for 1 to 2 weeks) may be helpful because infection may be present, but the tumor often must be excised if it persists.)

Lymphangioma

Probably congenital, but often not detected until years after birth. The lesion is benign yet slowly progressive and appears as a diffuse, multiloculated, cystic mass. This lesion is seen most commonly between birth and young adulthood, often before age 6 years. Hemorrhage into the cystic spaces may produce a "chocolate cyst." Lymphangiomas may enlarge, sometimes due to an upper respiratory tract infection. Concomitant eyelid, orbital, facial, nasal, or oropharyngeal lymphangiomas may be present. Surgical excision may be performed for cosmetic or functional purposes, but it often must be repeated, because it is difficult to remove the entire tumor with one surgical procedure. Lesions often stabilize in early adulthood. These lesions do not regress like the capillary hemangiomas.

Granuloma

May occur at any age, predominantly on the tarsal conjunctiva. No distinct clinical appearance, but patients may have an associated embedded foreign body, sarcoidosis, tuberculosis, or another granulomatous disease. Management often includes a course of topical corticosteroids or excisional biopsy.

Papilloma

Two types:

A. Viral [Frequently multiple pedunculated or sessile lesions in children and young adults. These lesions can occur on palpebral or bulbar conjunctiva. They are benign and are generally left untreated because of their high recurrence rate (which is often multiple) and their tendency for spontaneous resolution.]

B. Nonviral [Typically, a single sessile or pedunculated lesion found in older patients. These are located more commonly near the limbus and may represent precancerous lesions with malignant potential. Complete excisional biopsy flush with the surface is the preferred treatment. Supplemental cryotherapy may be applied.]

❖ **Note** *In dark-skinned individuals, papillomas may appear pigmented and may be mistaken for malignant melanoma (MM).*

Kaposi's Sarcoma

Malignant, subconjunctival nodule, usually red or purple. Patients should be evaluated for acquired immunodeficiency syndrome (AIDS) (See Section 14.1, Acquired Immunodeficiency Syndrome).

Conjunctival Intraepithelial Neoplasia (Dysplasia and Carcinoma in Situ)

Typically occurs in middle-aged to elderly people. The lesion is a leukoplakic or gray–white gelatinous lesion that usually begins at the limbus. Occasionally, a papillomatous, fernlike appearance develops. The lesions are usually unilateral and unifocal and may evolve into invasive squamous cell carcinoma if not treated early and successfully. They can spread over the cornea or, less commonly, invade the eye or metastasize. A complete excisional biopsy followed by supplemental cryotherapy to the remaining adjacent conjunctiva is the preferred treatment. Excision may require lamellar dissection into the corneal stroma and sclera in recurrent or long-standing lesions. Periodic follow-up examinations are required to detect recurrences.

Lymphoid Tumors (Range from Benign Reactive Lymphoid Hyperplasia to Lymphoma)

Occurs in young to middle-aged adults. Usually appears as a light pink, salmon-colored lesion. It may appear in the bulbar conjunctiva, where it is typically oval, or in the fornix, where it is usually horizontal, conforming to the contour of the fornix. Excisional or incisional biopsy is performed for immunohistochemical studies (may require nonfixed tissue). Symptomatic benign reactive lymphoid hyperplasia may be treated by excisional biopsy, low-dose radiation, cryotherapy, or topical steroid drops. Lymphomas should be completely excised, if that can be done without damage to the extraocular muscle or excessive sacrifice of conjunctiva. Otherwise an incisional biopsy is justified. Patients are referred to an internist or oncologist for systemic evaluation. Systemic lymphoma may or may not develop if it is not already present.

Epibulbar Osseous Choristoma

Congenital, benign, hard, bony mass, usually on the superotemporal bulbar conjunctiva. Surgical removal may be performed for cosmetic purposes.

Amyloid

Smooth, waxy, yellow masses seen especially in the lower fornix when the conjunctiva is involved. Often there are associated small hemorrhages. Definitive diagnosis is made with biopsy. Consider workup for systemic amyloidosis.

Amelanotic Melanoma

Pigmentation of conjunctival melanoma is variable. Look for bulbar or limbal lesions with significant vascularity to help make this difficult diagnosis.

Sebaceous Gland Carcinoma

Although usually involving the palpebral conjunctiva, this tumor can involve the bulbar conjunctiva as well when there is pagetoid invasion of the conjunctiva. This diagnosis should always be considered in older patients with refractory unilateral blepharoconjunctivitis.

Melanotic Lesions

Ocular or Oculodermal Melanocytosis

Congenital. Not a conjunctival lesion, but an episcleral lesion, as demonstrated (after topical anesthesia) by moving the conjunctiva back and forth over the area of pigmentation with a sterile, cotton-tipped swab. (Conjunctival pigmentation will move with the conjunctiva.) Typically, the lesion is unilateral, blue–gray, and is often accompanied by a darker ipsilateral iris and choroid. In oculodermal disease, also called nevus of Ota, the periocular skin is also pigmented. These lesions may become pigmented at puberty. Both conditions predispose to malignant melanoma of the uveal tract, orbit, and brain (most commonly in whites).

Primary Acquired Melanosis

Appears in middle-aged adults as flat, brown patches of pigmentation without small cysts within the conjunctiva. These tumors usually arise during or after middle age and almost always occur in whites. (Overall, approximately one fifth of these lesions will develop into malignant melanoma of the conjunctiva.) Malignant transformation should be suspected when an elevation or increase in vascularity in one of these areas develops. Management options include careful observation with photographic comparison for any change and incisional or excisional biopsy followed by cryotherapy for suggestive lesions.

Nevus

Commonly develops during puberty, most often within the palpebral fissure on the bulbar conjunctiva. It is usually well demarcated and may or may not be pigmented. The degree of pigmentation may also change with time. A key sign in the diagnosis is the presence of small cysts within the lesion. Benign nevi may enlarge; however, malignant melanoma may occasionally develop from a nevus, and enlargement may be an early sign of malignant transformation. Nevi of the palpebral conjunctiva are rare; primary acquired melanosis and malignant melanoma must be considered in such lesions. A baseline photograph of the nevus should be taken, and the patient should be observed every 6 to 12 months. Surgical excision is elective.

Malignant Melanoma

Typically occurs in middle-aged to elderly patients. The lesion is a nodular brown mass. The tumor is well vascularized, and a large conjunctival vessel can often be seen to be feeding the tumor. It may develop from a nevus or primary acquired melanosis, but it may also develop de novo. Check for an underlying ciliary body melanoma (dilated fundus examination, transillumination, and B-scan ultrasound). Intraocular and orbital extension may occur. Excisional biopsy (often with supplemental cryotherapy) is performed unless intraocular or orbital involvement is present. In advanced cases, exenteration is necessary.

Other Less Common Causes of Increased Pigmentation

Ochronosis with alkaptonuria: Autosomal recessive enzyme deficiency. Occurs in young adults with arthritis and dark urine. Pigment is at level of the sclera.

Argyrosis: Silver deposition causes black discoloration. Patients have a history of long-term use of silver nitrate drops.

Hemochromatosis (bronze diabetes): This condition can cause increased conjunctival pigmentation.

Ciliary staphyloma: Scleral thinning with uveal show.

Adrenochrome deposits: Long-term epinephrine or dipivifren (e.g., Propine) use.

Mascara deposits: Generally occurs in the inferior fornix and becomes entrapped in epithelium or cysts.

8.2 MALIGNANT MELANOMA OF THE IRIS

Malignant melanoma (MM) of the iris may occur as a localized or diffuse pigmented (melanotic) or nonpigmented (amelanotic) lesion.

Critical Signs

Unilateral brown or translucent iris mass lesion exhibiting slow growth. It is more common in the inferior one half of the iris and in light-skinned individuals. Rare in blacks.

Other Signs

A localized MM is generally >3 mm in diameter at the base and >1 mm in depth and sometimes has a prominent feeder vessel that ramifies to the mass. It may produce secondary glaucoma. Although nonspecific, it may cause a sector cortical cataract, ectropion iridis, spontaneous hyphema, seeding of tumor cells into the anterior chamber, or direct invasion of tumor into the trabecular meshwork.

A diffuse MM causes progressive darkening of the involved iris, loss of iris crypts, and increased intraocular pressure (IOP). Focal iris nodules may be present.

Differential Diagnosis

A. Melanotic masses
   • Nevi [Typically become clinically apparent at puberty, usually flat or minimally elevated (i.e. <1 mm) and uncommonly exceed 3 mm in diameter. Can cause ectropion iridis, sector cortical cataract, or secondary glaucoma. Generally not vascular. More common in the inferior one half of the iris. Nevi do not usually grow.]
   • Tumors of the iris pigment epithelium (Usually black, in contrast to melanomas, which are often brown or amelanotic.)
B. Amelanotic masses
   • Metastasis (Grows rapidly. More likely to be multiple or bilateral than is MM. Frequently liberates cells and produces a pseudohypopyon. Involves the superior and inferior halves of the iris equally.)
   • Leiomyoma (Transparent and vascular. May be difficult to distinguish from an amelanotic melanoma.)
   • Iris cyst (Unlike MM, most transmit light with transillumination.)
   • Inflammatory granuloma (e.g., sarcoidosis, tuberculosis, or juvenile xanthogranuloma) (Often have other signs of inflammation such as keratic precipitates, synechiae, and posterior subcapsular cataracts. A history of iritis or a systemic inflammatory disease may be elicited.)
C. Diffuse lesions
   • Congenital iris heterochromia (The darker iris is present at birth or in early childhood. It is nonprogressive and usually is not associated with glaucoma. The iris has a smooth appearance.)
   • Fuchs' heterochromic iridocyclitis (Asymmetry of iris color, mild iritis in the eye with the lighter-colored iris, usually unilateral. Often associated with a cataract and/or glaucoma.)

- Iris nevus syndrome (Corneal edema, peripheral anterior synechiae, iris atrophy, or an irregular pupil may be present along with multiple iris nodules and glaucoma.)
- Pigment dispersion [Usually bilateral. The iris is rarely heavily pigmented (although the trabecular meshwork may be), and iris transillumination defects are often present.]
- Hemosiderosis (A dark iris may result after iron-breakdown products from an old blood deposit on the iris surface. Patients have a history of a traumatic hyphema or vitreous hemorrhage.)

Workup
1. History: Previous cancer, ocular surgery or trauma? Weight loss? Anorexia?
2. Slit-lamp examination: Carefully evaluate the irides. Check IOP.
3. Gonioscopy of the anterior-chamber angle.
4. Dilated fundus examination using indirect ophthalmoscopy.
5. Transillumination (used to differentiate between epithelial cysts that transmit light and pigmented lesions that do not).
6. Photograph the lesion and accurately draw it in the chart, including dimensions. Ultrasound biomicroscopy may be helpful.

Treatment/Follow-up
1. Observe the patient through periodic examinations and photographs every 3 to 12 months, depending on suspicion of malignancy.
2. Surgical resection is indicated if growth is documented, the tumor interferes with vision, or it produces intractable glaucoma.
3. Diffuse iris MM with secondary glaucoma may require enucleation.
4. Avoid filtering surgery for glaucoma associated with possible MM because of the risk of tumor dissemination.

8.3 MALIGNANT MELANOMA OF THE CHOROID

Symptoms
Decreased vision, a visual field defect, floaters, light flashes, pain; may be asymptomatic.

Critical Signs
Gray–green or brown (melanotic) or yellow (amelanotic) choroidal mass that exhibits one or more of the following:

1. Growth.
2. Presence of subretinal fluid (i.e., retinal detachment).

3. Height >2 mm, especially with an abrupt elevation from the choroid.
4. Ill-defined, large areas of orange pigment over the lesion.
5. A mushroom shape with congested blood vessels in the dome of the tumor.

❖ **Note** *A diffuse choroidal malignant melanoma (MM) can appear as a minimally thickened dark choroid without a distinct mass.*

Other Signs
Overlying cystoid retinal degeneration, vitreous hemorrhage or vitreous pigment cells, drusen on the tumor surface, a choroidal neovascular membrane, proptosis (from orbital invasion). Choroidal MM rarely occurs in blacks and more commonly occurs in light-skinned individuals.

Differential Diagnosis
A. Pigmented lesions
  • Nevi (Melanotic or amelanotic choroidal lesions that rarely exhibit significant growth, are not mushroom-shaped, are generally <2 mm thick and show gradual elevation from the choroid. They may have an associated shallow retinal detachment or well-defined small areas of orange pigment on their surface, but surface drusen are more typical.)
  • Congenital hypertrophy of the retinal pigment epithelium (CHRPE) (Flat lesions that are often black, but may appear gray–green. The margins are often well delineated with a surrounding depigmented halo. Depigmented areas frequently appear on the surface of the lesion.)
  • Reactive hyperplasia of the retinal pigment epithelium (RPE) (Related to previous trauma or inflammation. Lesions are black, flat, have irregular margins, and may have associated white gliosis. Often multifocal.)
  • Age-related disciform macular degeneration [Subretinal blood can simulate a melanoma. This disease is typically bilateral in the posterior pole and associated with extensive exudate. Fluorescein angiography will assist in differentiation.]
  • Peripheral disciform degeneration (Peripheral, elevated, yellow-to-red mass with extensive exudation and hemorrhage. It may extend into the vitreous. The contralateral eye often shows peripheral RPE changes.)
  • Melanocytoma of the optic nerve (A black optic nerve lesion with fibrillated margins. It may grow slowly. Fluorescein angiography may allow differentiation.)
  • Choroidal detachment (Follows ocular surgery, trauma, or hypotony of another etiology. Dark peripheral multilobular fundus mass.)

(The ora serrata is often visible without scleral depression.) Localized suprachoroidal hemorrhage can be very difficult to differentiate from MM based on appearance alone because of its brown–black color. Transillumination will allow differentiation between serous choroidal detachment and MM but is not helpful when there is a hemorrhagic component. In these situations, fluorescein angiography is the study of choice, usually allowing differentiation between the two entities.

  B. Nonpigmented lesions

- Choroidal hemangioma (Red–orange, may be elevated, never mushroom-shaped.)
- Metastatic carcinoma [Cream or light brown, flat or slightly elevated, extensive subretinal fluid, may be multifocal or bilateral. Patient may have a history of cancer (especially breast or lung cancer)].
- Choroidal osteoma (Yellow–orange in color, generally close to the optic disc, pseudopodlike projections of the margin, often bilateral, typically occurs in young women in their teens or twenties. Ultrasound may show a calcified mass.)
- Posterior scleritis (Patients may have choroidal folds, pain, proptosis, uveitis, or anterior scleritis associated with an amelanotic mass. Look for the T-sign on ultrasound.)

Workup

1. History: Ocular surgery or trauma, cancer, anorexia, weight loss, or systemic illness?
2. Dilated fundus examination by using indirect ophthalmoscopy.
3. Fluorescein angiography.
4. Ultrasound A and B scans: Documents thickness and confirms clinical impression. With choroidal melanoma, the ultrasound usually shows low-to-moderate reflectivity with choroidal excavation.
5. Consider a fine-needle aspiration biopsy in selected cases, phosphorus 32 test, and computed tomography (CT) scan or magnetic resonance imaging (MRI) of the orbit and brain. We no longer perform phosphorus 32 tests.
6. If MM is confirmed:
   a. Blood work: lactate dehydrogenase (LDH), γ-glutamyl transferase (GGT), SGOT, SGPT, and alkaline phosphatase. If liver enzymes are elevated, consider a MRI or liver scan to rule out a liver metastasis.
   b. Chest radiograph.
   c. Complete physical examination by a medical internist.
7. Consider a carcinoembryonic antigen (CEA) assay if a choroidal metastasis is suspected.

Treatment

Depending on the results of the metastatic workup, the tumor characteristics, the status of the contralateral eye, and the age and general health of the patient, MM of the choroid may be managed by observation, photocoagulation, thermotherapy, radiotherapy, local resection, or enucleation.

PEDIATRICS

9.1 LEUKOCORIA

Definition

A white pupillary reflex

Etiology

- Retinoblastoma [A malignant tumor of the retina that appears as a white, nodular mass extending into the vitreous (endophytic), as a mass lesion underlying a retinal detachment (exophytic), or as a diffusely spreading lesion simulating uveitis (diffuse infiltrating). Iris neovascularization is common. Pseudohypopyon and vitreous seeding may occur. Cataract is uncommon, and the eye is normal in size. May be bilateral, unilateral, or multifocal. Diagnosis is usually made between 12 and 24 months of age. A family history may be elicited.]
- Toxocariasis [A nematode infection that may appear as a localized, white, elevated granuloma in the retina or as a diffuse endophthalmitis. Localized inflammation of ocular structures also may be seen. Vitreous traction bands associated with macular dragging may occur, traction retinal detachment may occur, and cataract may develop secondary to the inflammation. It is rarely bilateral and is usually diagnosed between ages 6 months and 10 years. Paracentesis of the anterior chamber may reveal eosinophils, and a serum enzyme-linked immunosorbent assay (ELISA) test for *Toxocara* organisms will be positive. The patient may have a history of contact with puppies and/or eating dirt.]
- Coats' disease (A retinal vascular abnormality resulting in small multifocal outpouchings of the retinal vessels, associated with yellow intraretinal and subretinal exudate. An exudative retinal detachment may account for the leukocoria. It usually develops in boys during the

first 2 decades of life; more severe cases occur in the first decade of life. Coats' disease is rarely bilateral, and there is no family history.)

- Persistent hyperplastic primary vitreous (PHPV) (A developmental ocular abnormality consisting of a varied degree of fibroglial and vascular proliferation in the vitreous cavity. It is usually associated with a slightly small eye. Other findings can include cataract, a fibrovascular membrane behind the lens that places traction on the ciliary processes, glaucoma, and retinal detachment. The condition is present at birth but may not be detected until later in childhood. It is rarely bilateral, and a negative family history is elicited.)
- Congenital cataract (Opacity of the lens present at birth; may be unilateral or bilateral. There may be a family history or an associated systemic disorder. See Section 9.7, Congenital Cataract)
- Retinal astrocytoma (A sessile to slightly elevated yellow–white retinal mass that may be calcified and is often associated with tuberous sclerosis, and rarely neurofibromatosis. May be associated with giant drusen of the optic nerve in patients with tuberous sclerosis.)
- Retinopathy of prematurity (ROP) (Predominantly occurs in premature children, who may have received supplemental oxygen therapy. Leukocoria is usually the result of a retinal detachment. See Retinopathy of Prematurity, Section 9.2.)
- Others (e.g., retinochoroidal coloboma, retinal detachment, familial exudative vitreoretinopathy, myelinated nerve fibers, uveitis, incontinenti pigmenti.)

Workup

1. History: Age at onset? Family history of one of the conditions mentioned? Prematurity? Contact with puppies or habit of eating dirt?
2. Complete ocular examination, including a measurement of corneal diameters (look for a small eye), an examination of the iris (look for neovascularization), and an inspection of the lens (look for a cataract). A dilated fundus examination and anterior vitreous examination are essential.
3. Any or all of the following may be helpful in diagnosis and planning treatment:
   a. B-scan ultrasound (retinoblastoma, PHPV, cataract).
   b. Intravenous fluorescein angiogram (Coats' disease, ROP, retinoblastoma).
   c. Computed tomography (CT) scan or magnetic resonance imaging (MRI) of the orbit and brain (retinoblastoma), particularly for bilateral cases or those with a family history.
   d. Serum ELISA test for toxocara (positive at 1:8 in the vast majority of infected patients.)
   e. Systemic examination (retinal astrocytoma, retinoblastoma).

f. Anterior chamber paracentesis (toxocariasis). Note that paracentesis in a patient with a retinoblastoma can possibly lead to tumor cell dissemination.
4. Consider examination under anesthesia (EUA) in young or uncooperative children, particularly when retinoblastoma, toxocariasis, Coats' disease, or ROP is being considered as a diagnosis.

See Congenital Cataract, Section 9.7, for a more specific cataract workup.

Treatment
- Retinoblastoma: Enucleation, irradiation, photocoagulation, cryotherapy, chemoreduction, chemothermotherapy, or occasionally other therapeutic modalities. Systemic chemotherapy is used in metastatic disease.
- Toxocariasis:
  1. Steroids (Topical, periocular depot injection, or systemic routes may be used, depending on the severity of the inflammation.)
  2. Consider a surgical vitrectomy when vitreoretinal traction bands form or when the condition does not improve or worsens with medical therapy.
  3. Consider laser photocoagulation of the nematode if it is visible.
- Coats' disease: Laser photocoagulation and/or cryotherapy to leaking vessels; surgery may be required for a retinal detachment.
- PHPV
  1. Cataract extraction.
  2. Possible vitreal membrane excision.
  3. Treat any amblyopia.
- Congenital cataract: See Section 9.7, Congenital Cataract.
- Retinal astrocytoma: Observation.
- ROP: See Section 9.2, Retinopathy of Prematurity.

Follow-up
Variable, depending on the diagnosis.

9.2 RETINOPATHY OF PREMATURITY (ROP)

Risk Factors
- Prematurity (especially <32 weeks of gestation).
- Birthweight <1,500 g (3 lb, 5 oz), especially <1250 g (2 lb, 12 oz).
- Supplemental oxygen therapy, hypoxemia, hypercarbia, concurrent illness, and possibly others.

Critical Signs
An avascular peripheral retina.

Other Signs
Extraretinal fibrovascular proliferation, plus disease (see classification later), vitreous hemorrhage, retinal detachment, and/or leukocoria, usually bilateral. Poor pupillary dilation despite mydriatic drops with engorgement of iris vessels. In older children and adults, decreased visual acuity, myopia, strabismus, retinal dragging, lattice-like vitreoretinal degeneration, or retinal detachment may occur.

Differential Diagnosis
- Familial exudative vitreoretinopathy (FEVR) (Appears similar to ROP, except FEVR is autosomal dominant, although family members may be asymptomatic; asymptomatic family members often show peripheral retinal vascular abnormalities. There usually is no history of prematurity or oxygen therapy.)
- Incontinentia pigmenti in girls.
- See Leukocoria, Section 9.1, for additional differential diagnoses.

Workup
Dilated retinal examination with scleral depression at gestational age 31 to 32 weeks (number of weeks after date of last menstrual period), or as soon as feasible before discharge from the hospital. Can dilate with phenylephrine, 2.5%, tropicamide, 0.5% to 1%, and homatropine, 2%.

Classification

LOCATION

Zone 1   Posterior pole: 2 times the disc–fovea distance, centered around the disc. (Poorest prognosis.)

Zone 2   From zone 1 to the nasal periphery, temporally equidistant from the disc.

Zone 3   The remaining temporal periphery.

EXTENT

Number of clock hours (30-degree sectors) involved.

SEVERITY

Stage 1   Flat demarcation line separating the vascular posterior retina from the avascular peripheral retina.

Stage 2   Ridged demarcation line.

Stage 3   Ridged demarcation line with extraretinal fibrovascular proliferation.

Stage 4A Extrafoveal retinal detachment.
Stage 4B Subtotal retinal detachment involving the macula.
Stage 5 Total retinal detachment.

"PLUS" DISEASE

Engorged veins and tortuous arteries in the posterior pole. If plus disease is present, a + is placed after the stage (e.g., stage 3+). Zone 1 ROP with plus disease indicates high risk for rapid progression ("rush" disease).

Treatment (Based on Severity)

Stages 1 and 2 No treatment necessary.

Stage 3 Laser photocoagulation or cryotherapy if threshold disease present, defined as at least five contiguous or eight accumulated clock hours of stage 3+ disease. Treatment of the avascular zone should be instituted within 72 hours.

Stages 4 and 5 Surgical repair of retinal detachment by scleral buckling, vitrectomy surgery, or both.

Follow-up

A. If the initial dilated fundus evaluation was abnormal, repeat examination every 2 weeks until the retina is fully vascularized or ROP regresses. If prethreshold disease is detected [(a) any stage less than threshold in zone 1, or (b) stage 2+ or 3 ROP in zone 2], then perform repeated examinations at least weekly, depending on the tempo of the disease. Once full vascularization or regression of the ROP is noted, follow up every 1 to 2 months at first and later every 6 to 12 months. Children who have had ROP have a higher incidence of myopia, strabismus, amblyopia, macular dragging, cataracts, glaucoma, and retinal detachment.

B. An untreated fully vascularized fundus needs examinations only at age 6 months to rule out myopia, strabismus, etc. Regression from stage 2 or 3 requires closer follow-up as described earlier.

C. If on the initial examination, the retina is normal, consider repeated examination in 2 to 3 months.

References

Committee for the Classification of Retinopathy of Prematurity. The international classification of retinopathy of prematurity. *Arch Ophthalmol* 1984;102:1130.

Cryotherapy for Retinopathy of Prematurity Cooperative Group. Multicenter trial of cryotherapy for retinopathy of prematurity: one-year outcome structure and function. *Arch Ophthalmol* 1990;108:1408.

McNamara JA, Tasman W, Brown GC, et al. Laser photocoagulation for stage 3+ retinopathy of prematurity. *Ophthalmology* 1991;98:576.

9.3 ESODEVIATIONS IN CHILDREN

Critical Signs

Either eye is turned inward (i.e., "cross-eyed"). The nonfixating eye turns outward to refixate straight ahead when the fixating eye is covered during the cover–uncover test (see Appendix 2).

Other Signs

Amblyopia, overaction of the inferior oblique muscles.

Types

A. Concomitant esotropic deviations [A manifest convergent misalignment of the eye (or eyes) in which the measured angle of esodeviation is nearly constant in all fields of gaze at distance fixation.]

- Congenital (infantile) esotropia [Manifests by age 6 months, the angle of esodeviation is usually large (>40 to 50 prism diopters) and equal at distance and near fixation. Refractive error is usually normal for age (slightly hyperopic). Amblyopia is often present in those who do not cross-fixate. The patient may have a family history of the condition, and often develops latent nystagmus and dissociated vertical deviation.]

- Accommodative esotropia (Convergent misalignment of the eyes associated with activation of the accommodative reflex. Average age of onset is 2.5 years.)

  Subtypes:

  1. Refractive accommodative esotropia [These children are hyperopic (farsighted) in the range of +3.00 to +10.00 diopters (average, +4.75). The measured angle of esodeviation is usually moderate (20 to 30 prism diopters) and is equal at distance and near fixation. Full hyperopic correction eliminates the esodeviation. The accommodative convergence/accommodation ratio (AC/A) is normal. Amblyopia is common.]

  2. Nonrefractive accommodative esotropia [The measured angle of esodeviation is greater at near fixation than at distance fixation. The refractive error is similar to that of normal children of similar age (slightly hyperopic). The AC/A ratio is high (>10 prism diopters). Amblyopia is common.]

  3. Partial or decompensated accommodative esotropia (Refractive and nonrefractive accommodative esotropias that demonstrate a significant reduction in the esodeviation when given full hyperopic correction, but still have a residual esodeviation. The residual esodeviation is the nonaccommodative component. This

condition often occurs when there is a delay between the onset of the accommodative esotropia and the use of full hyperopic correction.)

- Sensory-deprivation esotropia [An esodeviation that occurs in a patient with a monocular or binocular lesion or a condition that prevents good vision (e.g., corneal opacity, cataract, retinal scars, inflammations, tumors, optic neuropathy, anisometropia).]
- Divergence insufficiency (A convergent ocular misalignment that is greater at distance fixation than at near fixation. This is a diagnosis of exclusion and must be differentiated from divergence paralysis, which can be associated with pontine tumors, neurologic trauma, and other conditions.)

B. Incomitant esodeviations (The measured angle of esodeviation varies with the direction of gaze at distance fixation.)
- Serious neurologic disorder (Acute onset and new onset of nystagmus may suggest tumor, hydrocephalus, or other causes of increased intracranial pressure.)
- Medial rectus restriction (e.g., thyroid disease, medial orbital-wall fracture)
- Lateral rectus weakness [e.g., isolated sixth-nerve palsy (See Section 11.7, Isolated Sixth-Nerve Palsy), slipped or detached lateral rectus from trauma or previous surgery.

Differential Diagnosis
- Pseudoesotropia (The eyes appear esotropic; however, there is no ocular misalignment detected during cover–uncover testing. Usually, the child has a wide nasal bridge, prominent epicanthal folds, and/or a small interpupillary distance.)

See Strabismus Syndromes, Section 9.5.

Workup
1. History: Ascertain age of onset of crossing, frequency of crossing, history of glasses, and any history of patching or trauma.
2. Visual acuity of each eye separately, with correction and pinhole, to evaluate for amblyopia. Note any nystagmus.
3. Ocular motility examination; observe for restricted movements or oblique overactions.
4. Measure the distance deviation in all fields of gaze and the near deviation in the primary position (straight ahead) using prisms. See Appendix 2.
5. Manifest and cycloplegic refractions.
6. Pupillary, slit-lamp, and fundus examinations; look for causes of sensory deprivation.

7. If divergence insufficiency or paralysis or if acute-onset incomitant esotropia is present, a head CT scan (axial and coronal views) or an MRI and a neurologic evaluation are necessary to rule out an intracranial mass lesion.

8. With incomitant esodeviation, consider thyroid-function tests, edrophonium chloride (e.g., Tensilon) test or look for characteristics of strabismus syndromes (See Section 9.5, Strabismus Syndromes).

Treatment

In all cases, correct refractive errors of ≥+2.00 diopters, and treat any amblyopia by patching the better-seeing eye (see Amblyopia, Section 9.6).

• Congenital esotropia: When equal vision is obtained in the two eyes, corrective muscle surgery is usually performed.
• Accommodative esotropia: Glasses must be worn full time.
  1. If the patient is younger than 5 to 6 years, correct the hyperopia with the full cycloplegic refraction.
  2. If the patient is older than 5 to 6 years, push plus lenses during the manifest (noncycloplegic) refraction until distance vision blurs, and give the most plus lenses without blurring distance vision.
  3. If the patient's eyes are straight at distance with full correction, but still esotropic at near distance (high AC/A ratio), treatment options exist:
     a. Bifocals (executive type) +2.50 or +3.00 diopter add, with top of the bifocal crossing the lower pupillary border.
     b. Extraocular muscle surgery: there is no consensus on treatment.
• Nonaccommodative esotropia or decompensated accommodative esotropia: Muscle surgery is usually performed to correct any significant esotropia that remains when glasses are worn.
• Sensory-deprivation esotropia:
  1. Attempt to correct the cause of poor vision.
  2. Give the full cycloplegic correction.
  3. Muscle surgery to correct the manifest esotropia.
  4. All patients with very poor vision in one eye need to wear protective polycarbonate lens glasses at all times.

Follow-up

At each visit, evaluate for amblyopia and measure the degree of deviation with prisms (with glasses worn).

• If amblyopia is present, see Section 9.6, Amblyopia, for management.
• If amblyopia is not present, the child is reevaluated in 3 to 6 weeks after a new prescription is given or in 1 to 6 months if no changes are made and the eyes are straight.

- When a residual esotropia is present while the patient wears glasses, an attempt is made to add more plus power to the current prescription. Children younger than 6 years should receive a new cycloplegic refraction; plus lenses are pushed without cycloplegia in older children. The maximal additional plus lens that does not blur distance vision is prescribed. If the eyes cannot be straightened with more plus power, then a decompensated accommodative esotropia has developed (see preceding).
- Hyperopia (farsightedness) often decreases slowly after age 5 to 7 years, and the strength of the glasses may need to be reduced so as not to blur distance vision. If the strength of the glasses must be reduced to improve visual acuity and the esotropia returns, then this is a decompensated accommodative esotropia (see earlier).

9.4 EXODEVIATIONS IN CHILDREN

Critical Signs
Either eye is constantly or intermittently turned outward (i.e., "wall-eyed"). On the cover–uncover test, when the fixating eye is covered, the uncovered eye turns inward to fixate (See Appendix 2).

Other Signs
Amblyopia, overaction of the superior or inferior oblique muscles (producing an "A" or a "V" pattern), vertical deviation.

Types
- Intermittent exotropia (The most common type of exodeviation in children. Onset is usually from infancy to age 4 years, and it is often, but not always, progressive in frequency. Amblyopia is rare.)
  Phases:
  Phase 1 One eye turns out at distance fixation, spontaneously or when it is covered. Primarily occurs when the patient is fatigued, sick, or not concentrating. The eyes become straight within 1 to 2 blinks of the cover being removed. The eyes are straight at near fixation. Patient often has diplopia and closes one eye to relieve symptoms.
  Phase 2 Increasing frequency of exotropia at distance fixation. Exotropia begins to occur at near fixation.
  Phase 3 There is a constant exotropia at distance and near fixations.

- Sensory-deprivation exotropia (An eye that does not see well, for any reason, may turn outward.)
- Duane's syndrome, type 2 (Limitation of adduction of one eye, with globe retraction and narrowing of the palpebral fissure on attempted adduction. Rarely bilateral. See Section 9.5, Strabismus Syndromes.)
- Third-nerve palsy (Limitation of eye movement superiorly, medially, and inferiorly, usually with ptosis. See Section 11.5, Isolated Third-Nerve Palsy.)
- Orbital disease (e.g., tumor, orbital pseudotumor) (Proptosis and restriction of ocular motility are usually evident. See Section 7.1, Orbital Disease.)
- Myasthenia gravis [Ptosis and limitation of eye movement can vary throughout the day, positive edrophonium chloride (e.g., Tensilon) test. See Section 11.10, Myasthenia Gravis.]
- Convergence insufficiency (Usually occurs in patients older than 10 years. Blurred near vision, headaches when reading. An exodeviation at near fixation, but straight at distance fixation. Must be differentiated from convergence paralysis. See Section 15.6, Convergence Insufficiency.)

Differential Diagnosis
- Pseudoexotropia (The patient appears to have an exodeviation, but no movement is noted on cover–uncover testing despite good vision in each eye. A wide interpupillary distance or temporal dragging of the macula from retinopathy of prematurity, toxocariasis, or other retinal disorders may be responsible.)

Workup
1. Evaluate visual acuity of each eye, with correction and pinhole, to evaluate for amblyopia.
2. Perform motility examination; observing for restricted eye movements or signs of Duane's syndrome.
3. Measure the exodeviation in all fields of gaze at distance and in primary position (straight ahead) at near, using prisms (see Appendix 2).
4. Check for proptosis with Hertel exophthalmometry when appropriate.
5. Perform pupillary, slit-lamp, and fundus examinations; check for causes of sensory deprivation.
6. Manifest and cycloplegic refractions.
7. Consider an edrophonium chloride (e.g., Tensilon) test when myasthenia gravis is suspected.
8. Consider a CT scan (axial and coronal views) and/or an MRI of the orbit and brain, as needed.

Treatment

In all cases, correct significant refractive errors and treat amblyopia (see Section 9.6, Amblyopia).

- Intermittent exotropia:

    Phase 1: Follow up patient closely.

    Phase 2: Muscle surgery may be indicated to maintain normal binocular vision.

    Phase 3: Muscle surgery is often considered at this point. Bifixation and peripheral fusion can occasionally be attained.
- Sensory-deprivation exotropia:
    1. Correct the underlying cause, if possible.
    2. Treat any amblyopia.
    3. Muscle surgery may be performed for manifest exotropia.
    4. When one eye has very poor vision, protective glasses (polycarbonate lens glasses) should be worn at all times to protect the good eye.
- Duane's syndrome: See Section 9.5, Strabismus Syndromes.
- Third-nerve palsy: See Section 11.5, Third-Nerve Palsy.
- Convergence insufficiency: See Section 15.6, Convergence Insufficiency.

Follow-up

- If amblyopia is being treated, see Section 9.6, Amblyopia.
- If no amblyopia is present, then reexamine every 4 to 6 months. The parents and patient are told to return sooner if the deviation increases or becomes more frequent.

9.5 STRABISMUS SYNDROMES

Motility disorders that demonstrate typical features of a particular syndrome. Specific entities include the following:

Syndromes

- Duane's syndrome [A congenital motility disorder, usually unilateral, characterized by limited abduction, limited adduction, or both. The globe may retract and the eyelid fissure narrow on adduction. There is often a face-turn to allow the patient to use both eyes together. Duane's may be classified into three types:

Type 1: Limited abduction (most common).
Type 2: Limited adduction.
Type 3: Limited abduction and adduction.]
- Brown's syndrome (A motility disorder characterized by limitation of elevation in adduction. Elevation in abduction is normal. Typically, eyes are straight in primary gaze. Usually congenital, but may be acquired secondary to trauma, surgery, or inflammation in the area of the trochlea. Bilateral in 10% of patients.)
- Double-elevator palsy (Congenital unilateral limitation of elevation in all fields of gaze. There may be hypotropia of the involved eye when the other eye fixes in primary gaze. Ptosis or pseudoptosis may be present in primary gaze. The child may assume a chin-up position to maintain fusion in downgaze.)
- Mobius' syndrome (Congenital unilateral or bilateral limitation of horizontal eye movements with a unilateral or bilateral, partial or complete facial nerve palsy. Other cranial nerve palsies as well as deformities of the hands and/or feet may also occur.)
- Congenital fibrosis syndrome [Congenital stationary bilateral ptosis and external ophthalmoplegia with limited horizontal gaze. The eyes cannot be elevated to primary gaze (straight ahead) so the patient maintains a chin-up position.]

Workup
1. History: Age of onset? History of trauma? Family history? History of other ocular or systemic diseases?
2. Complete ophthalmic examination; including alignment in all fields of gaze. Note if a compensatory head posture is present. Look for retraction of globe and narrowing of interpalpebral fissure in adduction.
3. Pertinent physical examination, including cranial nerve evaluation.
4. Radiologic studies (e.g., MRI or CT scan) may be indicated for acquired, atypical, and/or progressive motility disturbances.

Treatment
1. Treatment is usually indicated for significant abnormal head position, or if a cosmetically noticeable horizontal or vertical deviation exists in primary gaze.
2. Surgery, when indicated, is dependent on the particular motility disorder, extraocular muscle function, and the degree of abnormal head position.

Follow-up
Follow-up is dependent on the condition or conditions being treated.

9.6 AMBLYOPIA

Symptoms

Usually asymptomatic or decreased vision in one eye.* A history of patching, strabismus, and/or muscle surgery as a child may be elicited.

Critical Sign

Poorer vision in one eye that is not improved with refraction and not entirely explained by an organic lesion. The decrease in vision develops during the first decade of life and does not deteriorate thereafter. Amblyopia occasionally occurs bilaterally as a result of bilateral visual deprivation such as in congenital cataracts.

Other Signs

Crowding phenomenon occurs when individual letters can be read better than a whole line. A neutral-density filter significantly reduces vision in organic disease, but generally does not in pure amblyopia.

❖ **Note** *Amblyopia, when severe, may cause a mild relative afferent pupillary defect.*

Etiology

- Anisometropia (A difference in refractive error between the two eyes.)
- Strabismus (The eyes are not straight. Vision is worse in the nonfixating eye. Strabismus can lead to, or be the result of, amblyopia.)
- Occlusion [Such as from ptosis; congenital or secondary (e.g., eyelid hemangioma) or iatrogenic (e.g., patching)].
- Organic [Such as a media opacity (e.g., cataract, corneal scar, persistent hyperplastic primary vitreous, retinal or macular lesion)].

Workup

1. History: Eye problem in childhood, particularly misaligned eyes? Patching or muscle surgery as a child?
2. Ocular examination to rule out an organic cause for the reduced vision. Carefully check the pupils, optic disc, and macula.
3. Cover–uncover test to evaluate eye alignment (see Appendix 2).
4. Refraction; cycloplegic in children too young to cooperate.

*Amblyopia occasionally occurs bilaterally as a result of bilateral visual deprivation (e.g., congenital cataracts, high refractive errors.)

Treatment/Follow-up

A. Patients younger than 9 to 11 years:
  1. Appropriate spectacle correction.
  2. Full-time patching over the eye with better vision for 1 week per year of age (e.g., 3 weeks for a 3-year-old), followed by a repeated eye examination. Pirate patches and patches worn over glasses are less effective than patches placed directly over the eye and adhering to the skin. If a patch causes local irritation, use tincture of benzoin on the skin before applying the patch and use warm water compresses on the patch before removal.
  3. Continue patching until the vision is equalized or shows no improvement after three compliant cycles of patching. If a recurrence of amblyopia is likely, then use part-time patching to maintain improved vision.
  4. If occlusion amblyopia (i.e., a decrease in vision in the patched eye) develops, patch the opposite eye for a short period (e.g., 1 day per year of age), and repeat the examination.
  5. In strabismic amblyopia, delay strabismus surgery until the vision in the two eyes is equal, or maximal vision has been obtained in the amblyopic eye.
B. Patients older than 11 years of age: A trial of patching may be considered if patching has never been done. Otherwise no treatment is available. Protective glasses (e.g., polycarbonate lenses) should be worn at all times if there is only one good eye.

9.7 CONGENITAL CATARACT

Presentation

A white fundus reflex (leukocoria), absent red pupillary reflex, or abnormal eye movements (nystagmus) in one or both eyes. Infants with bilateral cataracts may be noted to be visually inattentive.

Critical Sign

Opacity of the lens (see types, later).

Other Signs

Eye misalignment (strabismus), nystagmus, or a blunted red reflex may be present. In patients with a monocular cataract, the involved eye is often smaller. A cataract alone does not cause a relative afferent pupillary defect.

Types of Cataracts

A. Polar. Opacity of the lens capsule and adjacent cortex on the anterior or posterior pole of the lens.

B. Zonular (lamellar). White opacities that surround the nucleus with alternating clear and white cortical lamella like an onion skin.

C. Nuclear. Opacity within the embryonic/fetal nucleus.

D. Posterior lenticonus. A posterior protrusion, usually opacified, in the posterior capsule (most common cause of nontraumatic acquired cataract).

Etiology

- Idiopathic (most common).
- Familial, autosomal dominant.
- Galactosemia. (Cataract may be the sole manifestation when galactokinase deficiency is responsible. A deficiency of galactose-1-phosphate uridyl transferase may produce mental retardation and symptomatic cirrhosis along with cataracts. The typical oil-droplet opacity may or may not be seen.)
- Persistent hyperplastic primary vitreous. (PHPV) (Unilateral. The involved eye is usually slightly smaller than the normal fellow eye. Examination after pupil dilatation may reveal a plaque of fibrovascular tissue behind the lens with elongated ciliary processes extending to it. Progression of the lens opacity often leads to angle-closure glaucoma.)
- Rubella (Nuclear cataract, "salt-and-pepper" chorioretinitis, a smaller involved eye than the normal contralateral eye. Associated hearing defects and heart abnormalities are common.)
- Lowe's syndrome (oculocerebrorenal syndrome) (Opaque lens, congenital glaucoma, renal disease, and mental retardation. X-linked recessive. Patients' mothers may have small cataracts.)
- Others (Chromosomal disorders, systemic syndromes, other intrauterine infections, trauma, drugs, other metabolic abnormalities.)

Differential Diagnosis

See Leukocoria, Section 9.1.

Workup

1. History: Maternal illness or drug ingestion during pregnancy? Systemic or ocular disease in the infant or child? Radiation exposure or trauma? Family history of congenital cataracts?

2. Visual assessment of each eye alone, by using illiterate E's, pictures, or by following small toys or a light.

3. Ocular examination: Attempt to determine the visual significance of the cataract. Evaluate the size and location of the cataract and whether the retina can be seen with a direct ophthalmoscope when looking

through an undilated pupil. Cataracts 3 mm or more in diameter usually affect vision. A portable slit lamp is helpful when available, as is a retinoscope (a blunted retinoscopic reflex suggests the cataract is visually significant). Check for signs of associated glaucoma (e.g., large corneal diameter, corneal edema, breaks in Descemet's membrane) and examine the retina for abnormalities, if possible.

4. Cycloplegic refraction.
5. B-scan ultrasonography may be helpful when the fundus view is obscured.
6. Medical examination by a pediatrician looking for associated abnormalities.
7. Red blood cell (RBC) galactokinase activity (galactokinase levels) with or without RBC galactose-1-phosphate-uridyltransferase activity to rule out galactosemia. This test is performed routinely on all infants in the United States.
8. Other tests as suggested by the systemic or ocular examination: (The chance that one of these conditions is present in a healthy child is remote.)
   a. Blood: Calcium and phosphorus levels (hypocalcemia, hypoparathyroidism), glucose levels (hypoglycemia, diabetes mellitus).
   b. Urine: Amino acid quantitation (Alport's syndrome), amino acid content (Lowe's syndrome).
   c. Antibody titers for rubella.

Treatment

1. Referral to a pediatrician to treat any underlying disorder.
2. Treat associated ocular diseases (e.g., glaucoma, see Congenital Glaucoma, Section 9.10).
3. Cataract extraction, usually within days to weeks of discovery to prevent irreversible amblyopia, is performed in the following circumstances:
   a. Vision is obstructed, and the eye's visual development is at risk.
   b. The lens is responsible for intraocular disease (e.g., lens-related glaucoma, uveitis).
   c. Cataract progression threatens the health of the eye (e.g., in persistent hyperplastic primary vitreous).
4. After cataract extraction, treat amblyopia in children younger than 9 to 11 years.
5. A dilating agent (e.g., phenylephrine, 2.5%, t.i.d., homatropine, 2%, t.i.d., or scopolamine, 0.25%, qd) may be used as a temporizing measure, allowing peripheral light rays to pass around the lens opacity and reach the retina. This rarely is successful.
6. Unilateral cataracts that are not large enough to obscure the visual axis requiring removal may still result in amblyopia. Treat amblyopia in children younger than 9 to 11 years (see Amblyopia, Section 9.6).

Follow-up

Young children that do not undergo surgery are monitored closely for cataract progression and amblyopia. Older children are less likely to develop amblyopia even if the cataract progresses; they are followed up on a 6- to 12-month basis.

❖ **Note** *Children with rubella must be isolated from pregnant women.*

9.8 OPHTHALMIA NEONATORUM
(Newborn Conjunctivitis)

Critical Sign

Purulent, mucopurulent, or mucoid discharge from one or both eyes in the first month of life, with diffuse conjunctival injection.

Other Signs

Eyelid edema, chemosis.

Etiology

- Chemical [Seen within a few hours of instilling a prophylactic agent (e.g., silver nitrate), lasts no more than 24 to 36 hours. Rarely seen now that erythromycin is used routinely.]
- *Neisseria gonorrhoeae* (May see gram-negative intracellular diplococci on Gram's stain. Typically seen within the first few days.)
- *Chlamydia trachomatis* (May see basophilic intracytoplasmic inclusion bodies in conjunctival epithelial cells, polymorphonuclear leukocytes, or lymphocytes on Giemsa stain. Presentation in the second week of life is common.)
- Bacteria (Staphylococci, streptococci, and gram-negative species may be seen on Gram's stain.)
- Herpes simplex virus (May have typical herpetic vesicles on the eyelid margins, can see multinucleated giant cells on Giemsa stain.)

Differential Diagnosis

- Dacryocystis (Swelling and erythema of the inner canthus. Purulent discharge may be expressed from the punctum by rolling a finger from the lacrimal sac to the punctum. Nasal conjunctival injection may be present, but diffuse injection is typically not present. See Section 6.8, Dacryocystitis.)

- Nasolacrimal duct obstruction (Tearing, may have a mild mucopurulent discharge from the punctum, minimal-to-no conjunctival injection or eyelid swelling. See Section 9.9, Congenital Nasolacrimal Duct Obstruction.)
- Congenital glaucoma (Corneal enlargement >12.0 mm horizontally, photophobia, Haab's stria, corneal edema, buphthalmos, tearing not discharge. See Section 9.10, Congenital Glaucoma.)

Workup

1. History: Previous or concurrent venereal disease in the mother? Were cervical cultures performed during pregnancy? If so, obtain the results.
2. Ocular examination with a penlight and then a blue light after fluorescein instillation; look for corneal involvement.
3. Conjunctival scrapings for two slides: Gram and Giemsa stain.
   Technique: Irrigate the discharge out of the fornices, place a drop of topical anesthetic (e.g., proparacaine) in the eye, and scrape the palpebral conjunctiva of the lower eyelid with a flame-sterilized spatula after it cools off. Place the scrapings on the slides.
4. Conjunctival cultures for blood and chocolate agars. Chocolate agar should be placed in an atmosphere of 2% to 10% carbon dioxide immediately after being plated.
   Technique: Reanesthetize the eye if necessary. Moisten a calcium alginate swab (a cotton-tipped applicator is a less-desirable alternative) with liquid broth media, and vigorously rub it along the inferior palpebral conjunctiva. Plate it directly on the culture dish. Repeat the procedure for additional cultures.
5. Scrape the conjunctiva for the chlamydial immunofluorescent antibody test.
6. Viral culture: Moisten another cotton-tipped applicator and roll it along the palpebral conjunctiva. Break off the end of the applicator and place it into the viral transport medium.

Treatment

Initial therapy is based on the results of the Gram's and Giemsa stains, if they can be examined immediately. Therapy is then modified according to the culture results and the clinical response.

A. No information from stains, no particular organism suspected: Erythromycin ointment q.i.d. plus erythromycin elixir,* 50 mg/kg/day, for 2 to 3 weeks.
B. Suspect chemical (e.g., silver nitrate) toxicity: No treatment. Reevaluate in 24 hours.

---

*Erythromycin elixir is divided into four doses daily and placed into the baby's formula.

C. Suspect chlamydia: Erythromycin elixir, 50 mg/kg/day*, for 2 to 3 weeks, plus erythromycin ointment q.i.d. If confirmed by culture or immunofluorescent stain, treat the mother and her sexual partner or partners with one of the following:

Tetracycline, 250 to 500 mg p.o., q.i.d., or doxycycline, 100 mg p.o., b.i.d., for 7 days (for men and mothers who are neither breast-feeding nor pregnant)

or

Erythromycin, 250 to 500 mg p.o., q.i.d., for 7 days (for breast-feeding or pregnant women).

❖ **Note** *Inadequately treated chlamydial conjunctivitis in a neonate can lead to chlamydial otitis or pneumonia.*

D. Suspect *Neisseria gonorrhoeae: Treatment is not well established. We favor the following:*

1. Hospitalize and evaluate for disseminated gonococcal infection with careful physical examination (especially of joints). Blood and cerebrospinal fluid cultures are obtained if a culture-proven infection is present.
2. One dose of ceftriaxone, 125 mg i.m., or cefotaxime, 50 mg/kg i.v. or i.m., q 8 to 12 h for 7 days. In penicillin- or cephalosporin-allergic patients, an infectious disease consult is obtained.
3. Bacitracin ointment, q 2 to 4 h.
4. Topical saline lavage to remove any discharge, q.i.d.
5. All neonates with gonorrhea should also be treated for chlamydia with erythromycin elixir, 50 mg/kg/day* for 14 days.

❖ **Note** *If it is confirmed by culture, the mother and her sexual partner or partners should be treated in accordance with the sensitivity results for 7 days. If sensitivities not initially available, ceftriaxone is the first choice. Additionally, chlamydia should be treated as outlined earlier.*

E. Gram-positive bacteria on Gram's stain, with no suspicion of gonorrhea and no corneal involvement: Bacitracin ointment q.i.d. for 2 weeks.
F. Gram-negative bacteria on Gram's stain, but no suspicion of gonorrhea, and no corneal involvement: Gentamicin or tobramycin ointment q.i.d. for 2 weeks.
G. Bacteria on Gram's stain and corneal involvement: Hospitalize, workup, and treat as for Infectious Corneal Infiltrate/Ulcer, Section 4.12.

---

*Erythromycin elixir is divided into four doses daily and placed into the baby's formula.

H. Suspect herpes simplex virus: Vidarabine, 3% ointment (e.g., Vira-A) 5 times per day, then cut dosage in half for 1 week. Systemic acyclovir for systemic disease after pediatric consultation.

Follow-up

Initially, examine daily as an inpatient or outpatient. If the condition worsens (e.g., corneal involvement develops), reculture and hospitalize. As mentioned, therapy is tailored according to the clinical response and the culture results. The frequency of follow-up visits may be reduced once improvement is clearly demonstrated.

References

Ullman S, Roussel TJ, Forster RK. Gonococcal keratoconjunctivitis. *Surv Ophthalmol* 1987;32:199.

9.9 CONGENITAL NASOLACRIMAL DUCT OBSTRUCTION

Presentation

Persistent tearing, chronic mucopurulent discharge, matting of the eyelids, may be unilateral or bilateral.

Critical Signs

Wet-looking eye or tears flowing over the eyelid; moist or dried mucopurulent material on the eyelashes (predominantly medially), and reflux of mucoid or mucopurulent material from the punctum when pressure is applied over the lacrimal sac, where the lower eyelid abuts the nose.

Other Signs

Erythema (irritation) of the surrounding skin; redness and swelling of the medial canthus. Preseptal cellulitis or dacryocystitis may rarely develop.

❖ **Note** *Nasolacrimal duct obstruction may be associated with an otitis or pharyngitis.*

Etiology

Usually the result of an imperforate membrane at the distal end of the nasolacrimal duct.

Differential Diagnosis
- Conjunctivitis (Red eye, discharge. Usually acute. Follicles or papillae may or may not be present on the inferior tarsal conjunctiva. Tearing is not chronic.)
- Congenital anomalies of the upper lacrimal drainage system. (Atresia of the lacrimal puncta or canaliculus.)
- Mucocele of the lacrimal sac (Bluish, cystic, nontender mass located just below the medial canthal angle. Caused by both a distal and a proximal obstruction of the nasolacrimal apparatus.)
- Other causes of tearing [e.g., entropion/trichiasis, corneal defects, foreign body under the upper eyelid, congenital glaucoma (See Section 9.10, Congenital Glaucoma).]

Workup
1. Exclude other causes of tearing with slit-lamp or penlight examination. Make sure the corneal diameter is not large, and ruptures in Descemet's membrane are not present (congenital glaucoma).
2. Palpate over the lacrimal sac; reflux of mucoid or mucopurulent discharge from the punctum confirms the diagnosis.

Treatment
1. Digital pressure 2 to 4 times per day. The parent is taught to place his or her index finger over the child's common canaliculus (inner corner of the eye) and to apply pressure several times a day.
2. Use erythromycin ointment b.i.d., prn, to control mucopurulent discharge if present.
3. In the presence of acute dacryocystitis, a systemic antibiotic is needed (See Section 6.8, Dacryocystitis).

The majority of cases will open spontaneously with this regimen by age 1 year. If this is not the case:

4. Nasolacrimal duct probing is usually performed after age 13 months, earlier if recurrent or persistent infections of the lacrimal system develop or at the request of the parents. The majority of obstructions will be corrected after the initial probing; others may require repeated probings. If patency is not established after two probings, place silicone tubing in the nasolacrimal duct and leave it in place for weeks to months.

Follow-up
Follow up by phone calls. The child returns if the situation becomes worse, acute dacryocystitis is present, or if the parents are unsure.

9.10 CONGENITAL GLAUCOMA

Presentation

Photophobia, tearing, enlarged cornea, hazy cornea, most commonly in an infant; red eye may be present.

Critical Signs

Enlarged globe and corneal diameter (horizontal corneal diameter >12 mm before age 1 year is suggestive), corneal edema, increased intraocular pressure (IOP), increased cup/disc ratio, commonly bilateral.

Other Signs

Linear tears in Descemet's membrane of the cornea (Haab's stria), usually running horizontally or concentric to the limbus; corneal stromal scarring; conjunctival injection; myopic shift in refractive error.

Etiology

Majority of cases:
- Primary congenital glaucoma (Not associated with other ocular or systemic disorders.)

Less common:
- Sturge–Weber syndrome (Usually unilateral; may have a port-wine stain, cerebral calcifications, and seizures; not familial.)

Rare:
- Developmental anterior segment abnormality (e.g., Axenfeld's syndrome, Rieger's anomaly/syndrome, Peter's anomaly, others) (Bilateral. Abnormalities of the cornea, iris, and anterior-chamber angle.)
- Lowe's syndrome (oculocerebrorenal syndrome) (Cataract, glaucoma, and renal disease; X-linked recessive.)
- Rubella (Glaucoma, cataracts, "salt-and-pepper" chorioretinopathy, hearing and cardiac defects.)
- Aniridia (Iris hypoplasia, often with only a rudimentary iris stub visible on gonioscopy, cataracts, glaucoma, foveal hypoplasia, nystagmus.)
- Others (e.g., neurofibromatosis, homocystinuria, persistent hyperplastic primary vitreous, secondary glaucoma from anteriorly displaced lens–iris diaphragm.)

Differential Diagnosis

- Congenital megalocornea (Bilateral horizontal corneal diameter >13 mm with normal corneal thickness and endothelium. IOP and cup/disc ratio are normal.)

- Trauma from forceps during delivery (May produce tears in Descemet's membrane and localized corneal edema; however, the tears are typically vertical or oblique, and the corneal diameter is normal. Birth trauma is generally unilateral and may often be obtained from the history.)
- Congenital hereditary endothelial dystrophy (Bilateral corneal edema at birth with a normal corneal diameter and normal IOP.)
- Mucopolysaccharidoses and cystinosis (Some inborn errors of metabolism produce cloudy corneas in infancy or early childhood, but usually not at birth; the corneal diameter and IOP are normal.)
- Nasolacrimal duct obstruction (Tearing, sometimes with a mild mucopurulent discharge from the punctum. The cornea is clear and not enlarged. The IOP is normal. See Section 9.9, Congenital Nasolacrimal Duct Obstruction.)

Workup
1. History: Other systemic abnormalities? Rubella infection during pregnancy? Birth trauma?
2. Ocular examination, including a visual-acuity assessment of each eye separately (can the child fixate and follow?), a penlight examination to detect corneal enlargement and haziness, and retinoscopy to estimate refractive error. IOP measurement by Tonopen or Schiötz tonometry is attempted. A dilated fundus examination is performed to evaluate the optic disc and retina. Examination with a retinoscope or hand-held portable slit lamp is sometimes used in uncertain cases to look for tears in Descemet's membrane and corneal edema.
3. Examination under anesthesia (EUA) is performed in suggestive cases and in those for whom surgical treatment is planned. The horizontal corneal diameter and IOP are measured; retinoscopy, gonioscopy, and ophthalmoscopy are performed. Ultrasound is often used to measure axial length. At 40 gestational weeks, the mean axial length is 17 mm. This increases to 20 mm on average by age 1 year. Axial-length progression also may be monitored by successive cycloplegic refractions.

❖ **Note** *IOP may be reduced substantially by general anesthesia, particularly halothane; an IOP of ≥20 mm Hg under halothane anesthesia is suggestive of glaucoma. An exception is ketamine hydrochloride, which may increase IOP. In general, IOP is measured as soon as possible after general anesthesia is induced to achieve as accurate a measurement as possible.*

Treatment
Definitive treatment is usually surgical. Medical therapy is temporary and is started initially, pending surgery.

Medical (any or all of the following may be used.)
1. Topical β-blocker (e.g., levobunolol or timolol, 0.25% to 0.5%, b.i.d.).
2. Carbonic anhydrase inhibitor (e.g., acetazolamide, 5 to 10 mg/kg p.o., q 6 h).

❖ **Note** *Miotics are rarely effective in controlling and may increase IOP, but they sometimes are used to constrict the pupil in preparation for a surgical goniotomy.*

Surgical First choice, goniotomy (incising the trabecular meshwork with a blade under gonioscopic visualization) or trabeculotomy (opening Schlemm's canal into the anterior chamber). These procedures are often repeated if they are unsuccessful at first attempt.
Other Trabeculectomy.

❖ **Note** *Amblyopia may be superimposed on glaucoma and should be treated by patching (see Section 9.6, Amblyopia).*

Follow-up
Repeated examinations, under anesthesia when needed, are necessary to monitor corneal diameter, IOP, cup/disc ratio, and axial length. These patients must be followed up throughout life to monitor for progression.

9.11 Developmental Anterior Segment and Lens Anomalies

Unilateral or bilateral congenital abnormalities of the cornea, iris, anterior-chamber angle, and lens. Specific entities include the following:

- Megalocornea (A nonprogressive corneal enlargement. The horizontal corneal diameter is >13 mm in the newborn. There are two types:
  1. Simple megalocornea: Bilateral, clear corneas of normal thickness; sporadic or autosomal dominant.
  2. Anterior megalophthalmos: Bilateral; associated with abnormalities of the iris, angle, and lens; may be associated with glaucoma; X-linked recessive.)
- Microcornea [Horizontal corneal diameter <11 mm. May be isolated or associated with nanophthalmos (a small globe that is otherwise anatomically normal) and microphthalmos (a small globe with multiple anomalies).]

- Posterior embryotoxon (A prominent, anteriorly displaced Schwalbe's ring. A normal variant.)
- Axenfeld's anomaly (Posterior embryotoxon associated with iris strands that span the angle to insert into the prominent Schwalbe's ring. Fifty to sixty percent of patients develop glaucoma. Autosomal dominant or sporadic.)
- Rieger's anomaly (Axenfeld's anomaly plus iris thinning and abnormally shaped and displaced pupils. Fifty to sixty percent of patients develop glaucoma. Autosomal dominant or sporadic.)
- Rieger's syndrome (Rieger's anomaly associated with dental, craniofacial, and skeletal abnormalities. May be associated with short stature caused by growth hormone deficiency, cardiac defects, deafness, and mental retardation. Autosomal dominant or sporadic.)
- Peter's anomaly [Central corneal opacity, usually with iris strands that extend from the iris collarette to the margin of the corneal defect. The lens may be clear and normally positioned, cataractous and displaced anteriorly (making the anterior chamber shallow), or adherent to the corneal defect.]
- Microspherophakia (The lens is small and spherical in configuration. The lens can subluxate into the anterior chamber, causing a secondary glaucoma.)
- Anterior and posterior lenticonus (An anterior or posterior ectasia of the lens surface. Posterior occurring more commonly than anterior. Often associated with cataract. Usually unilateral.)
- Ectopia lentis (May be associated with Marfan's syndrome, homocystinuria, Weill–Marchesani syndrome, aniridia, and trauma. Simple ectopia lentis is either a sporadic or autosomal dominantly inherited condition with bilateral, usually superior, lens displacement. Glaucoma may occur because of displacement of the lens–iris diaphragm.)
- Ectopia lentis et pupillae (Lens displacement associated with pupillary displacement in the opposite direction. Glaucoma may occur. Autosomal recessive.)
- Aniridia (Bilateral, near-total absence of the iris. The pupil appears to occupy the entire area of the cornea. Glaucoma, foveal hypoplasia with poor vision, nystagmus, and corneal pannus can occur. At least two inheritance patterns are known to exist:
  1. Autosomal dominant in two thirds of patients. This type is not associated with Wilms' tumor.
  2. Sporadic in one third of patients. Twenty-five percent of children with sporadic aniridia will develop Wilms' tumor.)

Workup
  1. History: Family history of ocular disease? Associated systemic abnormalities?

2. Complete ophthalmic examination, including gonioscopy of the anterior-chamber angle and intraocular pressure (IOP) determination (may require examination under anesthesia [EUA]).
3. Complete physical examination by a primary care doctor with blood pressure determination (may be elevated with renal abnormalities).
4. Chromosomal karyotype in patients with sporadic cases of aniridia. (There is an increased incidence of Wilms' tumor in patients with a deletion of the short arm of chromosome 11.)
5. Renal ultrasound and possibly intravenous pyelography in patients with sporadic aniridia to monitor for Wilms' tumor. The frequency and duration of monitoring should be determined by a pediatrician and/or pediatric oncologist. One suggested schedule is to evaluate every 3 months up to age 5, and then every 6 months up to age 10, and then once per year up to age 16.

Treatment
1. Correct refractive errors and treat amblyopia if present (see Section 9.6, Amblyopia). Children with unilateral structural abnormalities often have improved visual acuity after amblyopia therapy.
2. Treat glaucoma if present. β-Blockers and carbonic anhydrase inhibitors may be used. Pilocarpine and epinephrine compounds are not as effective and are not used in primary therapy (see Primary Open-Angle Glaucoma, Section 10.1). Surgery is often used initially (see Congenital Glaucoma, Section 9.10).
3. Consider cataract extraction if a significant cataract exists and a corneal transplant if a dense corneal opacity exists.
4. Genetic counseling.
5. Systemic abnormalities (e.g., Wilms' tumor) are managed by pediatric specialists.

Follow-up
1. Ophthalmic examination every 6 to 12 months throughout life, checking for increased IOP and other signs of glaucoma.
2. If amblyopia exists, then follow-up may need to be more frequent (see Section 9.6, Amblyopia)

9.12 THE BLIND INFANT

An infant whose visual skills are far below those expected (e.g., an inability to fix on and follow objects after several months of age) may have an obvious or inconspicuous ocular or neuro-ophthalmic disorder. Obvious causes include bilateral central corneal opacities, congenital cataracts, or infectious retinal problems with macular scarring. The following are conditions that may not be obvious on clinical examination.

I. Conditions that usually produce a searching nystagmus:

A. Pupils react poorly to light:

- Any severe ocular disease or malformation [e.g., retinopathy of prematurity (ROP), cataracts, aniridia, optic nerve atrophy, optic nerve hypoplasia] diagnosed by examination.

- Leber's congenital amaurosis [May have a normal-appearing fundus initially, but by age 1 to 3 years, may develop narrowing of retinal blood vessels, optic disc pallor, and pigmentary retinal changes. The electroretinogram (ERG) is markedly abnormal or flat. Autosomal recessive.]

- Optic nerve hypoplasia [A small optic disc that can be difficult to detect when bilateral (compare disc to vessels). If unilateral, may be seen with strabismus, a relative afferent pupillary defect, and unilateral poor fixation instead of searching nystagmus. When present, a "double ring" sign (a pigmented ring at the inner and outer edge of peripapillary atrophy) is diagnostic. Usually idiopathic, but can be a result of maternal diabetes or quinine, phenytoin, alcohol, or lysergic acid diethylamide (LSD) use.]

❖ **Note** *Optic nerve hypoplasia is rarely associated with septo-optic dysplasia (de Morsier syndrome), which includes midline abnormalities of the brain and growth, thyroid, and other tropic hormone deficiencies. Growth retardation, seizures as a result of hypoglycemia, and diabetes insipidus may develop.*

- Congenital optic atrophy (Rare. Pale, normal-sized optic disc, often associated with mental retardation or cerebral palsy. Normal ERG. Autosomal recessive or sporadic.)

- Congenital stationary night blindness (Visual acuity may even be normal, nystagmus less common, associated with myopia. ERG is abnormal. Autosomal dominant, recessive, and X-linked forms exist.)

B. Pupils react briskly to light:

- Infantile nystagmus (Some patients with this condition have a severe visual deficit. The iris is normal. It may be accompanied by face turn, head nodding, or both.)

- Albinism with delayed maturation (Iris transillumination defects and foveal hypoplasia are seen.)

II. No nystagmus present and pupils react normally to light:

- Diffuse cerebral dysfunction (Infants do not respond to sound or touch and are neurologically abnormal. Vision may slowly improve with time.)

- Delayed maturation of the visual system (Normal response to sound and touch, and neurologically normal. The ERG is normal, and vision usually develops between age 4 and 12 months.)
- Extreme refractive error (Diagnosed on cycloplegic refraction.)
- Achromatopsia (Rod monochromatism) (Pupils react normally to light but have paradoxical pupils. Normal fundus, but photopic ERG is markedly attenuated or nonrecordable. Scotopic ERG is normal.)

Workup

1. History: Premature? Normal development and growth? Maternal infection, diabetes, or drug use during pregnancy? Family history of eye disease?
2. Evaluate the infant's ability to fixate on an object and follow it with each eye individually (cover one eye and then the other).
3. Pupillary examination, noting both equality and briskness.
4. Look carefully for nystagmus.
5. Penlight examination of the anterior segment; check especially for iris transillumination defects with a slit lamp.
6. Dilated retinal and optic nerve evaluation.
7. Cycloplegic refraction.
8. ERG, especially if Leber's congenital amaurosis is suspected.
9. Consider a CT scan and/or MRI of the brain in cases with other focal neurologic signs, seizures, failure to thrive, developmental delay, optic nerve hypoplasia, optic atrophy, or neurologically localizing nystagmus (e.g., see-saw, vertical, gaze paretic, vestibular). Consider including orbital cuts if optic atrophy is unilateral. Imaging is performed in these cases to rule out brain tumors, hydrocephalus, infarctions, evidence of trauma, and brain malformations such as septo-optic dysplasia.
10. Consider a sweep visual evoked potential (VEP) for vision measurement.
11. Consider eye-movement recordings to evaluate the nystagmus wave form, if available.

Treatment

1. Correct refractive errors and treat known or suspected amblyopia.
2. Parental counseling is necessary in all of these conditions with respect to the infant's visual potential, and likelihood of other siblings, etc.
3. Referral to educational services for the visually handicapped or blind may be helpful.
4. Genetic counseling.
5. If neurologic or endocrine abnormalities are found or suspected, the child should be referred to a pediatrician for appropriate workup and/or management.

GLAUCOMA

10.1 PRIMARY OPEN-ANGLE GLAUCOMA (POAG)*

Symptoms

Usually asymptomatic until the latter stages both because of the slowly progressive nature of the disease and because the individual visual fields of each eye overlap quite significantly when both eyes are open. For symptoms to occur, the individual field defects must overlap. Patients with early symptoms may complain that parts of a page are missing. The classic symptom of tunnel vision does not occur until both visual fields are markedly damaged. Typically, central fixation is preserved until late in the disease. In the end stages of glaucoma, the remaining visual field is usually a temporal island.

Critical Signs

1. Sixty to seventy percent of patients will have an intraocular pressure (IOP), greater than average (>22 mm Hg); 30% to 40% will have an IOP <21 mm Hg.
2. Open anterior-chamber angle on gonioscopic evaluation. No peripheral anterior synechiae (PAS).
3. Characteristic optic nerve appearance
   a. Documented thinning of the neurosensory rim over time
   b. Acquired pit of the optic nerve
   c. Notching in the rim

---

*Due to convention, the term "primary open angle glaucoma" will be used here. The entity is not truly "primary."

    d. Nerve-fiber layer hemorrhage that crosses the disc margin; i.e., Drance hemorrhage.

    e. Nerve fiber layer defect

    f. Cup/disc (C/D) asymmetry greater than 0.2 in the absence of a cause such as anisometropia

    g. Thinner rim superiorly or inferiorly than temporally, or thinner rim nasally than temporally.

    h. Bayoneting: quick angulation in the course of the blood vessels as they exit the nerve.

    i. Enlarged C/D ratio >0.6 (less specific)

4. Characteristic visual-field loss: Nasal step (respects the horizontal midline), paracentral scotoma, or an arcuate scotoma extending from the blind spot nasally (defects usually respect the horizontal midline, or are greater in one hemifield than the other). Late finding may show only a temporal island of vision remaining.

Other Signs

Large fluctuations in IOP, absence of microcystic corneal edema, an uninflamed eye.

Differential Diagnosis

- Ocular hypertension (Elevated IOP, with normal optic nerve and visual field. See Section 10.2, Ocular Hypertension.)
- Physiologic optic nerve cupping (Enlarged C/D, but no change over time, no neurosensory rim notching, no visual-field loss, and usually a normal IOP.)
- Secondary open-angle glaucoma [Lens-induced, inflammatory, exfoliative, pigmentary, steroid-induced, developmental anterior-segment abnormalities, angle recession, traumatic (as a result of direct injury, blood, or debris), glaucoma related to increased episcleral venous pressure (e.g., Sturge–Weber syndrome, carotid–cavernous fistulae), glaucoma related to intraocular tumors.]
- Secondary angle-closure glaucoma (e.g., iridocorneal endothelial (ICE) syndrome)
- Chronic angle-closure glaucoma (CACgl) (Findings of POAG except PAS are present on gonioscopy. CACgl has an insidious onset, and may be associated with secondary causes of PAS such as uveitis, central retinal vein occlusion (CRVO), and previous attack of angle closure leaving PAS.)
- Previous glaucomatous damage (e.g., from steroids, uveitis, glaucomatocyclitic crisis, trauma) in which the inciting agent has been removed.
- Optic atrophy [Chiasmal tumors, syphilis, ischemic optic neuropathy, drugs, retinal vascular or degenerative disease, others. IOP is usually not increased in these conditions, unless a secondary or unrelated glaucoma also is present. These conditions are differentiated by optic nerve

pallor in greater proportion than optic nerve cupping. Visual-field defects are usually larger than expected, given the degree of optic nerve cupping. Glaucomatous-appearing visual fields are possible. Altitudinal defects are less typical of glaucoma and are more characteristic of anterior ischemic optic neuropathies. Altitudinal defects that respect the vertical midline are more typical of intracranial pathology (tumor, hemorrhage, ischemia, etc.) in the visual pathways.]

- Congenital optic nerve defects (Myopic discs, colobomas, optic nerve pits. IOP is usually not increased in these conditions, unless a secondary or unrelated glaucoma also is present. Visual-field defects may be present, but do not progress.)
- Optic nerve drusen [Visual-field defects may remain stable or progress unrelated to IOP. Optic nerves are usually not cupped, and drusen are often visible on examination. Characteristic calcified lesions seen on B scan ultrasound testing and on computed tomography (CT).]

Workup
1. History: Presence of risk factors (e.g., family history of blindness or visual loss from glaucoma, hypertension, age, black race, myopia). Previous history of increased IOP or chronic steroid use? Medical problems such as asthma, congestive heart failure, heart block, renal stones, allergies?
2. Complete ocular examination including slit lamp, gonioscopy, and dilated fundus examination with special attention to the optic nerve.
3. Baseline documentation of the optic nerves (e.g., stereoscopic disc photos, red-free photographs, image analysis, or meticulous drawings) and formal visual-field testing [preferably automated (e.g., Humphrey or Octopus)]. Goldmann visual-field tests may be helpful in patients unable to take the automated tests adequately. Color vision testing indicated in those suspected of a neurologic disorder.
4. Atypical cases may warrant a further evaluation for other causes of optic nerve damage. Aspects that may warrant further evaluation include the following.
   a. Optic nerve pallor out of proportion to the degree of cupping.
   b. Visual-field defects greater than expected based on amount of cupping.
   c. Visual-field patterns not typical of glaucoma (defects respecting the vertical midline, hemianopic defects, enlarged blind spot, central scotoma, etc.).
   d. IOP within the average range (less than 21 mm Hg).
   e. Unilateral progression despite equal IOP in both eyes.
   f. Decreased visual acuity out of proportion to the amount of cupping or field loss.
   g. Color-vision loss, especially in the red–green axis.

If any of these are present, further evaluation may include:

a. History: Acute episodes of eye pain or redness? Steroid use? Acute visual loss? Ocular trauma? Surgery, systemic trauma, heart attack, or other event that may lead to hypotension.

b. Diurnal IOP curve consisting of multiple IOP checks during the course of the day.

c. Complete blood count, erythrocyte sedimentation rate, rapid plasma reagin (RPR), fluorescent treponemal antibody, absorbed (FTA-ABS), possibly anti-nuclear antibody (ANA).

d. If visual-field defect patterns are more indicative of neurologic disease or if other neurologic signs/symptoms are present, may consider CT (axial and coronal, preferably with contrast if no contraindications are present) or magnetic resonance imaging (MRI) of orbit and brain with gadolinium and fat suppression (if no contraindications are present).

e. Consider referral to the primary care doctor for a complete cardiovascular evaluation.

Treatment

A. General Considerations

1. Who to treat?

The clinician must evaluate the appropriateness of treatment for each individual case, because not all three elements of pressure, optic nerve damage, and visual-field loss may be present in every case. Treatment must be based on the patient's overall physical and social health. Some general guidelines are suggested.

a. Consideration should be given to the amount of damage already present, the rate of damage progression, and the estimated duration of time further damage may accumulate (i.e., an estimation of the patient's life expectancy).

b. Treatment decisions regarding patients with an IOP >27 mm Hg, without optic nerve or visual-field changes are difficult. Some clinicians may elect to monitor these patients with close observation because some patients may never get worse. Some clinicians may elect to treat these patients, given the statistical possibility that approximately 50% will develop visual-field loss in 5 to 10 years. Factors to consider when deciding whether to proceed with treatment include degree of IOP increase (e.g., the higher the IOP, the more likely they are to develop to visual loss), presence of risk factors (particularly family history of visual loss and black race), estimation of the duration of time damage may develop (i.e., the patient's life expectancy), and risks of the various treatment options.

2. What is the treatment goal?

   The goal of treatment is to enhance or at least maintain the patient's health. This is accomplished by halting optic nerve damage and not causing problems by the treatments. The only proven method of stopping or slowing optic nerve damage is reducing IOP. It appears necessary to reduce the IOP approximately 30% to have the best chance of preventing optic nerve damage. When optic nerve damage is marked, pressure reduction may need to be even greater for the destruction to be halted; some have suggested setting 15 mm Hg as the maximal tolerable IOP in such cases. Another method of calculating the IOP goal is the use of formula: [IOP d - (IOP d × IOP d)/100 = goal, where IOP d represents the level of pressure known to be associated with damage. Some have suggested that if IOP can be lowered below 40%, visual-field restoration can occur.

3. How to treat?

   Three main treatment options exist for glaucoma: medications, argon laser trabeculoplasty (ALT), and guarded filtration surgery (trabeculectomy). For many patients, medications are the first-line therapy. ALT is often an appropriate initial therapy, especially in elderly, ill, or demented patients with 2+, 3+, or 4+ posterior trabecular meshwork pigmentation. Surgery, as first-line therapy, is being investigated. Results of a prospective randomized, multi-center trial (CIGTS) are not yet available.

   The type and aggressiveness of treatment are determined by the amount of damage already present, the rate of destruction, and the anticipated duration of the disease. When the rate of destruction is rapid and damage is advanced, surgery is usually needed.

   Other treatment modalities, such as tube-shunt procedures (with either Molteno, Baerveldt, Krupin, Ahmed, or Schocket implants), laser cyclophotocoagulation of the ciliary body (with YAG laser, diode laser, or endolaser), cyclocryotherapy, and cyclodialysis are typically reserved for IOP uncontrolled by other methods such as medications, laser, and traditional filtering procedures.

B. Medications

   Unless there are extreme circumstances (such as an IOP >40 mm Hg or an impending risk to central fixation, treatment is started by using one type of drop in only one eye (one-eyed therapeutic trial). This is done by initiating therapy with the new medication in only one eye with reexamination in 3 to 6 weeks to check for effectiveness. Effectiveness is determined by comparing the difference in IOP in the two eyes before therapy with the differences in IOP after initiating therapy.

For example, if IOP is 30 mm Hg OD and 33 mm Hg OS before treatment, and after treatment of the right eye, the IOP was 20 mm Hg OD and 23 mm Hg OS, the drug is not having any effect. If the IOP after starting treatment is 25 mm Hg OD and 34 mm Hg OS, then the drug is having an effect.

1. β-Blockers (e.g., levobunolol or timolol 0.25% to 0.5% q.i.d. or b.i.d.; metipranolol, 0.3%; or carteolol, 1% b.i.d.), often effectively reduce IOP, but should be used with caution in patients with asthma/chronic obstructive pulmonary disease (COPD), heart block, congestive heart failure, depression, or myasthenia gravis. Betaxolol, 0.25% to 0.5% bid, is less likely to cause pulmonary complications. The pulse is usually checked before and after initiating therapy. Diabetics should be warned of the possibility of decreased sensitivity to the symptoms of hypoglycemia.

2. Selective α_2-receptor agonists (brimonidine, 0.2% t.i.d., or b.i.d. if used in conjunction with a β-blocker) are also often effective at reducing IOP. These agents should not be given to patients currently taking monoamine oxidase (MAO) inhibitors because of the possibility of hypertensive crisis. Commonly encountered side effects include allergy, dry mouth, dry eye, lethargy, mydriasis, and hypotension. Apraclonidine, 0.5% t.i.d., also may be used for short-term therapy (3 months), but tends to lose its effectiveness and has a relatively high allergy rate.

3. Topical carbonic anhydrase inhibitors (CAIs) (e.g., dorzolamide, 2%, or brinzolamide, 1% t.i.d., or b.i.d. if used in conjunction with a β-blocker) can be used to reduce IOP. These have the same potential side effects as systemic carbonic anhydrase inhibitors, except that metabolic acidosis, hypokalemia, gastrointestinal (GI) symptoms, weight loss, and paresthesias are usually not seen. More commonly seen side effects include burning, bitter taste, and topical allergy.

4. Prostaglandin agonists (e.g., latanoprost, 0.005% qhs) also can be added to further reduce IOP. This type of agent is contraindicated in patients with active uveitis, cystoid macular edema (CME), or pregnant women. Potential side effects include increase in melanin pigmentation in the iris, conjunctival injection, stinging sensation, increase in eyelash length, viral upper respiratory tract infection symptoms, and CME.

5. Miotics (e.g., pilocarpine q.i.d.) are generally used in low strengths initially (e.g., 0.5% to 1.0%) and then built up to higher strengths (e.g., 4%). Commonly not tolerated in patients older than 40 years because of accommodative spasm. Miotics are generally contraindicated in patients with retinal holes and should be used cautiously in patients at risk for retinal detachment (e.g.,

high myopes and aphakes). Pilocarpine is also available as a 4% gel used nightly or as an ocular insert replaced each week; the latter may be most useful in young patients. Long-acting agents, such as echothiophate iodide, are often the preferred medication in aphakic or pseudophakic glaucoma patients.

6. Sympathomimetics (dipivefrin, 0.1%, b.i.d., or epinephrine, 0.5% to 2.0%, b.i.d.) rarely reduce IOP to the degree of the other drugs, but have few systemic side effects other than red eyes. They may cause CME in aphakic patients and cardiac arrhythmias.

7. Systemic carbonic anhydrase inhibitors (e.g., methazolamide, 25 to 50 mg p.o., 2 to 3 times/day, acetazolamide, 125 to 250 mg p.o., 2 to 4 times daily, or acetazolamide, 500 mg sequel p.o., b.i.d.) should usually not be given to patients with a sulfa allergy and should be avoided in patients with a history of renal stones. Potassium levels must be monitored if the patient is taking other diuretic agents or digitalis. Side effects, such as fatigue, nausea, confusion, and paresthesias, are common. Rare, but severe, hematologic side effects (e.g., aplastic anemia) have occurred.

❖ **Note** *Digital punctal occlusion or passive eyelid closure should be used in every patient. All patients should be given specific instruction in this regard.*

C. Argon laser trabeculoplasty
In some patients, as defined earlier, ALT may be used as first-line therapy. Additionally, ALT may be considered first-line therapy in patients with demonstrated or suspected noncompliance. Approximately 10% of patients have some increase of pressure each year, so the average effective duration is around 5 years.

D. Guarded filtration surgery
Trabeculectomy may obviate the need for medications. Adjunctive use of antimetabolites during surgery may aid in the effectiveness of the surgery.

Follow-up

As mentioned earlier, patients are reexamined after starting a new medication to evaluate its efficacy; for β-blockers, latanaprost, and after ALT, it is usually best to recheck the patient in 3 to 6 weeks. With topical carbonic anhydrase inhibitors, α-agonists, and miotics, a steady state is achieved much more quickly, and recheck any time after 3 days is appropriate. When damage is severe, or IOP high, it may be necessary to see the patient within 1 to 3 days to assure that the desired effect has occurred. Once the IOP has been reduced adequately, patients are reevaluated in 3- to 6-month intervals for IOP and optic nerve checks. A goal of therapy is to reduce the IOP to a target pressure around 30% beneath the range at which glaucomatous progression occurred. This target pressure depends on the severity of disease and speed of progression, and it must be updated often.

Gonioscopy is performed yearly and after starting a new-strength cholinergic agent (e.g., pilocarpine). Formal visual fields of the same type (e.g.,, Humphrey, Octopus) are rechecked every 6 to 12 months. If loss is severe, or IOP reduction is not thought to be adequate, visual fields may need to be repeated more often, perhaps at 1- to 3-month intervals until the cause of the condition is defined. Once stabilized, repeated field examinations at yearly intervals usually suffice to monitor stability. Dilated retinal examinations should be performed yearly. If glaucomatous damage progresses, check patient compliance with medications before initiating additional therapy.

Patients must be questioned about side effects. They often do not associate eye drops with impotence, weight loss, or light-headedness, for example, and will not necessarily volunteer these and other significant symptoms. Specific questions appropriate for the agents used should be asked.
See the Drug Glossary for additional drug information.

References

Glaucoma Laser Trial Group. The glaucoma laser trial and glaucoma laser trial follow-up study: 7. Results. *Am J Ophthalmol* 1995;120:718–731.

10.2 OCULAR HYPERTENSION

Critical Signs
1. Asymptomatic increased intraocular pressure (IOP), generally >22 mm Hg.
2. Apparently normal anterior-chamber angle anatomy on gonioscopic evaluation.
3. Apparently normal optic nerve and visual field.

Differential Diagnosis
- Primary open-angle glaucoma (See Section 10.1, Primary Open-Angle Glaucoma).
- Secondary open-angle glaucoma [e.g., lens-induced, inflammatory, exfoliative, pigmentary, steroid-induced, developmental anterior-segment abnormalities, angle recession, traumatic (as a result of direct injury, blood, or debris), iridocorneal endothelial (ICE) syndrome, glaucoma

related to increased episcleral venous pressure (e.g., Sturge–Weber syndrome, carotid–cavernous fistulae), glaucoma related to intraocular tumors.]
- Chronic angle-closure glaucoma (CACgl) (Findings of primary open-angle glaucoma [POAG] except peripheral anterior synechiae [PAS] are present on gonioscopy. Patients with CACgl typically have an insidious onset, but may also be the result of acute angle closure glaucoma or uveitis.)

Workup
1. History and complete examination as with POAG. See Section 10.1, Primary Open-Angle Glaucoma.
2. We recommend obtaining baseline stereoscopic disc photos and automated visual-field testing (Humphrey, Octopus) or kinetic visual field (e.g., Goldmann). The purpose is to be able to detect changes over time. Visual fields must be normal. If any abnormalities are present, consider repeated testing in 2 to 4 weeks to exclude the possibility of learning-curve artifacts. If the defects are judged to be real, the diagnosis is not ocular hypertension alone. Some other additional entities are present.

Treatment
1. If there are no suggestive optic nerve or visual-field changes and IOP is <27 mm Hg, no treatment other than close observation is necessary.
2. In general, patients with an IOP >27 mm Hg are treated with medications even if no other optic nerve or visual-field changes are present. However, some clinicians may elect to monitor these patients with close observation. If treatment is elected, a therapeutic trial in one eye, as described for treatment of POAG. See Section 10.1, Primary Open-Angle Glaucoma.

Follow-up
1. For patients not undergoing treatment, close follow-up for the first few years is absolutely necessary. Patients should be monitored every 3 to 6 months for pressure and optic nerve examinations. Formal visual-field testing should be repeated every 6 to 12 months for the first 1 to 2 years to ensure no progression. After the first few years, patients should be checked every 6 to 12 months for IOP, and dilated fundus examination performed. Visual-field testing should be repeated every 1 to 2 years. Five to ten percent of patients with ocular hypertension will progress over 5 years to develop POAG. Because it is not known whether the patient will ever develop symptoms due to glaucoma, therapy must be used with caution.
2. For patients undergoing treatment, follow-up is the same as for patients with POAG. See Section 10.1, Primary Open-Angle Glaucoma.

10.3 Angle-Recession Glaucoma

Symptoms

Usually asymptomatic until the late stages, at which point unilateral visual-field or acuity loss may be noted. A history of trauma to the glaucomatous eye can usually be elicited. Glaucoma due to the angle-recession itself (not from the trauma that caused the angle-recession) usually takes approximately 20 years to develop after the trauma. Typically unilateral.

Critical Signs

Glaucoma [see critical signs of primary open-angle glaucoma (POAG), section 10.1] in an eye with characteristic gonioscopic findings. These findings include an uneven iris insertion with an area of torn or absent iris processes and posteriorly recessed iris to reveal a widened ciliary band. In some cases, these abnormalities and the angle recession extend for 360 degrees. Comparison with corresponding angle structures of the normal contralateral eye help in identification of recessed areas.

Other Signs

The scleral spur may appear abnormally white on gonioscopy because of the recessed angle; other signs of previous trauma may be present (e.g., cataract, iris sphincter tears).

Differential Diagnosis

See Primary Open-Angle Glaucoma, Section 10.1.

Workup

1. History: Trauma? Family history of glaucoma?
2. Complete ocular examination including measurement of intraocular pressure, slit-lamp, gonioscopic, and dilated examination with special attention to the optic nerve.
3. Baseline documentation of the optic discs (e.g., stereoscopic disc photos, red-free photographs, image analysis, or meticulous drawings).
4. Formal visual-field examination, preferably automated (e.g., Humphrey, Octopus) in cases suspicious for, or with definite, glaucoma.

Treatment

Similar to that for POAG (see Section 10.1, Primary Open-Angle Glaucoma), except miotics (e.g., pilocarpine) may be ineffective or even cause increase of intraocular pressure (IOP) as a result of a reduction of uveoscleral outflow. Argon laser trabeculoplasty is rarely effective in this condition.

Follow-up

Patients with angle recession without glaucoma are examined yearly. Those with glaucoma are examined according to the guidelines of Primary Open-Angle Glaucoma, Section 10.1. Follow-up should carefully monitor both eyes, as there is a high incidence of delayed open-angle glaucoma and steroid-responsive IOP in the uninvolved as well as the traumatized eye.

10.4 INFLAMMATORY OPEN-ANGLE GLAUCOMA

Symptoms

Pain, photophobia, decreased vision; symptoms may be minimal.

Critical Signs

Intraocular pressure (IOP) above the patient's baseline, often unilateral with a significant amount of aqueous white blood cells and flare, open angle on gonioscopy. Early in the course, there may not be the characteristic optic nerve and visual-field findings, but they may develop with time. See the critical signs of primary open-angle glaucoma (POAG) (see Section 10.1) for specific optic nerve and visual-field changes.

Other Signs

Miotic pupil, peripheral anterior synechiae (PAS), inflammatory precipitates on the posterior corneal surface or trabecular meshwork, conjunctival injection, ciliary flush.

❖ **Note** *Acute IOP increase is distinguished from chronic IOP increase by the presence of corneal edema, pain, and the perception of halos around light.*

Etiology
- Anterior uveitis
- Intermediate and posterior uveitis
- Panuveitis
- Keratouveitis (Corneal pathology present in addition to uveitis.)
- After trauma or intraocular surgery.

Differential Diagnosis
- Glaucomatocyclitic crisis (Posner–Schlossman syndrome) [Markedly increased IOP (usually 40 to 60 mm Hg), open angle and absence of synechiae on gonioscopy, mild anterior-chamber reaction with few fine keratic precipitates, and minimal-to-no conjunctival injection. Unilateral with recurrent attacks. See Section 10.12, Glaucomatocyclitic Crisis.]

- Acute angle-closure glaucoma (Angle closed in the involved eye and usually narrow in the contralateral eye, mid-dilated pupil that reacts poorly to light, iris bombé, corneal edema, mild anterior-chamber reaction without keratic precipitates. See Section 10.10, Acute Angle-Closure Glaucoma.)
- Pigmentary glaucoma (Acute increase in IOP, often after exercise or pupillary dilatation; pigment cells in the anterior chamber, on the trabecular meshwork, and along the posterior corneal surface. The angle is open, and radial iris transillumination defects are often present. See Section 10.6, Pigmentary Glaucoma.)
- Neovascular glaucoma (Iris and anterior-chamber angle neovascularization are present. See Section 10.13, Neovascular Glaucoma.)
- Fuchs' heterochromic iridocyclitis (Asymmetry of the iris color, mild iritis in the eye with the lighter colored iris, usually unilateral, often associated with cataract, glaucoma, or both. Conjunctival injection and ciliary flush are minimal. See Anterior Uveitis, Section 13.1.)

Workup
1. History: Previous attacks? Systemic disease [e.g., juvenile rheumatoid arthritis, ankylosing spondylitis, sarcoidosis, acquired immunodeficiency syndrome (AIDS)]? Previous corneal disease, especially herpetic keratitis? Recent dilating drops or a systemic anticholinergic agent (suggests angle-closure glaucoma)?
2. Slit-lamp examination: Assess the degree of conjunctival injection and aqueous cell and flare.
3. Measure IOP.
4. Gonioscopy of the anterior-chamber angle: Is the angle open? Synechiae present? Neovascular membrane present?
5. Evaluation of the optic nerve.

Treatment
1. Topical steroid (e.g., prednisolone acetate, 1%) q 1 to 6 h, depending on the severity of the anterior-chamber cellular reaction.

❖ **Note** *Topical steroids are not used, or are used with extreme caution, in patients with an infectious process, particularly a fungal or herpes simplex infection.*

2. Mydriatic/cycloplegic (e.g., cyclopentolate, 2%, scopolamine, 0.25% or atropine, 1% t.i.d.).
3. Topical β-blocker (e.g., timolol or levobunolol, 0.5%, b.i.d.) if not contraindicated (e.g., asthma, chronic obstructive pulmonary disease [COPD]).

One or more of the following pressure-reducing agents can be used in addition to the other treatments, depending on the IOP and the status of the optic nerve:

4. Topical α agonist (e.g., apraclonidine, 0.5%, or brimonidine, 0.2%, b.i.d. to t.i.d.).
5. Carbonic anhydrase inhibitor (e.g., methazolamide, 25 to 50 mg p.o., b.i.d. to t.i.d., or acetazolamide, 250 mg p.o., q.i.d., or 500 mg sequel p.o., b.i.d., or dorzolamide, 2.0%, or brinzolamide, 1%, t.i.d.).
6. Hyperosmotic agent when IOP is acutely increased (e.g., mannitol, 20%, 1 to 2 g/kg i.v. over 45 minutes; a 500-ml bag of mannitol, 20%, contains 100 g of mannitol).
7. Manage the underlying problem.
8. When IOP remains dangerously increased despite maximal medical therapy (a rare event), glaucoma filtering surgery with adjunct antifibrosis therapy may be indicated.

❖ **Note** *Miotics (e.g., pilocarpine) and prostaglandin agonists (e.g., latanoprost) are contraindicated in inflammatory glaucoma.*

Follow-up

Patients are seen every 1 to 7 days at first. The higher the IOP and the greater the amount of glaucomatous damage already present (e.g., the larger the optic nerve cup), the more frequent the follow-up. Steroids are tapered as the inflammation subsides. Antiglaucoma medications are discontinued as IOP returns to normal. Steroid-response glaucoma should always be considered in unresponsive cases (see Section 10.5, Steroid-Response Glaucoma).

10.5 STEROID-RESPONSE GLAUCOMA

Critical Signs

Increased intraocular pressure (IOP) with use of corticosteroids. Usually takes 2 to 4 weeks after starting topical steroids. May be seen after prolonged use of large doses of steroids in other forms (skin creams, nasal inhalers, etc.) or with subconjunctival depot injection of steroids. With systemic (oral or i.v.) steroid use, IOP may increase within a few days. On cessation of steroids, the IOP typically decreases to the level before the use of steroids. The rate of decrease relates to the duration of topical use and the severity of the pressure increase. The IOP increase is due to reduced outflow facility of the pigmented trabecular meshwork, and when this is severe, the IOP may remain increased for months after steroids are stopped. When systemic steroids are stopped, the IOP usually decreases to pretreatment levels within a few days.

Other Signs

Signs of primary open-angle glaucoma (POAG) may develop, including optic-nerve cupping and field loss in an eye with an open anterior-chamber angle.

❖ **Note** *Patients with POAG or a predisposition to develop glaucoma (i.e., family history, diabetes, black race, and high myopia) are more likely to develop a steroid response and subsequent glaucoma.*

Differential Diagnosis

- Inflammatory open-angle glaucoma (Increased IOP as a result of anterior-chamber inflammation. Because steroids are used to treat ocular inflammation, it may be difficult to determine the cause of the increased IOP. See Section 10.4, Inflammatory Open-Angle Glaucoma.)

Workup

1. History: Duration of steroid use? Previous steroid use or an eye problem from steroid use? Glaucoma or family history of glaucoma? Diabetes?
2. Complete ocular examination: Evaluate the degree of ocular inflammation and determine presence of iris or angle neovascularization (by gonioscopy), pigment suggestive of pigment-dispersion syndrome or pseudoexfoliation, blood in Schlemm's canal, peripheral anterior synechiae (PAS), etc. Measure IOP, and inspect the optic nerve.
3. Optic disc photographs are obtained, and formal visual-field (e.g., Humphrey, Octopus) examination performed when the optic nerve appears damaged or when the duration of IOP increase is prolonged or unknown.
4. If using topical steroids, may attempt discontinuation of steroid in one eye to see if IOP improves.

Treatment

Any or all of the following may be necessary to reduce IOP.

1. Discontinue the steroid or reduce the frequency of its administration (steroids should not be discontinued abruptly, but rather tapered).
2. Reduce the concentration or dosage of the steroid (e.g., topical prednisolone acetate, 1%, can be changed to topical prednisolone acetate, 0.12%).

3. Switch from a potent steroid with a greater propensity to produce a steroid response (e.g. prednisolone acetate) to one with a lesser propensity (e.g., fluorometholone or rimexalone).
4. Switch to a topical nonsteroidal antiinflammatory agent (nonsteroidal antiinflammatory drug; e.g., diclofenac, 0.1%).
5. Start antiglaucoma therapy. See Inflammatory Open-Angle Glaucoma, Section 10.4, for medical therapy options.

Notes
1. When a high IOP is found in a patient taking topical steroids for inflammatory glaucoma, it may be difficult to determine the cause of the increased IOP (i.e., whether it is the result of the inflammatory reaction or the steroids). If the inflammation is moderate to severe, we usually increase the steroids initially to reduce the inflammation while initiating antiglaucoma (e.g., topical β-blocker) therapy. If the inflammation subsides, but IOP remains increased, the glaucoma is assumed to be steroid-induced, and the outlined treatment regimen is followed.
2. When a dangerously high IOP that is uncontrollable with medication develops after a depot steroid injection, the steroid may need to be excised.

10.6 PIGMENT DISPERSION/PIGMENTARY GLAUCOMA

Definition
Pigment dispersion refers to a pathologic increase in the trabecular meshwork pigment, associated with characteristic midperipheral spokelike iris transillumination (TI) defects. Normally, the amount of pigment in the trabecular meshwork increases with aging, but does not exceed grade 2. Abnormal pigment dispersion is grade 3 to 4 trabecular pigmentation with increasing radial TI defects or increasing corneal endothelial pigmentation with time.

Symptoms
May be asymptomatic or the patient may experience episodes of blurred vision, eye pain, and colored halos around lights after exercise or pupillary dilatation. More common in young adult, myopic males (age 20 to 45 years). Usually bilateral, but asymmetric.

Critical Signs

Midperipheral, spokelike, iris TI defects corresponding to iridozonular contact; dense homogeneous pigmentation of the trabecular meshwork for 360 degrees (seen on gonioscopy)

Other Signs

A vertical pigment band on the corneal endothelium typically just inferior to the visual axis (Krukenberg's spindle); pigment deposition on the equatorial lens surface, on Schwalbe's line, and sometimes along the iris (which can produce iris heterochromia). The angle often shows a wide ciliary body band and is graded D or E 30 r or q (Spaeth classification, see Appendix 11), with 3+ to 4+ pigmentation of the posterior trabecular meshwork at the 12 o'clock position.

Pigmentary glaucoma is characterized by the pigment-dispersion syndrome plus glaucoma (optic nerve cupping, characteristic glaucomatous visual-field changes, and/or increased intraocular pressure [IOP]). Typically, large fluctuations in IOP can occur, during which pigment cells may be seen floating within the anterior chamber.

Differential Diagnosis

- Exfoliative glaucoma (Trabecular meshwork pigmentation is black, less homogeneous, and more prominent inferiorly. Iris TI defects may be present, but they are near the pupillary margin and are usually less prominent. White flaky material may be seen on the pupillary border and anterior lens capsule. The angle is narrower than in pigment-dispersion syndrome. A Sampolesi's line at 6 o'clock is pathognomonic. See Section 10.7, Exfoliative Glaucoma.)
- Inflammatory open-angle glaucoma (White blood cells and flare in the anterior chamber; typically no iris TI defects. Central corneal endothelial pigment deposits sometimes appear. Absence of grade 3 to 4 pigmentation of trabecular meshwork. Pigmentation is greater inferiorly. The presence of peripheral anterior synechiae (PAS) inferiorly is characteristic. See Section 10.4, Inflammatory Open-Angle Glaucoma.)
- Iris melanoma (Pigmentation of the angular structures accompanied by either a raised, pigmented lesion on the iris or a diffusely darkened iris. No iris TI defects. See Section 8.2, Malignant Melanoma of the Iris.)
- After irradiation (History of radiation, induces atrophy and depigmentation of the ciliary processes, with increased pigment deposition in outflow channels.)

Workup

1. History: Previous episodes of decreased vision or halos?
2. Slit-lamp examination, particularly checking for iris TI defects. Large defects may be seen by shining a small slit beam directly into the pupil

to obtain a red reflex, but scleral TI is required if the defects are not extremely marked. Look for a Krukenberg spindle on the corneal endothelium. Look for pigment on lens equator by angling the slit beam nasally and having the patient look temporally (pathognomonic for pigmentary glaucoma).
3. Measure IOP.
4. Gonioscopy of the anterior-chamber angle.
5. Evaluate the optic nerve.
6. Dilated retinal examination, with special attention to the periphery because of increased lattice degeneration in pigment dispersion.
7. Stereoscopic disc photographs.
8. Visual-field examination, preferably automated (e.g., Humphrey, Octopus).

Treatment
Depends on the IOP, status of the optic nerve, visual-field changes, and extent of the symptoms. Often patients with pigment dispersion without glaucoma or symptoms are observed carefully. A step-wise approach to control IOP is usually taken when mild-to-moderate glaucomatous changes are present. When advanced glaucoma is discovered on initial examination, maximal medical therapy may be instituted initially. (See Primary Open-Angle Glaucoma, Section 10.1.)

1. Miotic agents (a theoretic first line of therapy because they minimize iridozonular contact, which produces pigmentary release into the anterior chamber). However, because most patients are young and myopic, miotic drops, with resultant fluctuation in myopia, may not be practical. Additionally, approximately 14% of patients have lattice retinal degeneration and are thus predisposed to retinal detachment from the use of miotics. In some cases, pilocarpine inserts (e.g., Ocuserts) used once per week or pilocarpine 4% gel qhs are tolerated.

❖ **Note** *Miotics should be used cautiously because of the risk of retinal detachment in myopic patients.*

2. Other antiglaucoma medications may be appropriate (see Primary Open-Angle Glaucoma, Section 10.1).
3. Consider argon laser trabeculoplasty (ALT); these patients usually respond well. Younger patients respond better than older patients, in contrast to primary open-angle glaucoma (POAG).
4. Consider guarded filtration procedure when medical and laser therapy fail. These young myopic patients are at a greater risk of developing hypotony maculopathy.
5. Laser peripheral iridectomy has been recommended to reduce pigment dispersion, but it is still controversial.

Follow-up (as per POAG)

Every 1 to 6 months, with a formal visual-field test every 6 to 12 months, depending on the severity of the symptoms and the glaucoma.

10.7 EXFOLIATIVE GLAUCOMA (PSEUDOEXFOLIATIVE GLAUCOMA)

Definition

A systemic disease in which grayish white material is deposited on the lens, iris, and ciliary epithelium, and trabecular meshwork. Presence of exfoliative material increases the risk of glaucoma sixfold. Currently, the most common identifiable entity causing glaucoma in white persons.

Symptoms

Usually asymptomatic in its early stages.

Critical Signs

White, flaky material on the pupillary margin; anterior lens capsular changes (central zone of exfoliation material, often with rolled-up edges, middle clear zone, and a peripheral cloudy zone); peripupillary iris transillumination defects; and glaucoma (optic nerve cupping, glaucomatous visual-field loss, and/or increased intraocular pressure [IOP]). All of these signs are often asymmetric.

Other Signs

Irregular black pigment deposition on the trabecular meshwork more marked inferiorly than superiorly; pigment anterior to Schwalbe's line (Sampaolesi's line) seen on gonioscopy, especially inferiorly. Bilateral, but often asymmetric. Incidence increases with age. These patients are more prone to having narrow angles.

Differential Diagnosis

- Pigmentary glaucoma [Pigmented trabecular meshwork accompanied by midperipheral iris transillumination defects. There may be a vertical pigment band on the corneal endothelium (Krukenberg spindle or Zentmyer line). Pigment on lens capsule anterior to the equator. See Section 10.6, Pigmentary Glaucoma.]

- Capsular delamination (true exfoliation) [Trauma, exposure to intense heat (e.g., glass blower), or severe uveitis can cause a thin membrane to peel off the anterior lens capsule. Glaucoma uncommon.]
- Primary amyloidosis (Amyloid material can deposit along the pupillary margin or anterior lens capsule. Glaucoma can occur.)

Workup
1. History: Occupational exposure to heat?
2. Slit-lamp examination with IOP measurement; often need to dilate the pupil to see the anterior lens capsular changes. Pupil usually dilates poorly.
3. Gonioscopy of the anterior-chamber angle.
4. Optic nerve evaluation.
5. Stereo disc photographs.
6. Visual-field test, preferably automated (e.g., Humphrey, Octopus).

Treatment
1. For medical therapy, see Primary Open-Angle Glaucoma, Section 10.1.
2. Consider argon laser trabeculoplasty (ALT), which has a higher initial success rate in exfoliative than in primary open-angle glaucoma (POAG).
3. Consider guarded filtration procedure when medical or laser therapy fails.
4. The course of exfoliative glaucoma is usually not linear. Early, the condition may be relatively benign. However, the condition is associated with highly unstable IOP. When control starts to become increasingly difficult, the glaucoma may progress rapidly to cause advanced optic nerve damage, sometimes within a few months.

❖ **Note** *Cataract extraction does not eradicate the glaucoma. Cataract extraction may be complicated by weakened zonular fibers and synechiae between the iris and peripheral anterior lens capsule. The posterior capsule is easily ruptured.*

Follow-up
Every 1 to 3 months as with POAG, but with the awareness that damage in exfoliation syndrome can progress very rapidly, depending on the severity of the glaucoma.

❖ **Note** *Many patients have exfoliation syndrome without glaucoma. These patients are reexamined every 6 to 12 months because they are at risk for glaucoma, but they are not treated unless glaucoma develops.*

10.8 PHACOLYTIC GLAUCOMA

Definition
Leakage of lens material from a cataract through an intact lens capsule leads to trabecular meshwork outflow obstruction.

Symptoms
Unilateral pain, decreased vision, tearing, photophobia.

Critical Signs
Markedly increased intraocular pressure (IOP), accompanied by iridescent particles and white material within the anterior chamber or on the anterior surface of the lens capsule. A hypermature (liquefied) or mature cataract is typical.

Other Signs
Corneal edema, anterior-chamber cells and significant flare, pseudohypopyon, and severe conjunctival injection. Gonioscopy reveals an open anterior-chamber angle. Clumps of macrophages may be seen in inferior angle.

Differential Diagnosis
All of the following can produce an acute increase in IOP to high levels, but none displays iridescent particles and white material in the anterior chamber.

- Inflammatory glaucoma (Acute increased IOP as a result of severe anterior uveitis. See Section 10.4, Inflammatory Open-Angle Glaucoma.)
- Glaucomatocyclitic crisis (Recurrent idiopathic attacks of increased IOP with an open anterior-chamber angle and mild iritis. See Section 10.12, Glaucomatocyclitic Crisis.)
- Acute angle-closure glaucoma (Increased IOP as a result of sudden closure of the anterior-chamber angle, confirmed by gonioscopy. See Section 10.10, Acute Angle-Closure Glaucoma.)
- Lens-particle glaucoma ("Fluffed-up" lens material is seen in the anterior chamber; a history of traumatic lens damage or cataract extraction in the involved eye is characteristic. See Section 10.9, Lens-Particle Glaucoma.)
- Endophthalmitis (History of recent surgery or trauma, pain can be severe. See Section 13.10, Postoperative Endophthalmitis.)

- Glaucoma secondary to intraocular tumor (Unilateral cataract.)
- Others (e.g., traumatic glaucoma, ghost cell glaucoma, phacomorphic glaucoma, neovascular glaucoma.)

Workup

1. History: Recent trauma or ocular surgery? Recurrent episodes? Uveitis in the past?
2. Slit-lamp examination: Look for iridescent or white particles as well as cells and flare within the anterior chamber. Evaluate for cataract and increased IOP producing corneal edema.
3. Gonioscopy of the anterior-chamber angles of both eyes: Topical glycerin may be placed on the cornea after topical anesthesia to clear it temporarily if it is edematous.
4. Retinal and optic-disc examination if possible. Otherwise, B-scan ultrasound before cataract extraction to rule out an intraocular tumor or retinal detachment.
5. If the diagnosis is in doubt, a paracentesis can be performed to detect macrophages bloated with lens material on microscopic examination.

Treatment

The immediate goal of therapy is to reduce the IOP and to reduce the inflammation. The cataract should be removed promptly (within several days).

1. Topical β-blocker (e.g., levobunolol or timolol, 0.25% to 0.5%, in one dose initially, and then b.i.d.), α-agonist (e.g., brimonidine, 0.2%, b.i.d. to t.i.d., apraclonidine, 0.5%, t.i.d.), and/or topical carbonic anhydrase inhibitor (e.g. dorzolamide, 2%, or brinzolamide, 1% t.i.d.).
2. Carbonic anhydrase inhibitor (e.g., acetazolamide, 2 250-mg tablets p.o. in one dose, then 250 mg p.o., q.i.d.). Benefit of maintaining topical carbonic anhydrase inhibitor in addition to a systemic agent is controversial.
3. Topical cycloplegic (e.g., scopolamine, 0.25%, t.i.d.).
4. Topical steroid (e.g., prednisolone acetate, 1% q 15 min for four doses, then q 1 h).
5. Hyperosmotic agent if necessary and no contraindications are present (e.g., mannitol, 1 to 2 g/kg i.v. over 45 minutes; a 500-ml bag of mannitol 20% contains 100 g of mannitol).
6. The IOP usually does not respond adequately to medical therapy. Although it is preferable to reduce IOP before cataract extraction, adequate IOP control may not be possible. Cataract removal is generally performed within 24 to 36 hours. If the IOP cannot be controlled medically, the patient may need hospitalization and urgent cataract extrac-

tion. Glaucoma surgery is usually not necessary at the same time as cataract surgery.

Follow-up

If patients are not hospitalized, they should be reexamined the day after surgery. Patients are usually hospitalized after their cataract surgery so that their IOP can be monitored over the ensuing 24 hours. If the IOP returns to normal after the procedure, the patient should be rechecked within 1 week.

10.9 LENS-PARTICLE GLAUCOMA

Definition

Lens material, liberated by trauma or surgery, which obstructs aqueous outflow channels.

Symptoms

Pain, blurred vision, red eye, tearing, photophobia. History of recent ocular trauma or cataract surgery.

Critical Signs

White, fluffy pieces of lens cortical material in the anterior chamber, combined with increased intraocular pressure (IOP). A break in the lens capsule may be observed in posttraumatic cases.

Other Signs

Anterior-chamber cell and flare, conjunctival injection, or corneal edema. The anterior-chamber angle is open on gonioscopy.

Differential Diagnosis

See Phacolytic Glaucoma, Section 10.8. In phacolytic glaucoma, the cataractous lens has not been extracted or traumatized.

- Infectious endophthalmitis (Unless lens cortical material can be unequivocally identified in the anterior chamber, and there is nothing atypical about the presentation, endophthalmitis must be excluded. See Sections 13.10, Postoperative Endophthalmitis, and 13.11, Traumatic Endophthalmitis.)
- Phacoanaphylactic endophthalmitis (Follows trauma or intraocular surgery, producing anterior-chamber inflammation and sometimes a high IOP. The inflammation is often granulomatous, and fluffy lens material is not present in the anterior chamber.)

- Phacomorphic glaucoma (A cataractous lens becomes intumescent and physically closes the anterior chamber angle.)

Workup

1. History: Recent trauma or ocular surgery?
2. Slit-lamp examination: Search the anterior chamber for lens cortical material and measure the IOP.
3. Gonioscopy of the anterior-chamber angle.
4. Optic nerve evaluation: The degree of optic nerve cupping helps determine how long the increased IOP can be tolerated.

Treatment

1. Topical β-blocker (e.g., levobunolol or timolol, 0.25% to 0.5%, b.i.d.), topical α-agonist (e.g., brimonidine, 0.2%, b.i.d. to t.i.d., or apraclonidine, 0.5%, t.i.d.), topical carbonic anhydrase inhibitor (e.g., dorzolamide, 2%, or brinzolamide, 1%, b.i.d. to t.i.d.).
2. Carbonic anhydrase inhibitor (e.g., methazolamide, 25 to 50 mg p.o., b.i.d. to t.i.d., or acetazolamide, 250 mg p.o., q.i.d., or 500 mg sequel p.o., b.i.d.). Benefit of maintaining topical carbonic anhydrase inhibitor in addition to a systemic agent is controversial.
3. Topical cycloplegic (e.g., scopolamine, 0.25%, t.i.d.).
4. Topical steroid (e.g., prednisolone acetate, 1%, q.i.d.).
   - If IOP is markedly increased (e.g., >45 mm Hg in a previously healthy eye or less in a patient with previous optic nerve damage), a hyperosmotic agent is added to acutely reduce the pressure (e.g., mannitol, 1 to 2 g/kg i.v. over 45 minutes; a 500-ml bag of mannitol 20% contains 100 g of mannitol).
   - If medical therapy fails to control the IOP, the residual lens material must be removed surgically.

Follow-up

Depending on the IOP and the health of the optic nerve, patients are reexamined in 1 to 7 days.

10.10 ACUTE ANGLE-CLOSURE GLAUCOMA

Symptoms

Pain, blurred vision, colored halos around lights, frontal headache, nausea and vomiting.

Critical Signs

Closed angle in the involved eye, acutely increased intraocular pressure (IOP), corneal microcystic edema. Shallow anterior chamber in both eyes.

Other Signs

Conjunctival injection; fixed, mid-dilated pupil.

Etiology

- Pupillary block [Anatomically predisposed in eyes with narrow anterior-chamber angle recess, anterior iris insertion of the iris root, or both; common in Asians, Eskimos, and hyperopes. May be precipitated by topical mydriatics or rarely miotics, systemic anticholinergics (e.g., antihistamines or antipsychotics), accommodation (e.g., reading), or dim illumination (e.g., movie theater). The angle is narrow or occludable in the contralateral eye.]
- Angle crowding as a result of an abnormal iris configuration (e.g., high peripheral iris roll or plateau iris syndrome angle closure occurs despite a patent peripheral iridectomy. See Section 10.11, Plateau Iris)

❖ **Note** *A secondary mechanical cause of angle-closure glaucoma should be suspected when the anterior-chamber angles are asymmetric, i.e., one angle is narrow but the other is deep.*

Differential Diagnosis

Other causes of acute IOP increase, but with an open angle.

- Glaucomatocyclitic crisis (Posner–Schlossman syndrome) (Recurrent IOP spikes in one eye, mild cell and flare with or without fine keratic precipitates; the eye is generally not inflamed and not painful. See Section 10.12, Glaucomatocyclitic Crisis.)
- Inflammatory open-angle glaucoma (Moderate to severe anterior-chamber reaction. See Section 10.4, Inflammatory Open-Angle Glaucoma.)
- Retrobulbar hemorrhage or inflammation (Proptosis and restriction of ocular motility. See Section 3.11, Traumatic Retrobulbar Hemorrhage.)
- Traumatic (hemolytic) glaucoma (History of trauma, red blood cells in the anterior chamber. See Section 3.7, Hyphema and Microhyphema.)
- Pigmentary glaucoma (Deep anterior chamber. Pigment cells floating in the anterior chamber, often after exercise or pupillary dilatation; radial iris TI defects. See Section 10.6, Pigmentary Glaucoma.)

Other causes of acute IOP increase, with closed angle.

- Secondary angle-closure glaucomas
  1. Neovascular or inflammatory membrane pulling the angle closed (Abnormal misdirected blood vessels along the pupillary margin,

the trabecular meshwork, or both are seen. See Section 10.13, Neo-vascular Glaucoma)
2. Mechanical closure of the angle secondary to anterior displacement of the lens–iris diaphragm:
   a. Lens-induced [Pupillary block as a result of a large lens (phaco-morphic).]
   b. Choroidal detachment (serous or hemorrhagic) (Generally follows surgery; diagnose by indirect ophthalmoscopy, B-scan ultrasonography or both.)
   c. Choroidal swelling after extensive retinal laser surgery or after placement of a tight encircling band in retinal-detachment surgery
   d. Posterior-segment tumor (e.g., choroidal or ciliary body melanoma. See Section 8.3, Malignant Melanoma of the Choroid.)
   e. Aqueous misdirection syndrome (See Section 10.16, Malignant Glaucoma)
3. Peripheral anterior synechiae (PAS) (IOP increase is not acute; caused by uveitis, laser trabeculoplasty, iridocorneal endothelial syndrome, others.)

Workup
1. History: Family history? Retinal problem? Recent laser treatment or surgery? Medications?
2. Slit-lamp examination: Look for keratic precipitates, posterior synechiae, iris neovascularization, a swollen lens, anterior-chamber cells and flare or iridescent particles, and a shallow anterior chamber. Glaukomflecken (small anterior subcapsular lens opacities) indicate prior attacks.
3. Measure IOP.
4. Gonioscopy of both anterior-chamber angles: Corneal edema can usually be cleared by using topical hyperosmolar agents (e.g., glycerin). Compression gonioscopy may help determine if the trabecular blockage is reversible and may break an acute attack. Gonioscopy of the involved eye after IOP is reduced is essential in determining whether the angle has opened and whether neovascularization is present.
5. Careful examination of the fundus looking for signs of central retinal vein occlusion, hemorrhage, and optic nerve cupping. If cupping is pronounced, treatment is more urgent.

Treatment
Depends on severity and duration of attack. Severe, permanent damage may occur within several hours. If visual acuity is hand movements or worse, IOP reduction is truly urgent, and medications should include all topical glaucoma medications not contraindicated, intravenous acetazolamide, and intravenous osmotics. If IOP is <50, and vision loss is less

severe, parenterel/oral agents are usually not needed. See Neovascular Glaucoma, Section 10.13, Postoperative Glaucoma, Section 10.15, and Malignant Glaucoma (Aqueous Misdirection), Section 10.16, for specific treatment of these conditions.

1. Topical β-blocker (e.g., levobunolol or timolol, 0.5%) in one dose (use with caution with concurrent asthma or chronic obstructive pulmonary disease [COPD]).
2. Topical steroid (e.g., prednisolone acetate, 1%) q 15 to 30 min for four doses, then hourly.
3. Topical apraclonidine, 1.0%, or brimonidine, 0.2%, for one dose.
4. Carbonic anhydrase inhibitor (e.g., acetazolamide, 250 to 500 mg i.v., or two 250-mg tablets p.o., in one dose) if IOP decrease is considered urgent.
5. When acute angle-closure glaucoma is the result of
   a. Phakic pupillary block or angle crowding: Pilocarpine, 1% to 2%, q 15 min for 2 doses, and pilocarpine, 0.5%, in the contralateral eye for one dose.
   b. Aphakic or pseudophakic pupillary block or mechanical closure of the angle: Do not use pilocarpine. A mydriatic and cycloplegic agent (e.g., cyclopentolate, 2%, and phenylephrine, 2.5%, q 15 min for four doses) is used when laser or surgery is not initially used because of corneal edema, inflammation, or both.
6. In cases of phacomorphic glaucoma, the lens should be removed as soon as the eye is quieted with steroids and the IOP maximally controlled.
7. Address systemic problems: pain, vomiting, etc.
   Recheck the IOP and visual acuity in 1 hour.
   • If IOP does not decrease and vision does not improve, repeat topical medications and give i.v. mannitol, 1 to 2 g/kg i.v. over 45 minutes (a 500-ml bag of mannitol 20% contains 100 g of mannitol). Oral isosorbide is usually not tolerated and should be used only if patient is not nauseated.
   • If IOP does not decrease after two courses of maximal medical therapy, a laser peripheral iridectomy (PI) should be considered, if there is an adequate view of the iris.
   • If IOP still does not decrease after the second round of medication and a second attempt at a laser PI, then a surgical PI is needed and, in some cases, a guarded filtration procedure.
   • If the IOP decreases significantly and the angle is determined to be open by gonioscopy, definitive treatment is performed once the cornea is clear and the anterior chamber is quiet (see the following). In most cases, this requires waiting 1 to 5 days or more for the inflammation to resolve. The attack cannot be considered broken

unless the IOP decreases lower than that of the fellow eye. Patients are discharged on the following medications and followed up daily.

Prednisolone acetate, 1%, 4 to 8 times per day to quiet the eye. This should not be continued longer than necessary.

Acetazolamide, 500 mg sequel p.o., b.i.d.

Topical β-blocker (e.g., levobunolol or timolol, 0.5%, b.i.d.)

Pilocarpine, 1% to 2%, q.i.d. (in cases of phakic pupillary block or angle crowding).

❖ **Note** *Some believe that once the attack is broken, only pilocarpine and prednisolone acetate are sufficient if normal outflow is reestablished (i.e., the angle is open again).*

8. If IOP is still increased or the angle is still closed, surgery is needed.
9. If indicated by gonioscopy, PI to the fellow eye should be performed within 1 or 2 weeks.

Definitive Treatment

A. Pupillary block (all forms) or angle crowding
   1. Laser PI (YAG PI) to the involved eye.
   2. Laser PI to the contralateral eye if it is occludable. If corneal edema prohibits laser in the involved eye at the time of initial treatment, the contralateral eye can be lasered first. An untreated fellow eye has a 40% to 80% chance of developing acute angle-closure in 5 to 10 years.
   3. Surgical iridectomy if a laser PI is not possible.
   4. Consider a guarded filtration procedure (trabeculectomy), with a tightly sutured scleral flap, when the IOP remains high despite an iridectomy and maximal medical treatment, especially in presence of significant optic nerve cupping.

B. Secondary or mechanical angle closure
   1. Consider argon laser gonioplasty to open the angle, particularly in cases that are the result of extensive retinal laser surgery, a tight encircling band from retinal-detachment surgery, or nanophthalmos.
   2. Consider goniosynechialysis for chronic angle closure less than 6 months in duration.
   3. Treat the underlying problem. Systemic steroids may be required to treat serous choroidal detachments secondary to AIDS or other choroidal inflammation.

Follow-up

After definitive treatment of one or both eyes, patients are reevaluated in weeks to months initially, and then less frequently. Visual fields (e.g.,

Humphrey, Octopus) and stereo disc photographs are obtained for baseline purposes.

❖ **Notes**
1. *The patient's cardiovascular status and electrolyte balance must be considered when contemplating osmotic agents, carbonic anhydrase inhibitors, and β-blockers.*
2. *When mechanical angle-closure glaucoma is suspected, a B-scan ultrasound or ultrasound biomicroscopy may be helpful in diagnosis.*
3. *If a repeated attack of angle closure occurs despite a patent iridectomy, a plateau iris syndrome may be present (see Section 10.11, Plateau Iris Syndrome).*
4. *The appearance of the cornea usually worsens when the IOP decreases, with increasing thickness and folds.*
5. *Vision needs to be monitored carefully. Worsening sight is a sign of increasing urgency of pressure reduction.*
6. *The patient should be instructed to alert relatives about the occurrence of angle-closure attacks. Primary angle-closure glaucoma is a highly inheritable condition and 1/3 to 1/2 of the first-degree relatives will be expected to have occludable anterior-chamber angles.*
7. *Angle-closure glaucoma may be seen without an increased IOP. The diagnosis should be suspected in a patient who had pain and reduced acuity and is noted to have*
   a. *An edematous, thickened cornea in one eye*
   b. *Normal or markedly asymmetric pressure in both eyes*
   c. *Shallow anterior chambers in both eyes*
   d. *Occludable anterior-chamber angle in the fellow eye (gonioscopy may not be helpful in an eye with corneal haziness due to stromal thickening).*

10.11 PLATEAU IRIS

Symptoms
Usually asymptomatic, unless acute angle-closure glaucoma develops (decreased vision, throbbing pain, nausea, and vomiting; see Section 10.10, Acute Angle-Closure Glaucoma).

Critical Signs
Flat iris plane and normal anterior-chamber depth centrally, convex peripheral iris with an anterior iris apposition seen on gonioscopy. With acute

angle-closure associated with a plateau iris, the axial anterior-chamber depth may be normal, but the peripheral iris bunches up to occlude the angle (see Section 10.10, Acute Angle-Closure Glaucoma).

Types

Plateau iris configuration   Because of the anatomic configuration of the angle, these patients may develop acute angle-closure glaucoma from only a mild degree of pupillary block. These angle-closure attacks may be cured by peripheral iridectomy (PI), because it relieves the pupillary block.

Plateau iris syndrome   The peripheral iris can bunch up in the anterior-chamber angle and obstruct aqueous outflow without any element of pupillary block. The diagnosis can be by gonioscopy or ultrasound biomicroscopy when angle-closure glaucoma occurs despite a patent PI.

Differential Diagnosis

- Acute angle-closure glaucoma associated with pupillary block (The central anterior-chamber depth is decreased, and the entire iris has a convex appearance. See Section 10.10, Acute Angle-Closure Glaucoma.)
- Aqueous misdirection syndrome (Marked diffuse shallowing of the anterior chamber, often after cataract extraction or glaucoma surgery. See Section 10.16, Malignant Glaucoma.)
- For other disorders, see Acute Angle-Closure Glaucoma, Section 10.10.

Workup

1. Slit-lamp examination: Specifically check for the presence of a patent PI and the critical signs listed previously.
2. Measure intraocular pressure (IOP).
3. Gonioscopy of both anterior-chamber angles.
4. Undilated optic nerve evaluation.
5. Can be confirmed with ultrasound biomicroscopy.

❖ **Note** *If dilatation must be performed in a patient suspected of having a plateau iris, then warn the patient that this may provoke an acute angle-closure attack. May use phenylephrine (Neo-Synephrine), 2.5%, to dilate if dapiprazole, 0.5%, is available for reversal. If an anticholinergic agent is needed to dilate, then use only tropicamide, 0.5%. Recheck the IOP every few hours until the pupil returns to normal size. Have the patient notify you immediately if symptoms of acute angle-closure develop.*

Treatment

1. Treat acute angle-closure glaucoma medically if present (see Section 10.10, Acute Angle-Closure Glaucoma).

2. A laser PI is performed within 1 to 3 days if the angle-closure attack can be broken medically. If the attack cannot be controlled, a laser or surgical PI may need to be done as an emergency.
3. One week after the laser PI, the eye should be dilated with a weak mydriatic (e.g., tropicamide, 0.5%). If the IOP increases, plateau iris syndrome is diagnosed and should be treated with a weak miotic (e.g., pilocarpine, 0.5% to 1%, 3 to 4 times per day, long term) or with an iridoplasty.
4. If angle-closure glaucoma develops spontaneously despite a patent PI, then the plateau iris syndrome exists and should be treated as described previously.
5. Consider a laser iridoplasty to break an acute attack not responsive to medical treatment and PI.
6. If the patient's IOP does respond to a laser PI (i.e., with plateau iris configuration, not syndrome by definition), then a prophylactic laser PI may be indicated in the contralateral eye within 1 to 2 weeks.

Follow-up
1. Subsequent to a PI for an attack of acute angle-closure glaucoma, patients are reevaluated in 1 week, 1 month, and 3 months, and then yearly if no problems have developed. Examination should include IOP and gonioscopy at each visit; look for a narrowing angle recess or increasing angle closure. The PI should be examined for patency.
2. Patients suspected of having a plateau iris configuration who have never had an acute angle-closure attack are examined every 6 months. At each visit, IOP is measured and gonioscopy is performed; look for peripheral anterior synechiae formation and further narrowing of the anterior-chamber angle. Dilation should cautiously be performed periodically (about every 2 years) to assure that the PI remains adequate to prevent angle closure.

10.12 GLAUCOMATOCYCLITIC CRISIS
(Posner–Schlossman Syndrome)

Symptoms
Mild pain, decreased vision, observation of rainbows around lights. Often, a history of similar episodes is obtained. Usually unilateral in young to middle-aged patients.

Critical Signs
Markedly increased intraocular pressure (IOP) (usually 40 to 60 mm Hg), open angle without synechiae on gonioscopy, minimal conjunctival injection (white eye), very mild anterior-chamber reaction (few aqueous cells and little flare).

Other Signs
Corneal epithelial edema, ciliary flush, pupillary constriction, iris hypochromia, few fine keratic precipitates on the corneal endothelium or trabecular meshwork.

Differential Diagnosis
- Inflammatory open-angle glaucoma (Significant amount of aqueous cells and flare, conjunctival injection, and pain. Synechiae may be present. May be bilateral. See Section 10.4, Inflammatory Open-Angle Glaucoma.)
- Acute angle-closure glaucoma (Closed angle in the involved eye and usually a narrow angle in the contralateral eye; painful, conjunctival injection; corneal edema; patient may have history of recent dilatation with drops or use of systemic anticholinergic medication. See Section 10.10, Acute Angle-Closure Glaucoma.)
- Pigmentary glaucoma [Acute increase in IOP, often after exercise or pupillary dilatation, pigment cells in the anterior chamber, open angle, radial iris transillumination defects, vertical base down triangle of pigmented cells on the posterior corneal surface (Krukenberg's spindle), and pigment in the trabecular meshwork seen on gonioscopy. See Section 10.6, Pigmentary Glaucoma.]
- Neovascular glaucoma (Iris and/or angle neovascularization is present. See Section 10.13, Neovascular Glaucoma.)
- Fuchs' heterochromic iridocyclitis (Asymmetry of iris color, mild iritis in the eye with the lighter-colored iris, usually unilateral, often associated with cataract, glaucoma, or both. The increase in IOP is rarely as acute. See Anterior Uveitis, Section 13.1.)
- Others (e.g., herpes simplex and herpes zoster keratouveitis.)

Workup
1. History: Recent dilating drops, systemic anticholinergic agents, or exercise? Previous attacks? Corneal or systemic disease?
2. Slit-lamp examination: Assess the degree of conjunctival injection and aqueous cell and flare. Measure IOP.
3. Gonioscopy of the anterior-chamber angle: Angle open? Synechiae, neovascular membrane, or keratic precipitates present?
4. Optic nerve evaluation.
5. Stereo optic disc photos and formal visual-field testing (e.g., Humphrey or Octopus).
6. Retinal examination: Vasculitis? Snowbanking of pars planitis?

Treatment
1. Topical β-blocker (e.g., timolol or levobunolol, 0.5%, b.i.d.), topical α-agonist (e.g., brimonidine, 0.2%, b.i.d. to t.i.d., or apraclonidine, 0.5%,

t.i.d.), topical carbonic anhydrase inhibitor (e.g., dorzolamide, 2%, or brinzolamide, 1%, b.i.d. to t.i.d.).
2. Topical steroid (e.g., prednisolone acetate, 1%, q.i.d.).
3. Substitute a systemic carbonic anhydrase inhibitor (e.g., methazolamide, 25 to 50 mg p.o., b.i.d. to t.i.d., or acetazolamide, 500 mg sequel p.o., b.i.d.) for a topical carbonic anhydrase inhibitor if IOP is significantly increased.
4. Hyperosmotic agents (e.g., mannitol, 20%, 1 to 2 g/kg i.v. over 45 minutes) are used acutely when the IOP is determined to be dangerously high for the involved optic nerve. A 500-ml bag of mannitol, 20%, contains 100 g of mannitol.
5. Consider a cycloplegic agent (e.g., cyclopentolate, 1%, t.i.d.) if the patient is symptomatic.

Follow-up
Patients are seen every few days at first, and then weekly until the episode resolves. Attacks usually subside within a few hours to a few weeks. Medical or surgical therapy may be required, depending on the baseline level of IOP between attacks. If the IOP decreases to levels that are not associated with disc or visual-field damage, then no treatment is necessary. Steroids are tapered rapidly if they are used for 1 week or less, and slowly if they are used for longer. Note that both eyes are at risk of developing chronic open-angle glaucoma.

10.13 NEOVASCULAR GLAUCOMA

Definition
Glaucoma caused by a fibrovascular membrane, overgrowing the anterior-chamber angle structures. Initially, the angle may appear open, but blocked by the membrane. The fibrovascular membrane eventually contracts, causing peripheral anterior synechiae (PAS) formation and secondary angle-closure glaucoma. Rarely, may have neovascularization of the angle without neovascularization of the iris at the pupillary margin. The etiology of the fibrovascular membrane is ischemia from a variety of causes.

Symptoms
May be asymptomatic or patient may complain of pain, red eye, photophobia, and decreased vision.

Critical Signs

Stage 1 Abnormal, nonradial, misdirected blood vessels along the pupillary margin, the trabecular meshwork, or both. No signs of glaucoma.

Stage 2 Stage 1 plus increased intraocular pressure (IOP) (open-angle neovascular glaucoma).

Stage 3 Partial or complete angle-closure glaucoma caused by a fibrovascular membrane covering the trabecular meshwork. PAS and florid iris neovascularization are common.

Other Signs

Mild anterior-chamber cells and flare, conjunctival injection, corneal edema when an acute increase in IOP occurs, hyphema, eversion of the pupillary margin allowing visualization of the iris pigment epithelium (ectropion uvea), optic nerve cupping, visual-field loss.

Etiology

- Diabetic retinopathy
- Central retinal vein occlusion, particularly the ischemic type
- Central retinal artery occlusion
- Ocular ischemic syndrome (carotid occlusive disease)
- Others (Branch retinal vein occlusion, chronic uveitis, chronic retinal detachment, intraocular tumors, trauma, other ocular vascular disorders, and radiation therapy, chronic long-standing increased IOP.)

Differential Diagnosis

- Inflammatory glaucoma (Increased IOP, abundant anterior-chamber cells and marked flare, and dilated normal iris blood vessels may be seen. No neovascular vessels. Normal iris blood vessels run radially, have a sense of direction, and are usually symmetrical 360 degrees around the pupillary margin. The angle is open. See Section 10.4, Inflammatory Open-Angle Glaucoma.)
- Primary acute angle-closure glaucoma (No signs of new iris blood vessels. Usually a shallow anterior chamber with a closed or narrow angle in both eyes. See Section 10.10, Acute Angle-Closure Glaucoma.)

Workup

1. History: Determine the underlying etiology.
2. Complete ocular examination, including IOP measurement and gonioscopic evaluation of the anterior-chamber angle to determine what degree of the angle is closed, if any. A dilated retinal evaluation is essential in determining the cause of the iris neovascularization.
3. Fluorescein angiogram as needed to identify an underlying retinal abnormality or in preparation for retinal laser treatment (panretinal photocoagulation).

4. Carotid noninvasive studies to rule out carotid disease when no retinal pathology can be found accountable for the neovascularization.

5. B-scan ultrasound is indicated when the retina cannot be visualized to rule out an intraocular tumor or retinal detachment.

Treatment

1. Reduce inflammation and pain: Topical steroid (e.g., prednisolone acetate, 1%, q 1 to 6 h) and a cycloplegic (e.g., atropine, 1%, t.i.d.). Atropine may reduce IOP when the angle is closed by increasing uveoscleral outflow.

2. Reduce the IOP if it is increased. Any or all of the following medications are used:

    a. Topical β-blocker (e.g., levobunolol or timolol, 0.5%, b.i.d.)

    b. Topical α agonists (e.g., apraclonidine, 0.5%, or brimonidine, 0.2%, b.i.d. to t.i.d.)

    c. Systemic or topical carbonic anhydrase inhibitor (e.g., methazolamide, 25 to 50 mg p.o., 2 to 3 times per day, or acetazolamide, 500 mg p.o., b.i.d., dorzolamide, 2%, or brinzolamide, 1%, b.i.d. to t.i.d.).

❖ **Note** *Miotics (e.g., pilocarpine) are contraindicated because of the effects on the blood–aqueous barrier. Epinephrine compounds (e.g., dipivefrin) are generally ineffective and are not often used.*

3. If retinal ischemia is thought to be responsible for the iris neovascularization, then treat with panretinal photocoagulation (PRP). If the retina cannot be visualized, then treat with cryoablation. These procedures are used if the angle is open or if filtration surgery (regardless of whether the angle is open or closed) is going to be performed.

4. Goniophotocoagulation (laser photocoagulation of new vessels in the angle) may be used in addition to the previously described treatment in patients with significant angle neovascularization, but minimal-to-no angle closure. This procedure may reduce the risk of angle closure during the interval required for the PRP to take effect (often several weeks), but this is not well established.

5. Glaucoma filtration surgery may be performed when the neovascularization is inactive and the IOP cannot be controlled with medical therapy. Tube-shunt procedures or YAG laser cyclophotocoagulation may be helpful to control IOP in some patients with active neovascularization. It is often best to perform panretinal photocoagulation before attempting filtration surgery.

In eyes without useful vision, topical steroids and cycloplegics may be adequate therapy. The pain in neovascular glaucoma is not primarily a function of the IOP, and reducing IOP may not be needed if the goal is only pain control. β-Blockers, retrobulbar alcohol injection, or enucleation may be required to reduce pain (see The Blind, Painful Eye, Section 15.9).

6. Treat the underlying disorder; see the appropriate section.

Follow-up
The presence of iris neovascularization, especially when accompanied by high IOP, requires urgent therapeutic intervention, usually within 1 to 2 days. Angle closure can proceed relatively rapidly (within days to weeks).

❖ **Note** *Iris neovascularization without glaucoma is managed in a similar manner as to that described; however, there is no need for antiglaucomatous therapy unless IOP increases.*

10.14 IRIDOCORNEAL ENDOTHELIAL (ICE) SYNDROME

Definition
Three overlapping syndromes—essential iris atrophy, Chandler's, and iris nevus (Cogan–Reese)—that share an abnormal corneal endothelial cell layer, which can grow across the anterior chamber angle. Secondary angle closure can result from contraction of this tissue.

Symptoms
Asymptomatic in its early stages. Later, the patient notes an irregular iris appearance, blurred vision, or pain in one eye. Patients are typically young to middle-aged adults. Familial cases are extremely rare.

Critical Signs
Corneal endothelial changes (fine, hammered-metal appearance) localized, irregular peripheral anterior synechiae (PAS) that often extend beyond Schwalbe's line, deep central anterior chamber, unilaterality, and iris alterations as follows:

Essential iris atrophy   Marked iris thinning often leading to iris holes and displacement and distortion of the pupil.
Chandler's syndrome   Mild iris thinning and pupil distortion. The corneal changes are most marked in this variant. Patients often have corneal edema even at normal intraocular pressure (IOP).
Cogan–Reese syndrome   Pigmented nodules on the iris surface, variable iris atrophy. The iris changes may also be seen in Chandler's and essential iris atrophy.

Other Signs

Corneal edema, elevated IOP, optic nerve cupping, or visual-field loss. Typically unilateral, although mild corneal changes consistent with this syndrome are sometimes found in the contralateral eye. However, the glaucoma is nearly always unilateral.

Differential Diagnosis

- Axenfeld–Rieger syndrome [Prominent, anteriorly displaced Schwalbe's line (posterior embryotoxon), peripheral iris strands extending to Schwalbe's line, iris thinning with atrophic holes, may have dental, craniofacial, and skeletal abnormalities. Bilateral and congenital. See Section 9.11, Developmental Anterior-Segment and Lens Anomalies.]
- Posterior polymorphous dystrophy (Bilateral. Endothelial vesicles or bandlike lesions, occasionally associated with iridocorneal adhesions, corneal edema, and glaucoma. See Section 4.24, Corneal Dystrophies.)
- Fuchs' endothelial dystrophy (Bilateral corneal edema and endothelial guttata. The iris and anterior-chamber angle are normal. See Section 4.25, Fuchs' Endothelial Dystrophy.)
- Iris melanoma (Pigmented iris lesion or lesions noted to enlarge over time. See Section 8.2, Malignant Melanoma of the Iris.)
- Prior uveitis (Pigmented keratic precipitates, posterior synechiae, cataract)

Workup

1. Family history: ICE syndrome is not inherited; Axenfeld–Rieger syndrome and posterior polymorphous dystrophy are often autosomal dominant.
2. Slit-lamp examination: Assess the cornea and iris and measure IOP.
3. Gonioscopy of the anterior-chamber angle.
4. Optic nerve examination.
5. Slit-lamp photos and stereoscopic disc photographs.
6. Visual-field test, preferably automated (e.g., Humphrey, Octopus).
7. Consider obtaining corneal endothelial specular microscopy.

Treatment

No treatment is needed unless glaucoma or corneal edema is present, at which point one or more of the following treatments is used:

1. Antiglaucomatous medications for corneal edema or glaucoma (see Primary Open-Angle Glaucoma, Section 10.1). The IOP may need to be reduced beneath a critical level to rid the cornea of edema. This critical level may become lower as the patient ages.
2. Hypertonic saline solutions (e.g., sodium chloride, 5% drops, q.i.d., and ointment qhs) may help to reduce corneal edema.
3. Consider filtering procedure when medical therapy fails to maintain the IOP low enough to prevent corneal edema or progression of optic nerve

damage. Argon laser trabeculoplasty (ALT) and laser peripheral iridectomy (PI) are ineffective. Tube-shunt procedures may be required for refractory cases, but results with this procedure are poor.

4. Consider a corneal transplant in cases of advanced chronic corneal edema in the presence of good IOP control.

Follow-up

Depends on the level of IOP and state of the nerve. If asymptomatic with healthy optic nerve, may see every 12 months. If glaucoma is present, then every 1 to 3 months, depending on the severity of the glaucoma.

10.15 POSTOPERATIVE GLAUCOMA

Early Postoperative Glaucoma

Intraocular pressure (IOP) tends to start to increase about 1 hour after cataract extraction and generally returns to normal within 1 week. Etiologies include retained viscoelastic, pupillary block, hyphema, pigment dispersion, and generalized inflammation. Most normal eyes can tolerate an IOP <30 mm Hg for this duration. However, eyes with preexisting optic nerve damage require antiglaucoma medications (e.g., levobunolol, 0.5%, b.i.d., timolol, 0.5%, b.i.d., brimonidine, 0.2%, b.i.d. to t.i.d., dorzolamide, 2%, t.i.d., brinzolamide, 1%, t.i.d., or methazolamide, 25 to 50 mg p.o., b.i.d. to t.i.d.) for any significant pressure increase. Most eyes with an IOP >30 mm Hg should likewise be treated. If inflammation is excessive, increase the topical steroid dose to q 30 to 60 min while awake and consider topical nonsteroidal antiinflammatory drug (NSAID) (e.g., diclofenac, q.i.d.; see Inflammatory Open-Angle Glaucoma, Section 10.4).

Pupillary Block

Differential diagnosis of pupillary block

Early postoperative period (within 2 weeks)
- Inflammation secondary to prostaglandin release, blood, fibrin, etc.
- Hyphema
- Failure to filter after filtration surgery due to tight scleral flap, blocked sclerostomy (iris, vitreous, blood, fibrin, etc.)
- Malignant glaucoma (aqueous misdirection)
- Suprachoroidal hemorrhage
- Anterior chamber lens with vitreous loss: vitreous plugs the pupil if iridectomy is not performed

Late postoperative period (after 2 weeks)
- Pupillary block glaucoma
- Failing bleb (after filtering surgery)
- Suprachoroidal hemorrhage
- Uveitis, glaucoma, hyphema syndrome
- Malignant glaucoma (when cycloplegics are stopped)
- Steroid-induced glaucoma

Signs

Increased IOP, shallow or partially flat anterior chamber, absence of a patent peripheral iridectomy (PI). Iris typically has marked anterior bowing (iris bombé). Evidence of iris adhesions to lens or intraocular lens (IOL).

Treatment of Pupillary Block

A. If the cornea is clear and the eye is not significantly inflamed, then a PI is performed, usually by YAG laser. Because the PI tends to close, it is often necessary to perform two or more iridectomies. They need to be larger than in the eye with primary angle closure glaucoma.

B. If the cornea is hazy, the eye is inflamed, or a PI cannot be performed immediately, then:

    1. Mydriatic agent (e.g., cyclopentolate, 2%, and phenylephrine, 2.5%, q 15 min for four doses).

    2. Carbonic anhydrase inhibitor (e.g., acetazolamide, two 250-mg tablets p.o. or 500 mg i.v.).

    3. Topical β-blocker (e.g., timolol, 0.5%), one dose.

    4. Topical α-agonist (e.g., brimonidine, 0.2%, or apraclonidine, 1.0%), one dose.

    5. Topical steroid (e.g., prednisolone acetate, 1%, q 15 to 30 min for four doses). If the IOP is too high, some clinicians recommend dosing the steroid q 30 to 60 min while awake for 1 day with the return the next day.

    6. PI, preferably YAG laser, as soon as available and when the eye is less inflamed. If the cornea is edematous and cloudy, topical glycerin may be used to clear it temporarily.

    7. A surgical PI may be needed.

    8. If angle has become closed, a guarded filtration procedure or tube shunt may be needed.

Uveitis, Glaucoma, Hyphema (UGH) Syndrome

Signs

Anterior-chamber cells and flare and increased IOP, often with a hyphema. Usually secondary to irritation from a malpositioned anterior- or posterior-chamber intraocular lens; often with a vitreous wick.

Treatment of UGH Syndrome
1. Atropine, 1%, t.i.d.
2. Topical steroid (e.g., prednisolone acetate, 1%, q.i.d. or more often if the uveitis is severe) and consider topical NSAID (e.g., diclofenac, q.i.d.).
3. Systemic carbonic anhydrase inhibitor (e.g., acetazolamide, 250 mg p.o., q.i.d., or 500 mg sequel p.o., b.i.d., or methazolamide, 25 to 50 mg p.o., b.i.d. to t.i.d.) or may consider topical carbonic anhydrase inhibitor (e.g., dorzolamide, 2%, or brinzolamide, 1%, t.i.d.).
4. Topical β-blocker (e.g., timolol or levobunolol, 0.5%, b.i.d.), α-agonist (e.g., brimonidine, 0.2%, b.i.d. to t.i.d., or apraclonidine, 0.5%, t.i.d.).
5. Consider argon laser treatment to control the hemorrhage if a bleeding site can be identified.
6. Consider surgical repositioning, replacement, or removal of the intraocular lens, especially if peripheral anterior synechiae (PAS) are forming or cystoid macular edema persists.
7. Consider YAG vitreolysis if discrete strands can be seen.

❖ **Note** *Functional patency of iridectomy is difficult to determine. A helpful way to distinguish UGH syndrome from malignant glaucoma is injection of fluorescein (as for a retinal angiogram) into antecubital vein with pupillary block glaucoma; fluorescein is not seen entering the anterior chamber or structures except after about 30 seconds as it diffuses through the blood vessels. In malignant glaucoma, the fluorescein streams into the retrolental space.*

Ghost Cell Glaucoma

Degenerated red blood cells (RBCs) pass from the vitreous into the anterior chamber and obstruct the trabecular meshwork. These cells are tan. Often occurs after a large vitreous hemorrhage with a posterior capsular opening, allowing easy access of the RBCs into the anterior chamber. Usually occurs 1 to 4 weeks after the vitreous hemorrhage.

Treatment of ghost cell glaucoma
1. Medical treatment: see Primary Open-Angle Glaucoma (Section 10.1)
2. Anterior chamber irrigation
3. Posterior vitrectomy to clear the blood, if medical management fails

Malignant Glaucoma

See Section 10.16.

Steroid-Response Glaucoma

See Section 10.5.

Follow-up for Postoperative Glaucoma

Patients should generally not be sent out of the office or emergency room with an IOP >35 to 40 mm Hg. If the patient is monocular or has significant optic nerve damage, then the IOP should be even lower. For aphakic/pseudophakic pupillary block, be certain that the angle is open and the block is relieved (by using gonioscopy). If these criteria are met, the patient must be reevaluated in 1 to 7 days, depending on the particular situation.

10.16 MALIGNANT GLAUCOMA
(Aqueous Misdirection)

Symptoms

May be very mild in the early stages. Late, may develop moderate pain, red eye, photophobia; often occurs after surgical treatment of angle-closure glaucoma; also occurs in association with shallow anterior chamber after surgery without a patent peripheral iridectomy (PI), as with tube-shunt operations, and may be induced by miotics (even without surgery).

Critical Signs

Shallow or flat anterior chamber and increased intraocular pressure (IOP) in the presence of a patent PI and in the absence of a choroidal detachment. Absence of iris bombé.

Etiology

It is believed that aqueous is misdirected and accumulates within the vitreous, displacing the vitreous forward, pushing the ciliary processes, the crystalline lens, the intraocular implant, or the anterior vitreous face anteriorly, causing secondary angle closure.

Differential Diagnosis (Table 10-1)

- Pupillary block glaucoma (Iris bombé, adhesions of iris to other anterior chamber structures. See Pupillary Block, Section 10.15)
- Acute angle-closure glaucoma (No history of surgery; other eye has shallow anterior chamber and narrow angle. See Section 10.10, Acute Angle-Closure Glaucoma.)
- Choroidal detachment (Shallow or flat anterior chamber, but the IOP is typically low. A choroidal detachment is seen on funduscopic examination or by B-scan ultrasound in most cases. See Section 12.21, Choroidal Detachment.)
- Suprachoroidal hemorrhage (Sudden onset of shallow or flat anterior chamber, excruciating pain, increased IOP early. Dark, nonserous

TABLE 10-1. *Postoperative Complications of Glaucoma Surgery*

Diagnosis	Intraocular Pressure	Anterior Chamber	Iris Bombé	Pain	Bleb
Inflammation	Mildly elevated	Deep	No	Possible	Varies
Hyphema	Mild–moderately elevated	Varies	Not early	Possible	Varies
Failure to filter	Moderately elevated	Deep	No	Moderate	Falling
Malignant glaucoma	Early: moderately elevated	Shallow everywhere	No	Moderate	Falling or absent
	Late: moderate– markedly elevated	Grade 2 or 3			
Suprachoroidal hemorrhage	Early: markedly elevated, later falling to mild or moderately elevated	Grade 1 and 2 flat	No	Excruciating	Varies
Pupillary block	Early, moderately elevated, may become markedly elevated	Grade 1–3 flat	Yes	None or mild	None
Serous choroidal detachment	Low	Grade 1–3 flat	No	Ache	Frequently present

choroidal detachment seen on funduscopic examination or B-scan ultrasound.)

Workup
1. History: Previous eye surgery?
2. Slit-lamp examination: Determine if a patent PI is present. Pupillary block is unlikely in the presence of a patent PI, unless it is plugged, bound down, or plateau iris syndrome is present. Is iris bombé present?
3. Gonioscopy of the anterior-chamber angle.
4. Dilated retinal examination unless a phakic angle closure is likely.
5. Consider B-scan ultrasound to rule out a choroidal detachment and suprachoroidal hemorrhage if they cannot be ruled out by ophthalmoscopy.

Treatment
1. If an iridectomy is not present or it is not certain whether an existing one is patent, pupillary block cannot be ruled out, and a PI should be performed (see Acute Angle-Closure Glaucoma, Section 10.10).

If signs of malignant glaucoma are still present with a patent PI:

2. Atropine, 1%, and phenylephrine, 2.5%, q.i.d. topically.
3. Carbonic anhydrase inhibitor (e.g., acetazolamide, 500 mg i.v. or two 250-mg tablets p.o., then 250 mg p.o., q.i.d.).
4. Hyperosmotic agent (e.g., mannitol, 20%, 1 to 2 g/kg i.v. over 45 minutes; a 500-ml bag of mannitol 20% contains 100 g of mannitol).
5. Topical β-blocker (e.g., timolol or levobunolol, 0.5%, b.i.d.).
6. Topical apraclonidine, 1.0%, or brimonidine, 0.2%, b.i.d.

If the attack is broken (the anterior chamber deepens and the IOP returns to normal), maintain atropine, 1% once per day, indefinitely.

If steps 1 through 6 are unsuccessful, consider one or more of the following:

7. YAG laser disruption of the anterior hyaloid face and posterior capsule if the patient is aphakic or pseudophakic. May attempt through a pre-existing large PI if phakic.
8. Argon laser treatment of the ciliary processes.
9. Core vitrectomy and reformation of the anterior chamber.
10. Lensectomy with disruption of the anterior hyaloid and/or vitrectomy.

❖ **Note** *A choroidal detachment may be present, yet undetectable. Therefore a sclerotomy to drain a choroidal detachment may be advisable before vitrectomy.*

11. PI in the contralateral eye if the angle appears occludable; generally performed at a later date.

Follow-up

Variable, depending on the therapeutic modality used. PI is generally performed in an occludable contralateral eye 1 week after treatment of the involved eye.

10.17 POSTOPERATIVE COMPLICATIONS OF GLAUCOMA SURGERY

Bleb Infection (Blebitis)

See Section 10.18

Increased Postoperative Intraocular Pressure (IOP) after Trabeculectomy

Grade of Shallowing of Anterior Chamber

 I. Peripheral iris–cornea contact.
 II. Entire iris in contact with cornea.
 III. Lens (or pseudophakia or vitreous face)–corneal contact.

Differential Diagnosis (Table 10-1)
 1. If the anterior chamber is deep (formed), consider the following:
 • Occlusion of the filtration opening *internally*: by an iris plug, hemorrhage, fibrin, vitreous or viscoelastic material.
 • Occlusion of filtration *externally*: by a tight trabeculectomy flap (sutured tightly or scarred).

❖ **Note** *Diagnosis is made by careful slit-lamp examination and gonioscopy.*

 2. If the anterior chamber is flat or shallow and IOP is increased, consider the following:
 • Suprachoroidal hemorrhage (sudden onset of severe pain, commonly 1 to 5 days after surgery, with injection, variable IOPs [15 to 45 mm Hg], hazy cornea, shallow chamber.) Diagnosis confirmed by indirect ophthalmoscopy or B-scan ultrasound.
 • Malignant glaucoma (See Section 10.16, Malignant Glaucoma)
 • Pupillary block (See Section 10.15, Pupillary Block)

Treatment
 1. If the bleb is not formed and the anterior chamber is deep, point pressure with an applicator on the edge of the bleb should be used to try to determine if the sclerostomy will drain.
 2. If the trabeculectomy flap is too tight, argon or suture lysis may be indicated.
 3. If sclerostomy is blocked with iris, pressure of the globe of any sort is contraindicated. Intracameral injection of acetylcholine, slowly, can pull the iris out of the sclerostomy if used before 12 to 24 hours postoperatively. If this fails, and sclerostomy is completely blocked by iris, and acetylcholine fails, transcorneal, mechanical retraction of the iris may work. If sclerostomy is blocked with vitreous, it may occasionally be photodisrupted of the sclerostomy with a Nd:YAG laser. If blood or fibrin plugs the sclerostomy, time may clear the problem.
 4. For suprachoroidal hemorrhage, if the IOP is mildly increased and the chamber is formed, observation with medical management is indicated. If the flat chamber persists, the IOP remains increased, there is corneal–lenticular touch, or the pain is intolerable, surgical drainage of the choroidal hemorrhage is necessary.

5. Medical therapy may be needed if these measures are not successful. (See Primary Open Angle Glaucoma, Section 10.1)
6. If all of these fail, reoperation may be necessary.

Low Postoperative Intraocular Pressure after Filtering Procedure

Low pressures (5 to 9 mm Hg range) are not desirable. IOP <8 mm Hg is associated with increased incidence of flat anterior chamber, choroidal detachment, and suprachoroidal hemorrhage. IOP <4 mm Hg is even more likely to be associated with problems, including macular hypotony and corneal edema.

Differential Diagnosis and Treatment (Table 10-1)
1. Very large filtering bleb with a formed (deep) chamber (overfiltration): It is desirable to have a large bleb in the first few weeks after trabeculectomy. However, if it still present 6 to 8 weeks after surgery, the patient is symptomatic, IOP is decreasing, and/or anterior chamber is shallowing, consider shell tamponade or autologous blood injections into the bleb. If IOP is stable and anterior chamber is deep, leave alone.
2. Large bleb with a flat chamber: Treatment is indicated when recognized and includes cycloplegics (atropine, 1%, t.i.d.), and careful observation. If the anterior chamber becomes more shallow (e.g., grade I becoming grade II), IOP decreases as bleb flattens, or is associated with development of choroidal detachment, the anterior chamber should be reformed with a viscoelastic material.
3. No bleb with flat chamber: Check carefully for a wound leak by Seidel testing (see Appendix 4). If positive, aqueous suppressants, patching, or surgical closure may be necessary. If Seidel negative, look for a cyclodialysis cleft by gonioscopy or for serous choroidal detachments. Cyclodialysis clefts are managed by cycloplegics, laser or cryotherapy closure, or surgical closure. Serous choroidal detachments are often observed and are not frequently drained, unless associated with recurrent flat anterior chamber and persistent hypotony.

10.18 BLEBITIS

Description

Infection of the filtering bleb. May occur any time after glaucoma filtering procedures (days to years).

Mild: Bleb infection but NO anterior chamber or vitreal involvement

Moderate: Bleb infection with anterior chamber inflammation but NO vitreal involvement

Severe: Bleb infection with anterior chamber and vitreal involvement. See Postoperative Endophthalmitis, Section 13.10.

Symptoms

Red eye and discharge early. Later, aching pain, photophobia, decreased vision, mucous discharge.

Signs

Mild: Bleb appears milky, with loss of translucency. Microhypopyon within loculations of the bleb, intraocular pressure (IOP) after rising. Turbid fluid in bleb possibly with frank purulent material in or leaking from the bleb, intense conjunctival injection.

Moderate: Findings of *Mild* with anterior chamber cell and flare, possibly an anterior chamber hypopyon, with no vitreal inflammation.

Severe: Findings of *Moderate* with vitreal involvement. Same appearance of endophthalmitis except with bleb involvement.

Differential Diagnosis

- Episcleritis [Sectorial inflammation (rarely superior) but no inflammation of bleb. See Section 5.6, Episcleritis.]
- Conjunctivitis (Little to no decrease in vision, no pain or photophobia. Bacterial conjunctivitis can progress to blebitis if not promptly treated. See Section 5.1, Conjunctivitis.)
- Anterior uveitis (Anterior segment findings similar except there will be no inflammation of the bleb. See Section 13.1, Anterior Uveitis.)
- Endophthalmitis (Similar anterior segment findings as blebitis, except with vitreous cells and inflammation. May have more intense pain, eyelid edema, chemosis, greater decrease in vision, hypopyon, and fibrinous reaction than blebitis. See Section 13.10, Postoperative Endophthalmitis)
- Ischemic bleb (In immediate postoperative period after the use of antimetabolites. Conjunctiva is opaque with sectorial conjunctival injection. The view of the fluid in the bleb may be obscured.)

Workup

1. Slit-lamp examination with close examination of the bleb, anterior chamber, and vitreous. Search for hole in the bleb. Look for microhypopyon by using gonioscopy.
2. Culture bleb and perform anterior chamber tap for *Moderate;* for *Severe,* see Postoperative Endophthalmitis, Section 13.10.

❖ **Note** *Commonly isolated organisms have been* Staphylococcus epidermidis, Staphylococcus aureus, *and other Gram positives in the first days to weeks after surgery. If blebitis occurs months to years later,* Streptococcus, Haemophilus influenzae, S. aureus, Moraxella, Pseudomonas *and* Serratia *are more common.*

3. B-scan ultrasound of the vitreous may reveal inflammation if visualization is difficult.

Treatment
1. Mild: Intensive topical antibiotics with either of two regimens
   a. Fortified cefazolin or vancomycin and fortified gentamicin, amikacin, or tobramycin alternating every half hour for the first 24 hours. A loading dose of one drop of each every 5 minutes ×4 is often given.
   b. Fluoroquinolones (e.g., ciprofloxacin or ofloxacin) every hour after a loading dose.
   c. Reevaluate in 6 to 12 hours and again at 12 to 24 hours. Must not be getting worse.
   d. Start steroids 24 hours after antibiotics started and blebitis resolving.
2. Moderate: same approach as mild blebitis, plus cycloplegics and more careful monitoring.
3. Severe: admit and treat as endophthalmitis (See Section 13.10, Postoperative Endophthalmitis).

Follow-up
Daily until infection is resolving. Admission to the hospital is indicated for noncompliance or worsening of infection.

NEURO-OPHTHALMOLOGY

11.1 ANISOCORIA

See Fig. 11-1.

Definition/Etiology
A. The abnormal pupil is constricted.
- Unilateral use of a miotic (green-top) eye drop (e.g., pilocarpine).
- Iritis (Eye pain, redness, and anterior-chamber cells and flare.)
- Horner's syndrome (Mild ptosis is usually present on the side of the small pupil; positive cocaine test.)
- Argyll Robertson (syphilitic) pupil [The pupil is irregular in shape, reacts poorly or not at all to light, but constricts normally during convergence. Although the disease is typically bilateral, a mild degree of anisocoria is often present. Should have positive syphilis serology (fluorescent treponemal antibody, absorbed [FTA-ABS] or MHA-TP).]
- Long-standing Adie's pupil (The pupil is initially dilated, but over time may constrict. At the slit lamp, it can be seen to react slowly and irregularly to a bright light. It is supersensitive to pilocarpine 0.125%*
B. The abnormal pupil is dilated.
- Iris sphincter muscle damage from trauma (Torn pupillary margin or iris transillumination defects seen on slit-lamp examination.)
- Adie's tonic pupil (The pupil is irregular, reacts minimally to light and slowly to convergence, but is supersensitive to weak

---

*Note: pilocarpine, 0.125%, is prepared by diluting one part pilocarpine 1% with 7 parts balanced salt solution.

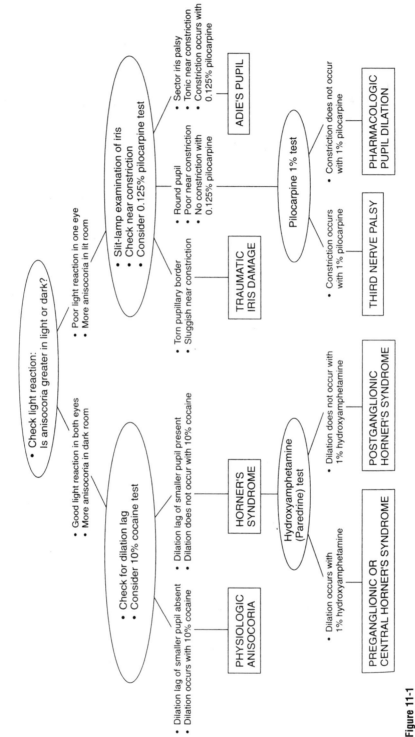

Figure 11-1

Flow diagram for the workup of anisocoria. (Modified from Thompson HS, Pilley SEJ. *Surv Oph-thalmol* 1976;24:45–48, with permission.)

cholinergic agents such as pilocarpine, 0.125%,* or metha-
choline, 2.5%.)
- Third-nerve palsy [Associated ptosis and extraocular muscle
  palsies. The pupil will not react to weak cholinergic agents, but will
  constrict to regular-strength miotic drops (e.g., pilocarpine, 1%).]
- Unilateral use of a mydriatic (red-top, dilating) eye drop (e.g.,
  atropine) [If the drop has been instilled recently, the pupil will not
  react to pilocarpine, 1%, drops. If the effect of the drop is wearing
  off (e.g., atropine was used 1 to 2 weeks previously), the eye may
  be dilated and partly reactive to pilocarpine.]

C. Physiologic anisocoria (Pupil size disparity is the same in light as in
dark, and the pupils react normally to light. The size difference is usually, but not always ≤1 mm in diameter.)

Workup
1. History: When was the anisocoria first noted? Any associated symptoms or signs? History of ocular trauma? Use of any eye drops or ointments? History of syphilis? History of decreased vision? Old photographs?
2. Ocular examination: Try to determine which is the abnormal pupil by
   observing the pupillary size. Younger patients tend to have pupillary
   diameters of 4 to 5 mm on average, whereas elderly patients often have
   slightly smaller pupils. If it is uncertain which is the abnormal pupil,
   compare pupil sizes in light and in dark. Anisocoria greater in light suggests the abnormal pupil is the larger pupil; anisocoria greater in dark
   suggests the abnormal pupil is the smaller pupil. Test the pupillary reaction to light. Test convergence if the light reaction is abnormal. Look for
   ptosis, evaluate ocular motility, and examine the pupillary margin with
   a slit lamp.
   - If the abnormal pupil is small, a diagnosis of Horner's syndrome
     may be confirmed by a cocaine test (see Section 11.2, Horner's syn-
     drome). In the presence of ptosis and an unequivocal increase in
     anisocoria in dim illumination, a cocaine test is unnecessary because
     the diagnosis is made clinically.
   - If the abnormal pupil is large and there is no sphincter muscle dam-
     age or signs of third-nerve palsy (extraocular motility deficit, pto-
     sis), the pupils are tested with one drop of pilocarpine, 0.125%*.
     Within 10 to 15 minutes, an Adie's pupil will usually have con-
     stricted significantly more than the fellow pupil (see Section 11.4,
     Adie's Tonic Pupil).

*Note: pilocarpine, 0.125%, is prepared by diluting one part pilocarpine 1% with 7 parts balanced
salt solution.

❖ **Note** *Soon after the development of an Adie's pupil, the pupil may not react to a weak cholinergic agent.*

- If the pupil does not constrict with pilocarpine, 0.125%, or pharmacologic dilatation is suspected, pilocarpine, 1%, is instilled in both eyes. A normal pupil constricts sooner and to a greater extent than the pharmacologically dilated pupil. An eye that recently received a strong mydriatic agent such as atropine usually will not constrict at all.

See Horner's Syndrome, Section 11.2; Argyll Robertson Pupil, Section 11.3; Adie's Tonic Pupil, Section 11.4; and Isolated Third-Nerve Palsy, Section 11.5, for more information regarding diagnosis and treatment of the specific entity causing anisocoria.

11.2 HORNER'S SYNDROME

Symptoms
Droopy eyelid, pupil size disparity; often asymptomatic.

Critical Signs
Anisocoria that is greater in dim illumination (especially during the first few seconds the room light is dimmed) because of a small pupil that does not dilate as well as the normal, larger pupil; usually, mild ptosis and lower eyelid elevation ("reverse ptosis") occur on the same side as the small pupil.

Other Signs
All of the following may occur on the side affected by Horner's syndrome: Lower intraocular pressure, lighter iris color in congenital cases (iris heterochromia), loss of sweating ability (anhidrosis), increase in accommodation (older patients can be noted to hold their reading card closer in the Horner's eye). Light and near reactions are intact.

Differential Diagnosis
See Anisocoria, Section 11.1.

Etiology
First-order neuron disorder   Stroke (e.g., vertebrobasilar artery insufficiency or infarct); tumor; rarely, severe osteoarthritis of the neck with bony spurs.

Second-order neuron disorder   Tumor (e.g., lung carcinoma, metastasis, thyroid adenoma, neurofibroma). Patients with arm pain should be suspected of having a Pancoast tumor. In children, consider neuroblastoma, lymphoma, or metastasis.

Third-order neuron disorder   Headache syndrome (e.g., cluster, migraine, Raeder's paratrigeminal syndrome), internal carotid dissection, herpes zoster virus, otitis media, and Tolosa–Hunt syndrome.

Congenital Horner's syndrome   Trauma (e.g., during delivery).

Workup

1. If the diagnosis is uncertain, it may be confirmed with a cocaine test: One drop of cocaine, 10%, is placed into each eye and then repeated 1 minute later. Check the pupils in 15 minutes. If no change in pupillary size is noted, repeat one set of drops and recheck the pupils in another 15 minutes. A Horner's pupil dilates less than the normal pupil.
2. Hydroxyamphetamine, 1% (e.g., Paredrine), is used to distinguish a third-order neuron disorder from a first- and second-order neuron disorder: Place one drop of hydroxyamphetamine, 1%, into each eye, repeating the drop 1 minute later. Check the pupils in 30 minutes. Failure of the Horner's pupil to dilate to an equivalent degree as the fellow eye indicates a third-order neuron lesion.

❖ **Notes**
- *Hydroxyamphetamine should not be administered within 24 hours of cocaine or they will interfere with each other's action.*
- *Both tests are thought to require an intact corneal epithelium and no prior eye-drop administration for accurate results.*

3. Determine the duration of the Horner's syndrome from the patient's history and an examination of old photographs. New-onset Horner's syndrome requires a more extensive diagnostic workup. An old Horner's syndrome is more likely to be benign.
4. History: Headaches? Arm pain? Previous stroke? Previous surgery that may have damaged the sympathetic chain, including cardiac, thoracic, thyroid or neck surgery? History of head or neck trauma?
5. Physical examination (especially check for supraclavicular nodes, thyroid enlargement, or a neck mass).

Depending on the duration of Horner's syndrome and the results of the hydroxyamphetamine test, any or all of the following tests may be ordered: (A more aggressive work-up is performed for new-onset Horner's syndromes, first- or second-order neuron disorders, and those with a history or physical examination that might indicate a tumor. Some physicians workup all Horner's syndrome patients.)

6. Computed tomography (CT) scan of the chest to evaluate lung apex for possible mass (e.g., Pancoast tumor).

7. Magnetic resonance imaging (MRI) of the brain and neck.
8. Complete blood count (CBC) with differential.
9. Magnetic resonance angiography (MRA) of head/neck and carotid Doppler ultrasound if carotid artery dissection possible (especially with neck pain). Carotid angiogram if MRA and Doppler equivocal.
10. Lymph node biopsy when lymphadenopathy is present.

Treatment
1. Treat the underlying disorder if possible. (Carotid dissection usually requires urgent anticoagulation to prevent thrombosis: consider neurovascular surgical consultation.)
2. Ptosis surgery may be performed as needed.

Follow-up
Acute Horner's syndromes should be worked up as soon as possible to rule out life-threatening causes. Chronic Horner's syndromes can be evaluated with less urgency. With the exception of possible amblyopia in children, which occurs only when the eyelid covers the visual axis, there are no ocular complications that necessitate close follow-up.

11.3 ARGYLL ROBERTSON PUPILS

Symptoms
Usually asymptomatic.

Critical Signs
Small, irregular pupils that exhibit "light-near" dissociation (react poorly or not at all to light but constrict normally during convergence). By definition, vision is normal.

Other Signs
The pupils do not dilate well. May initially be unilateral, but always becomes bilateral, although possibly asymmetric.

Etiology
Tertiary syphilis.

Differential Diagnosis
See Anisocoria, Section 11.1.

Other causes of "light-near" dissociation:

- Bilateral optic neuropathy or severe retinopathy (Visual acuity is reduced, pupil size is normal.)
- Adie's tonic pupil (Unilateral or bilateral irregularly dilated pupil that constricts slowly and unevenly to light. Normal vision. See Section 11.4, Adie's Tonic Pupil.)
- Dorsal midbrain (Parinaud's) syndrome (Bilateral, normal to large pupils. Accompanied by convergence–retraction nystagmus and supranuclear upgaze palsy. See Sections 11.4, Adie's Tonic Pupil, and 11.19, Nystagmus.)

Workup
1. Test the pupillary reaction to light and convergence: To test the reaction of the pupil to convergence, patients are asked to look first at a distant target and then at their own finger, which the examiner holds in front of them and slowly brings in toward their face.
2. Slit-lamp examination: look for interstitial keratitis.
3. Dilated fundus examination: Search for chorioretinitis, papillitis, and uveitis.
4. Fluorescent treponemal antibody, absorbed (FTA-ABS) or MHA-TP, rapid plasma reagin (RPR) or Venereal Disease Research Laboratories test (VDRL).
5. Consider a lumbar puncture if the diagnosis of syphilis is established (see Section 14.2, Acquired Syphilis).

Treatment
The decision to treat is based on whether active disease is present and whether the patient has been treated appropriately in the past. See Acquired Syphilis, Section 14.2, for treatment indications and specific antibiotic therapy.

Follow-up
This is not an emergency, but a diagnostic workup and determination of syphilitic activity should be undertaken within a few days of detecting Argyll Robertson pupils.

11.4 ADIE'S TONIC PUPIL

Symptoms
Difference in the size of the pupils, blurred vision; may be asymptomatic.

Critical Signs
An irregularly dilated pupil exhibiting minimal or no reaction to light, slow constriction to convergence, and slow redilatation. It is typically

unilateral at first and is found most often in young women. The pupil demonstrates supersensitivity to weak cholinergic agents (e.g., pilocarpine, 0.125%*.

Other Signs

It may develop acutely and may become bilateral. The pupil dilates normally to mydriatic agents. Deep tendon reflexes (knees and ankles) are often absent (Adie's syndrome). The involved pupil may become smaller than the normal pupil over time.

❖ **Note** *Supersensitivity may not be present soon after the development of an Adie's pupil and may need to be tested a few weeks later.*

Etiology

Idiopathic, orbital trauma or infection, herpes zoster infection, diabetes, autonomic neuropathies, Guillain–Barré syndrome, others.

Differential Diagnosis

See Anisocoria, Section 11.1.

❖ **Note** *Parinaud's syndrome may produce bilateral mid-dilated pupils that react poorly to light but constrict normally during convergence (i.e., not tonic). Eyelid retraction and paralysis of upgaze with retraction nystagmus may additionally be present. A pinealoma or other midbrain abnormality must be ruled out by MRI.*

Workup

See Anisocoria, Section 11.1, for a general workup when the diagnosis is uncertain.

1. Observe the suspect pupil with the slit lamp, shining a bright light on it. The Adie's pupil will contract slowly and irregularly.
2. Test for a supersensitive pupil: Have the patient fixate at a distance, and measure the pupil size of each eye. Instill one drop of pilocarpine, 0.125%*, in each eye, and recheck the pupil size in 10 to 15 minutes. The tonic pupil constricts significantly more than the contralateral pupil in Adie's syndrome.

❖ **Note** *The dilute pilocarpine test may occasionally be positive in an Argyll Robertson pupil and in familial dysautonomia.*

---

*Note: pilocarpine, 0.125%, is prepared by diluting one part pilocarpine 1% with 7 parts balanced salt solution.)

3. If Adie's pupil or supersensitivity or both are present and the patient is younger than 1 year, refer him or her to a pediatric neurologist to rule out familial dysautonomia (Riley–Day syndrome).

Treatment

Pilocarpine, 0.125%, b.i.d. to q.i.d., for cosmesis and to aid in accommodation, if desired.

Follow-up

If the diagnosis is established with certainty, follow-up is routine.

11.5 ISOLATED THIRD-NERVE PALSY

Symptoms

Double vision that disappears when one eye is closed; droopy eyelid, with or without pain.

Critical Signs

A. External ophthalmoplegia (i.e., motility impaired)
   1. Complete palsy: Limitation of ocular movement in all fields of gaze except temporally.
   2. Incomplete palsy: Partial limitation of ocular movement.
   3. Superior-division palsy: Ptosis and an inability to look up.
   4. Inferior-division palsy: Inability to look nasally or inferiorly; pupil is involved.
B. Internal ophthalmoplegia (i.e., pupil reaction impaired)
   1. Pupil-involving: A fixed, dilated or minimally reactive pupil.
   2. Pupil-sparing: Pupil not dilated and normally reactive to light.
   3. Relative pupil-sparing: Pupil partially dilated and sluggishly reactive to light.

Other Signs

An exotropia or hypotropia. Aberrant regeneration [elevation of the upper eyelid with gaze down or nasally; sometimes pupil constriction (usually segmental) when looking up, down, or nasally].

❖ **Note** *Aberrant regeneration may occur spontaneously (primary regeneration) without a preceding third-nerve palsy. This is usually caused by a cavernous sinus tumor or aneurysm.*

Etiology

A. *Pupil-involving:*

More common   Aneurysm (particularly a posterior communicating artery aneurysm).

Less common   Ischemic microvascular disease (typically a result of diabetes or hypertension), tumor, trauma, congenital.

Rare   Uncal herniation, cavernous sinus mass lesion, pituitary apoplexy, orbital disease, herpes zoster, leukemia. In children, ophthalmoplegic migraine.

B. *Pupil-sparing:* Ischemic microvascular disease; rarely cavernous sinus syndrome, giant cell arteritis (GCA).

C. *Relative pupil-sparing:* Ischemic microvascular disease; less likely aneurysm.

D. *Aberrant regeneration present:* Trauma, aneurysm, tumor, congenital. Not microvascular.

Differential Diagnosis

- Myasthenia gravis [Diurnal variation of symptoms and signs, pupil not involved, increased eyelid droop after sustained upgaze, weak orbicularis oculi muscle, positive edrophonium chloride (e.g., Tensilon) test. See Section 11.10, Myasthenia Gravis.]
- Thyroid eye disease (Eyelid lag, stare, injection over the rectus muscles, proptosis, resistance on forced duction testing, abnormal CT scan of the orbits, no ptosis. See Section 7.2, Thyroid Eye Disease.)
- Chronic progressive external ophthalmoplegia (CPEO; Bilateral, slowly progressive ptosis and limitation of ocular motility, pupil spared, often no double vision. See Section 11.11, Chronic Progressive External Ophthalmoplegia.)
- Orbital inflammatory pseudotumor (Pain and proptosis are usually present. See Section 7.3, Orbital Inflammatory Pseudotumor.)
- Internuclear ophthalmoplegia (Unilateral or bilateral adduction deficit with horizontal nystagmus of opposite abducting eye. No ptosis. Lesion in ipsilateral brainstem medial longitudinal fasciculus. See Section 11.12, Internuclear Ophthalmoplegia.)
- Skew deviation (Supranuclear brainstem lesion producing asymmetric, mainly vertical ocular deviation not consistent with single cranial nerve defect. See Section 11.12, Internuclear Ophthalmoplegia.)
- Parinaud's syndrome/Dorsal midbrain lesion (Inability to look up; pupils react slowly to light and briskly to convergence; no ptosis; eyelid-retraction and convergence-retraction nystagmus may or may not be present. Bilateral.)
- GCA (Extraocular muscle ischemia causing nonspecific motility deficits. Pupil not involved. Age older than 50, associated systemic symptoms. See Section 11.16, Giant Cell Arteritis.)

Workup

1. History: Onset and duration of diplopia? Recent trauma? Pertinent medical history [e.g., diabetes, hypertension, known cancer or central nervous system (CNS) mass, recent infections].

2. Complete ocular examination: Check for pupillary involvement, the directions of motility restriction (in both eyes), ptosis, a visual-field defect (visual fields by confrontation), proptosis, resistance to retropulsion, orbicularis muscle weakness and eyelid fatigue with sustained upgaze. Look carefully for signs of aberrant regeneration (discussed previously).

3. Full neurologic examination: Carefully assess the other cranial nerves on both sides. (The ipsilateral fourth nerve can be assessed by focusing with the slit lamp on a superior conjunctival blood vessel and asking the patient to look down and nasally. The eye should intort, and the blood vessel should turn down and toward the nose.)

4. Immediate imaging study of the brain (preferably MRI) to rule out mass/aneurysm is indicated for
   a. Pupil-involving (relatively or completely involved) third-nerve palsies.
   b. Pupil-sparing third-nerve palsies only in the following groups of patients:
      - Patients younger than 50 years (unless there is known long-standing diabetes or hypertension.)
      - Patients with incomplete third-nerve palsies (i.e., with sparing of some muscle function) because this condition may be evolving into a pupil-involving third-nerve palsy. (These patients may alternatively be monitored closely over 5 to 7 days for development of pupil involvement.)
      - Patients whose third-nerve palsy is over 3 months in duration, but has not improved.
      - Patients with an additional cranial nerve or neurologic abnormalities.
   c. All patients who develop aberrant regeneration, with the exception of regeneration after traumatic third-nerve palsies.

❖ **Note** *Imaging is generally not required in pupil-sparing third-nerve palsies that do not fit these criteria, especially when patients have known vasculopathic risk factors such as diabetes or hypertension.*

5. Cerebral angiography is indicated for all patients older than 10 years with pupil-involving third-nerve palsies and whose imaging study is normal or shows a mass consistent with an aneurysm.

6. CBC with differential in children.

7. Edrophonium chloride (e.g., Tensilon) test when myasthenia gravis is suspected and the pupil is not involved (see Section 11.10, Myasthenia Gravis).
8. For suspected ischemic disease: check blood pressure, fasting blood sugar, glycosylated hemoglobin.
9. Immediate erythrocyte sedimentation rate (ESR) if GCA is possible (see Section 11.16, Giant Cell Arteritis).

Treatment
1. Treat the underlying abnormality.
2. If the third-nerve palsy is causing symptomatic diplopia, an occlusion patch may be placed over the involved eye. Patching is generally not performed in children younger than 9 to 11 years because of the risk of amblyopia. Children should be monitored closely for the development of amblyopia in the deviated eye.

Follow-up
A. *Pupil-sparing:* Observe daily for 5 to 7 days from onset of symptoms for delayed pupil involvement, and then recheck every 4 to 6 weeks. Patients should regain the function lost from their third-nerve palsy within 3 months. If the palsy does not reverse by this time, or if an additional neurologic abnormality or evidence of aberrant regeneration develops, an immediate MRI is obtained. Refer to internist for management of vasculopathic disease risk factors.
B. *Pupil-involving:* If imaging and angiography are negative, follow as in pupil-sparing case earlier.

11.6 ISOLATED FOURTH-NERVE PALSY

Symptoms
Binocular vertical diplopia (double vision that disappears when one eye is occluded; one image appears on top of or up and to the side of the second image with both eyes open), difficulty reading, sensation that objects appear tilted; may be asymptomatic.

Critical Signs
Deficient inferior movement of an eye when attempting to look down and in. The three-step test isolates a palsy of the superior oblique muscle (see the following discussion).

Other Signs

The involved eye is higher (hypertropic) when patient looks straight ahead. The hypertropia increases when looking in the direction of the uninvolved eye or tilting the head toward the ipsilateral shoulder. The patient often maintains a head tilt toward the contralateral shoulder to eliminate double vision.

Etiology

More common   Trauma; vascular infarct (often the result of underlying diabetes or hypertension); congenital, idiopathic, or demyelinating disease.

Rare   Tumor, hydrocephalus, aneurysm, giant cell arteritis (GCA).

Differential Diagnosis

All of the following may produce binocular vertical diplopia, hypertropia, or both.

- Myasthenia gravis [Double vision worse toward the end of the day when fatigued, usually accompanied by ptosis, positive edrophonium chloride (e.g., Tensilon) test. See Section 11.10, Myasthenia Gravis.]
- Thyroid eye disease (May have proptosis, eyelid lag, stare, or injection over the involved rectus muscles. Positive forced duction test. See Section 7.2, Thyroid Eye Disease.)
- Orbital inflammatory disease (pseudotumor) (Pain and proptosis are common. See Section 7.3, Orbital Inflammatory Pseudotumor.)
- Orbital fracture (History of trauma. Can cause entrapment or fibrosis of the inferior rectus muscle. Positive forced duction test. See Section 3.10, Orbital Blow-out Fracture.)
- Skew deviation (The three-step test does not isolate a particular muscle. Rule out a posterior fossa or brainstem lesion by MRI of the brain. See Section 11.12, Internuclear Ophthalmoplegia.)
- Incomplete third-nerve palsy (Inability to look down and out, usually with adduction weakness. Intortion on attempted downgaze. Three-step test will not isolate superior oblique. See Section 11.5, Isolated Third-Nerve Palsy.)
- Brown's syndrome [Limitation of elevation in adduction due to restriction of superior oblique tendon. May be congenital or acquired (e.g., trauma, inflammation). Positive forced duction test. See Section 9.5, Strabismus Syndromes.]
- GCA (Extraocular muscle ischemia causing nonspecific motility deficits or neural ischemia mimicking cranial nerve palsy. Age older than 50 years, associated systemic symptoms. See Section 11.16.)

Workup

1. History: Onset and duration of the diplopia? Misaligned eyes or head tilt since early childhood? Trauma? Stroke?

2. Examine old photographs to determine whether the head tilt is long standing, indicating an old or congenital fourth-nerve palsy.

❖ **Note** *A congenital fourth-nerve palsy can be distinguished from an acquired fourth-nerve palsy by measuring the vertical fusional amplitudes. A patient with an acquired fourth-nerve palsy will have a normal vertical fusional amplitude of 1 to 3 prism diopters. On the other hand, a patient with a congenital fourth-nerve palsy has greater than 1 to 3 prism diopters (often up to 10 to 15 prism diopters) of fusional amplitude. This is detected by using vertical prism bars. If a patient can fuse greater than 1 to 3 prism diopters, then the fourth-nerve palsy is congenital.*

3. Three-step test:
   Step 1 Determine which eye is deviated upward in primary gaze (looking straight ahead). This is best seen with the cover–uncover test (see Appendix 2). The higher eye comes down after being uncovered.
   Step 2 Determine whether the upward deviation is greater when the patient looks to the left or to the right.
   Step 3 Determine whether the upward deviation is greater when tilting the head to the left shoulder or right shoulder.
   As mentioned previously, patients with a superior oblique muscle paresis have a hyperdeviation that is worse when turning the elevated eye nasally and when tilting the head toward the shoulder ipsilateral to the elevated eye.
   Patients with a bilateral fourth-nerve palsy demonstrate hypertropia of the right eye when looking left, hypertropia of the left eye when looking right, and a V-pattern esotropia (the eyes cross more when looking down).
4. Perform the double Maddox rod test* if a bilateral fourth-nerve palsy is suspected.
5. Edrophonium chloride (e.g., Tensilon) test if myasthenia gravis is suspected (see Section 11.10, Myasthenia Gravis).
6. CT scan head and orbits (axial and coronal views) for suspected orbital disease.

---

*A white Maddox rod is placed before one eye and a red Maddox rod is placed before the other eye in a trial frame, aligning the axes of each rod along the 90-degree vertical mark. While looking at a white light in the distance, the patient is asked if both the white and red lines seen through the Maddox rods are horizontal and parallel to each other (sometimes placing a six-prism diopter base-down in front of one eye helps the patient determine if the lines are parallel, but this should not be performed in the presence of hypertropia). When the lines are not horizontal and parallel, the patient is asked to rotate the Maddox rod(s) until they are parallel. If he or she rotates the top of this vertical axis outward (away from the nose) for more than 10 degrees total for the two eyes, then a bilateral superior oblique muscle paresis exists.

7. Blood pressure measurement, fasting blood sugar, and glycosylated hemoglobin. Immediate erythrocyte sedimentation rate (ESR) if GCA is possible.
8. MRI of the brain for:
    a. A fourth-nerve palsy accompanied by other cranial nerve or neurologic abnormalities (i.e., not an isolated palsy).
    b. All patients younger than 40 years with no definite history of significant head trauma, and patients aged 40 to 55 years with no vasculopathic risk factors or trauma.

Treatment
1. Treat the underlying disorder.
2. An occlusion patch may be placed over one eye or fogging plastic tape can be applied to one lens of patient's spectacles to relieve symptomatic double vision. Patching is generally not performed in children younger than 9 to 11 years because of the risk of amblyopia.
3. Prisms in spectacles may be prescribed for small stable hyperdeviations.
4. Strabismus surgery may be indicated for bothersome double vision in primary or reading position, for a manifest head tilt, or to improve appearance. We generally wait at least 6 months after the onset of the palsy for the deviation to stabilize and because many palsies resolve spontaneously.

Follow-up
Congenital fourth-nerve palsy   (i.e., head tilt in old photographs, enlarged vertical fusion amplitude) Routine.
Acquired fourth-nerve palsy   As per the underlying disorder identified in the workup. If the workup is negative (the lesion is presumed vascular or idiopathic), then reexamine the patient in 1 to 3 months. If the palsy does not resolve in 3 months or if an additional neurologic abnormality develops, appropriate imaging studies of the brain are indicated. Patients are instructed to return immediately if they notice any changes (e.g., ptosis, worsening diplopia, sensory abnormality).

11.7 ISOLATED SIXTH-NERVE PALSY

Symptoms
Binocular horizontal diplopia (double vision producing side-by-side images; single vision is restored when one eye is closed or covered), worse for distance than near, most pronounced in the direction of the paretic lateral rectus muscle.

Critical Sign

One eye does not turn outward (temporally).

Other Signs

Lack of restriction on forced-duction testing. (See Appendix 5 for forced-duction test description.) No proptosis.

Etiology

ADULTS

More common   Vasculopathic (diabetes, hypertension, atherosclerosis), trauma, idiopathic.

Less common   Increased intracranial pressure, cavernous sinus mass (e.g., meningioma, aneurysm, metastasis), multiple sclerosis, sarcoidosis/vasculitis, after myelography or lumbar puncture, stroke (usually with other neurologic deficits), meningeal inflammation/infection (e.g., Lyme disease, tertiary syphilis), giant cell arteritis (GCA).

CHILDREN

Benign postviral condition, trauma, increased intracranial pressure (multiple causes; e.g., obstructive hydrocephalus), pontine glioma, Gradenigo's syndrome (petrositis causing sixth- and often seventh-nerve involvement, with or without eighth- and fifth-nerve involvement on the same side. Associated with complicated otitis media.)

Differential Diagnosis

All of the following may produce limitation of abduction.

*   Thyroid eye disease (Proptosis, injection of blood vessels over the restricted muscle, restriction on forced-duction testing. See Section 7.2, Thyroid Eye Disease.)
*   Myasthenia gravis [Symptoms worse toward the end of day with fatigue, orbicularis oculi weakness and ptosis may or may not be present, positive edrophonium chloride (e.g., Tensilon) test. See Section 11.10, Myasthenia Gravis.]
*   Orbital inflammatory disease (pseudotumor) (Proptosis, pain, restriction on forced-duction testing. See Section 7.3, Orbital Inflammatory Pseudotumor.)
*   Orbital trauma (Medial wall fracture causing entrapment of the ipsilateral medial rectus muscle, restriction on forced-duction testing. See Section 3.10, Orbital Blow-out Fracture.)
*   Duane's syndrome, type 1 (Congenital; narrowing of the palpebral fissure and retraction of the globe on adduction. See Section 9.5, Strabismus Syndromes.)

- Mobius' syndrome (Congenital; bilateral facial paralysis present. See Section 9.5, Strabismus Syndromes.)
- Convergence spasm (The pupils constrict on attempted abduction.)
- GCA (Extraocular muscle ischemia, age older than 50, associated systemic symptoms. See Section 11.16, Giant Cell Arteritis.)

Workup

ADULTS

1. History: Do the symptoms fluctuate during the day? History of cancer, diabetes, or thyroid disease?
2. Complete neurologic and ophthalmic examinations; pay careful attention to the function of the other cranial nerves and the appearance of the optic disc. It is especially important to evaluate the fifth cranial nerve; corneal sensation (supplied by the first division) can be tested by touching a wisp of cotton or a tissue to the corneas *before* applying topical anesthetic.
3. Check blood pressure, fasting blood sugar, and glycosylated hemoglobin.
4. MRI of the brain is indicated for the following patients:
   a. Younger than 40 years,
   b. Sixth-nerve palsy accompanied by severe pain or any other neurologic or neuro-ophthalmic sign,
   c. Any history of cancer. Consider MRI for patients aged 40 to 55 years with no history of vasculopathic disease.
5. Immediate erythrocyte sedimentation rate (ESR) if GCA is possible (see Section 11.16, Giant Cell Arteritis.).
6. Consider rapid plasma reagin (RPR), fluorescent treponemal antibody, absorbed (FTA-ABS), Lyme titer.

CHILDREN

1. History: Recent illness or trauma? Neurologic symptoms, lethargy, or behavioral changes? Chronic ear infections?
2. Complete neurologic and ophthalmic examinations as described for adults.
3. Otoscopic examination to rule out complicated otitis media.
4. MRI of the brain in all children.

Treatment
1. Any underlying problem revealed by the workup is treated.
2. An occlusion patch may be placed over one eye or fogging plastic tape applied to one spectacle lens to relieve symptomatic diplopia. In patients younger than 9 to 11 years, patching is avoided, and these patients are monitored closely for the development of amblyopia (see Section 9.6, Amblyopia).

3. Prisms in glasses may be fit for chronic stable deviations (e.g., after stroke). Consider strabismus surgery for stable deviation that persists more than 6 months.

Follow-up

Reexamine every 6 weeks after the onset of the palsy until it resolves. MRI of the head is indicated if any neurologic signs or symptoms develop during the follow-up period, the abduction deficit increases, or the isolated sixth-nerve palsy does not resolve in 3 to 6 months.

11.8 ISOLATED SEVENTH-NERVE PALSY

Symptoms

Weakness or paralysis of one side of the face, inability to close one eye, excessive drooling.

Critical Signs

Weakness or paralysis of the facial musculature on one side.

Central lesion   Weakness or paralysis of lower facial musculature only. (Upper eyelid closure and forehead wrinkling intact.)
Peripheral lesion   Weakness or paralysis of upper and lower facial musculature.

Other Signs

Flattened nasolabial fold, droop of corner of the mouth, ectropion, or lagophthalmos. May have ipsilateral decreased taste on anterior two thirds of tongue, decreased basic tear production, or hyperacusis. May have an injected eye with a corneal epithelial defect.

Synkinesis   Simultaneous movement of muscles supplied by different branches of the facial nerve or simultaneous stimulation of visceral efferent fibers of facial nerve [e.g., corner of mouth contracts when eye closes, excessive lacrimation when eating ("crocodile" tears)]. Due to aberrant regeneration and therefore implies chronicity.

Etiology

CENTRAL LESIONS

- Cortical: lesion of contralateral motor cortex or internal capsule (e.g., stroke, tumor). (Loss of voluntary facial movement; emotional facial movement sometimes intact. May also have ipsilateral hemiparesis.)

- Extrapyramidal: Lesion of basal ganglia (e.g., parkinsonism, tumor, vascular lesion of basal ganglia). (Loss of emotional facial movement; volitional facial movement intact. Not a true facial paralysis.)
- Brain stem: Lesion of ipsilateral pons (e.g., multiple sclerosis, stroke, tumor) (Often with ipsilateral sixth-nerve palsy, contralateral hemiparesis. Occasionally with cerebellar signs.)

PERIPHERAL LESIONS

- Cerebellopontine angle (CPA) masses (e.g., acoustic neuroma, facial neuroma, meningioma, cholesteatoma, metastasis). (Gradually progressive onset, although sometimes acute. May have facial pain or twitching. May have eighth-nerve dysfunction including hearing loss, vertigo, or dysequilibrium.)
- Trauma
  1. Temporal bone fracture [History of head trauma. May have Battle's sign (ecchymoses over mastoid region), cerebrospinal fluid otorrhea, hearing loss, vertigo, or vestibular nystagmus.]
  2. Other [Accidental or iatrogenic (e.g., facial laceration, local anesthetic block, parotid or mastoid surgery).]
- Otitis
  1. Acute otitis media
  2. Chronic suppurative otitis media
  3. Malignant otitis externa (*Pseudomonas* infection in diabetic or elderly patients. Begins in external auditory canal but may progress to osteomyelitis, meningitis, or abscess.)
- Ramsay–Hunt syndrome (herpes zoster oticus) (Viral prodrome followed by ear pain; vesicles on pinna, external auditory canal, tongue, face, or neck. Progresses over 10 days. May have sensorineural hearing loss, tinnitus, or vertigo.)
- Guillain–Barré syndrome (Viral syndrome followed by progressive motor weakness or paralysis or cranial-nerve palsies or both. Loss of deep tendon reflexes. May have bilateral facial palsies.)
- Lyme disease (May have rash, fever, fatigue, arthralgias, myalgias, or nausea. There may or may not be a history of tick bite. See Section 14.4, Lyme Disease.)
- Sarcoidosis (May have uveitis, parotitis, skin lesions, or lymphadenopathy. May have bilateral facial palsies. See Section 13.4, Sarcoidosis.)
- Parotid neoplasm (Slowly progressive paralysis of all or portion of facial musculature. Parotid mass with facial pain.)
- Metastasis [History of primary tumor (e.g., breast, lung, prostate) with multiple cranial nerve palsies in rapid succession. Can be the result of basilar skull metastasis or carcinomatous meningitis.]
- Bell's palsy (Idiopathic seventh-nerve palsy. Most common, but other etiologies must be ruled out. May have viral prodrome followed by ear

pain, facial numbness, decreased tearing or taste. Facial palsy may be complete or incomplete and progress over 10 days. May be recurrent, rarely bilateral. Possible familial predisposition.)

- Others (e.g., diabetes mellitus, botulism, human immunodeficiency virus (HIV), syphilis, Epstein–Barr virus, acute porphyrias, nasopharyngeal carcinoma, collagen–vascular disease)

Workup

1. History: Onset and duration of facial weakness? First bout or recurrence? Facial or ear pain? Trauma? Stroke? Recent infection? Hearing loss, tinnitus, dizziness, or vertigo? History of sarcoidosis or cancer?

2. Thorough neurologic examination. Determine if facial palsy is central or peripheral, complete or incomplete. Assess taste with bitter or sweet solution on anterior two thirds of tongue on affected side. Carefully assess other cranial nerves, especially the fifth, sixth, and seventh. Look for motor weakness, cerebellar signs.

3. Complete ocular examination. Check ocular motility and look for nystagmus. Assess orbicularis strength bilaterally, degree of ectropion, and Bell's phenomenon. Examine cornea carefully for signs of exposure (superficial punctate keratitis, abrasion, or ulcer). Perform Schirmer's test to assess basic tear production (see Dry Eye Syndrome, Section 4.2, for explanation of Schirmer's test). Check for signs of uveitis.

4. Otolaryngologic examination. Examine ear and oropharynx for vesicles, masses, or other lesions. Palpate parotid for mass or lymphadenopathy. Check hearing.

5. CT scan if history of trauma to rule out basilar skull fracture. Axial and coronal cuts with attention to temporal bone.

6. MRI or CT scan of brain if any other associated neurologic signs or with history of cancer. If sixth-nerve involvement, pay attention to brainstem. If eighth-nerve involvement, pay attention to CPA. If multiple cranial nerves involved, pay attention to base of skull.

7. Chest radiograph and angiotensin-converting enzyme level if sarcoidosis suspected.

8. Lyme titer, Epstein–Barr virus titer, rapid plasma reagin (RPR), HIV test, CBC with differential, as needed, depending on suspected etiology.

9. Rheumatoid factor, erythrocyte sedimentation rate (ESR), antinuclear antibody (ANA), antineutrophil cytoplasmic antibody if collagen–vascular disease suspected.

10. Echocardiogram, Holter monitor, carotid noninvasive studies in patients with a history of stroke.

11. Lumbar puncture (LP) in patients with history of primary neoplasm to rule out carcinomatous meningitis (repeat up to 3 times if negative to increase sensitivity).

Treatment/Follow-up
A. Treat the underlying disease as follows:
  - Stroke: Refer to neurologist.
  - CPA masses, temporal bone fracture, nerve laceration: Refer to neurosurgeon.
  - Otitis: Refer to otolaryngologist.
  - Ramsay–Hunt syndrome: If seen within 72 hours of onset, start acyclovir, 800 mg, 5 times per day for 7 to 10 days (contraindicated in pregnancy and renal failure, see Drug Glossary). Refer to otolaryngologist.
  - Guillain–Barré syndrome: Refer to neurologist. May require urgent hospitalization for rapidly progressive motor weakness or respiratory distress.
  - Lyme disease: Refer to infectious disease specialist. May need LP. Treated with oral doxycycline, penicillin, or i.v. ceftriaxone.
  - Sarcoidosis: Treat uveitis if present (See Section 13.4, Sarcoidosis). Consider brain MRI or LP or both to rule out CNS involvement; if present, refer to neurologist. Refer to internist for systemic evaluation. May require oral prednisone for systemic or CNS disease.
  - Metastatic disease: Refer to oncologist. Systemic chemotherapy, radiation, or both may be required.
B. In idiopathic/Bell's palsy, 86% of patients recover completely with observation only within 2 months. Options for treatment (controversial) include
  1. Facial massage or electrical stimulation of facial musculature.
  2. Oral steroids (e.g., prednisone, 60 mg p.o., daily for 4 days, tapering to 5 mg daily over 10 days). Consider in patients with complete palsy.
  3. Surgical decompression of facial nerve by otolaryngologist. If not resolved after 3 months, order MRI of brain to rule out mass lesion.
C. The primary ocular complication of facial palsy is corneal exposure, which is managed as follows (See also Section 4.4, Exposure Keratopathy):
  1. Mild exposure keratitis: Artificial tears, q.i.d., with lubricating ointment qhs.
  2. Moderate exposure keratitis: Preservative-free artificial tears every 1 to 2 hours, moisture chamber during the day with lubricating ointment, or tape tarsorrhaphy qhs. Consider a temporary tarsorrhaphy.
  3. Severe exposure keratitis: Temporary or permanent tarsorrhaphy. For expected chronic facial palsy, consider eyelid gold weight or spring implants to facilitate eyelid closure.

D. Recheck all patients at 1 and 3 months and more frequently if corneal complications arise.
E. In nonresolving facial palsy with repeatedly negative workup, consider referral to neurosurgeon or plastic surgeon for facial nerve graft, cranial nerve reanastomosis, or temporalis muscle transposition for patients who strongly desire facial reanimation.

11.9 Cavernous Sinus/Superior Orbital Fissure Syndrome
(Multiple Ocular Motor Nerve Palsies)

Symptoms
Double vision, eyelid droop, facial pain or numbness.

Critical Signs
Limitation of eye movement corresponding to any combination of a third-, fourth-, or sixth-nerve palsy on one side; facial pain or numbness or both corresponding to one or more branches of the fifth cranial nerve; a droopy eyelid and a small pupil (Horner's syndrome); the pupil also may be dilated if the third cranial nerve is involved. All signs involve the same side of the face when one cavernous sinus/superior orbital fissure is involved.

Other Signs
Proptosis may be present when the superior orbital fissure is involved.

Etiology
• Arteriovenous fistula [carotid–cavernous ("high-flow") or dural–cavernous ("low-flow")] [Proptosis, chemosis, dilated and tortuous ("corkscrew") episcleral and conjunctival blood vessels. Intraocular pressure is often increased. Enhanced ocular pulsation ("pulsatile proptosis") may be present, sometimes discernible on slit-lamp examination or during applanation. A bruit may even be heard by the patient, and sometimes by the physician if the globe or temple region is auscultated. Reversed, arterialized flow in the superior ophthalmic vein (SOV) is detectable with orbital color Doppler ultrasound; orbital CT scan or MRI may show an enlarged SOV. High-flow fistulas have an abrupt onset and are most commonly caused by trauma or rupture of an intracavernous aneurysm, whereas low-flow fistulas have a more insidious presentation, most commonly in hypertensive women older than 50 years.]

- Tumors within the cavernous sinus [May be primary intracranial neoplasms with direct involvement (e.g., meningioma, pituitary adenoma, craniopharyngioma); or metastatic tumors to the cavernous sinus, either local (e.g., nasopharyngeal carcinoma, perineural spread of a periocular squamous cell carcinoma) or distant metastasis (e.g., breast, lung, lymphoma).]

❖ **Note** *Previously resected tumors may invade the cavernous sinus years after resection.*

- Intracavernous aneurysm (Usually not ruptured. If aneurysm does rupture, the signs of a carotid–cavernous fistula develop.)
- Mucormycosis (Must be suspected in all diabetics, particularly those in ketoacidosis, and any debilitated or immunocompromised individual with multiple cranial nerve palsies, with or without proptosis. Onset is typically acute. Nasal discharge of blood may be present, and nasal examination may reveal a black, crusty material. This condition is life threatening.)
- Pituitary apoplexy (Acute onset of the critical signs listed previously; often bilateral with severe headache, decreased vision, and possibly bitemporal hemianopsia or blindness. An enlarged sella turcica or an intrasellar mass, usually with acute hemorrhage, is seen on CT scan or MRI of the brain.)
- Herpes zoster (Patients with the typical zoster rash may develop ocular motor nerve palsies as well as a middilated pupil that reacts better to convergence than to light.)
- Cavernous sinus thrombosis (Proptosis, chemosis, and eyelid edema. Usually bilateral. Fever, nausea, vomiting, and an altered level of consciousness often develop. May result from spread of infection from the face, mouth, throat, sinus, or orbit. Less commonly noninfectious, resulting from trauma or surgery.)
- Tolosa–Hunt syndrome (Acute idiopathic inflammation of the superior orbital fissure or anterior cavernous sinus. Orbital pain often precedes restriction of eye movements. Recurrent episodes are common. This is a diagnosis of exclusion.)
- Others (e.g., sarcoidosis, Wegener's granulomatosis, mucocele, tuberculosis, and other infections.)

Differential Diagnosis
- Myasthenia gravis [Eyelid droop and limitation of eye movements, especially with fatigue; weakness of the orbicularis oculi muscle; positive edrophonium chloride (e.g., Tensilon) test. No pupillary abnormality, no pain, no proptosis.]
- Chronic progressive external opthalmoplegia (CPEO) (Slowly progressive, painless, bilateral limitation of eye movements with ptosis. The pupils are normal, and the orbicularis oculi muscles are usually weak.)

- Orbital lesions (e.g., tumor, thyroid disease, pseudotumor) [Proptosis and resistance to retropulsion are usually present, in addition to motility restriction. Forced-duction tests are abnormal (see Appendix 5). May have an afferent pupillary defect if the optic nerve is involved.]

❖ **Note** *Orbital apex syndrome combines the superior orbital fissure syndrome with optic nerve dysfunction, and most commonly results from an orbital lesion.*

- Brainstem disease (Tumors and vascular lesions of the brainstem can produce multiple ocular motor nerve palsies. MRI of the brain is best for making this diagnosis.)
- Carcinomatous meningitis (Diffuse seeding of the leptomeninges by metastatic tumor cells can produce a rapidly sequential bilateral cranial nerve disorder. Diagnosis is made by serial lumbar punctures.)
- Skull-base tumors, especially nasopharyngeal carcinoma (Most commonly affects the sixth cranial nerve, but the second, third, fourth, and fifth cranial nerves may be involved as well. Typically, one cranial nerve after another is affected by invasion of the base of the skull. The patient may have cervical lymphadenopathy, nasal obstruction, ear pain or popping caused by serous otitis media or blockage of the eustachian tube, weight loss, or proptosis.)
- Progressive supranuclear palsy (Vertical limitation of eye movements; initially, downward gaze restriction, dementia, and rigidity of the neck and trunk. All eye movements are eventually lost.)
- Rare [Myotonic dystrophy, the bulbar variant of the Guillain–Barré syndrome (Miller–Fisher variant), intracranial sarcoidosis, others.]

Workup

1. History: Diabetes? Hypertension? Recent trauma? Prior cancer (including skin cancer)? Weight loss? Ocular bruit? Recent infection? Severe headache? Diurnal variation of symptoms?
2. Ophthalmic examination: Pay special attention to pupils, extraocular motility, Hertel exophthalmometry, and resistance to retropulsion.
3. Examine the periocular skin for malignant lesions.
4. CT scan (axial and coronal views) or MRI of the sinuses, orbit, and brain, or both.
5. Consider color Doppler imaging if arteriovenous fistula is suspected.

If the CT scan and MRI are normal, consider any or all of the following:

6. Serial lumbar puncture (3 times if first 2 are negative to increase sensitivity) to rule out carcinomatous meningitis in patients with a history of primary carcinoma.

7. Nasopharyngeal examination with or without a blind nasopharyngeal biopsy to rule out nasopharyngeal carcinoma.
8. Lymph node biopsy when lymphadenopathy is present.
9. CBC with differential, erythrocyte sedimentation rate (ESR), antinuclear antibody (ANA), rheumatoid factor to rule out infection, malignancy, and systemic vasculitis. Antineutrophilic cytoplasmic antibody if Wegener's granulomatosis is suspected.
10. Cerebral arteriogram is rarely required to rule out an aneurysm or arteriovenous fistula because most of these are seen by noninvasive imaging studies.
11. If cavernous sinus thrombosis is being considered, obtain two to three sets of peripheral blood cultures, and also culture the presumed primary source of the infection.

Treatment/Follow-up

ARTERIOVENOUS FISTULA

1. Many dural fistulas will close spontaneously, with intermittent ipsilateral carotid massage, or after arteriography. Others may require neurosurgical or interventional neuroradiologic techniques.
2. Treat secondary glaucoma with aqueous suppressants [i.e., topical β-blocker (e.g., timolol or levobunolol, 0.25% to 0.5%, b.i.d.), or topical α_2-agonist (e.g., brimonidine, 0.2%, or apraclonidine, 0.5%, t.i.d.), or both, with or without a carbonic anhydrase inhibitor (e.g., topical dorzolamide, 2%, t.i.d., or methazolamide, 50 mg, p.o., b.i.d.)]. Drugs that increase outflow facility (e.g., epinephrine, latanoprost, and pilocarpine) are generally not so effective because the intraocular pressure is increased as a result of increased episcleral venous pressure. (See Section 10.1, Primary Open-Angle Glaucoma.)

METASTATIC DISEASE TO THE CAVERNOUS SINUS

Often requires systemic chemotherapy (if a primary is found) with or without radiation therapy to the metastasis. Refer to an oncologist.

INTRACAVERNOUS ANEURYSM

Refer to a neurosurgeon for workup and possible treatment.

MUCORMYCOSIS

1. Immediate hospitalization, as this is a rapidly progressive and possibly life-threatening disease.
2. Consult an infectious disease specialist and an otolaryngologist as required.
3. Begin amphotericin B, 0.25 to 0.30 mg/kg, i.v., in D5W slowly over 3 to 6 hours on the first day, 0.5 mg/kg, i.v., on the second day, and then

up to 0.8 to 1.0 mg/kg, i.v., daily. The duration of treatment is determined by the clinical condition.

❖ **Note** *Renal status and electrolytes must be checked before initiating therapy with amphotericin B, and then monitored closely during treatment. (See Drug Glossary.)*

4. Early surgical debridement of all necrotic tissue (possibly including orbital exenteration), plus irrigation of the involved areas with amphotericin B, is often necessary to eradicate the infection.
5. Treat the underlying medical condition, with appropriate consultation as required.

PITUITARY APOPLEXY

Refer immediately to neurosurgeon for surgical consideration. These patients are often quite ill.

HERPES ZOSTER

See Section 4.16, Herpes Zoster Virus.

CAVERNOUS SINUS THROMBOSIS

1. For possible infectious cases (usually caused by *Staphylococcus aureus*), hospitalize the patient and treat with intravenous antibiotics for several weeks. One possible regimen:
   Nafcillin, 1 to 2 g, i.v., q4h, or cefazolin, 1 g, i.v. q8h (or vancomycin 1 g, i.v., q12h if the patient is penicillin allergic);
   plus
   Ceftazidime, 1 to 2 g, i.v., q8h.
   Modify therapy based on blood culture and antibiotic sensitivity results.
2. Intravenous fluid replacement is usually required.
3. For aseptic cavernous sinus thrombosis, consider systemic anticoagulation (heparin followed by warfarin) or aspirin, 325 mg, p.o., daily. Systemic anticoagulation therapy may require collaboration with a medical internist.
4. Exposure keratopathy is treated with lubricating ointment (e.g., Refresh PM, t.i.d. and qhs). (See Section 4.4, Exposure Keratopathy.)
5. Treat secondary glaucoma as described previously for arteriovenous fistulas.

TOLOSA–HUNT SYNDROME

Prednisone, 60 to 100 mg, p.o. daily for 2 to 3 days, and then a short taper (e.g., over 5 to 10 days) as the pain subsides. If pain persists after 72 hours, stop steroids and initiate reinvestigation to rule out other disorders.

❖ **Note** *Other infectious or inflammatory disorders also may respond to steroids initially, so these patients need to be monitored closely. (See Drug Glossary for systemic steroid guidelines.)*

REFERENCES

Kohn R, Hepler R. Management of limited rhino-orbital mucormycosis without exenteration. *Ophthalmology* 1985;92:1440–1444.
Levine SR, Twyman RE, Gilman S. The role of anticoagulation in cavernous sinus thrombosis. *Neurology* 1988;38:517–522.

11.10 MYASTHENIA GRAVIS

Symptoms
Droopy eyelid or double vision or both that is worse toward the end of the day or when the individual is fatigued; may have weakness of facial muscles, proximal limb muscles, and difficulty swallowing or breathing.

Critical Signs
Worsening of eyelid droop with sustained upgaze or double vision with continued eye movements, weakness of the orbicularis muscle on the affected side (cannot close the eyelid as forcefully as on the unaffected side), no pupillary abnormalities.

Other Signs
Upward twitch of ptotic eyelid when shifting gaze from inferior to primary position (Cogan's lid twitch). Can have complete limitation of ocular movements.

Etiology
Autoimmune disease; sometimes triggered by underlying thyroid dysfunction. May be associated with occult thymoma or antecedent infection. Increased incidence of other autoimmune disease (e.g., lupus, multiple sclerosis, rheumatoid arthritis). All age groups can be affected.

Differential Diagnosis
- Eaton–Lambert syndrome (A myasthenia-like paraneoplastic condition associated with carcinoma, especially lung cancer. Isolated eye signs do not occur, although eye signs may accompany systemic signs of weakness. Unlike myasthenia, muscle strength increases after exercise. Electromyography distinguishes between the two conditions.)

- Myasthenia-like syndrome due to medication (e.g., penicillamine, aminoglycosides)
- Chronic progressive external ophthalmoplegia (CPEO) [No diurnal variation of symptoms or relation to fatigue; usually a negative edrophonium chloride (e.g., Tensilon) test, but not always. See Section 11.11, Chronic Progressive External Ophthalmoplegia.]
- Kearns–Sayre syndrome (CPEO and retinal pigmentary degeneration in a young person; heart block develops a few years later. See Section 11.11, Chronic Progressive External Ophthalmoplegia.)
- Third-nerve palsy (Pupil may be involved, no orbicularis weakness, no fatigability, no diurnal variation. See Section 11.5, Isolated Third-Nerve Palsy.)

❖ **Note** *Myasthenia does not respect the boundaries of specific cranial nerves, and the pupil is never involved.*

- Horner's syndrome (Miosis accompanies the ptosis. Pupil does not dilate well in darkness. See Section 11.2, Horner's Syndrome.)
- Levator muscle dehiscence or disinsertion (High eyelid crease on the side of the droopy eyelid, no variability of eyelid droop, no orbicularis weakness.)
- Thyroid eye disease (No ptosis. May have eyelid retraction or eyelid lag, may or may not have exophthalmos, no diurnal variation of double vision. See Section 7.2, Thyroid Eye Disease.)
- Orbital inflammatory disease (pseudotumor) (Proptosis, pain with ocular movements, inflammation. See Section 7.3, Orbital Inflammatory Pseudotumor.)
- Myotonic dystrophy (May have ptosis and rarely, gaze restriction. After a handshake, these patients are often unable to release their grip. May have a Christmas tree cataract.)

Workup
1. History: Do the signs fluctuate with the time of the day and fatigue? Any systemic weakness? Difficulty swallowing, chewing, or breathing? Medications?
2. Have the patient focus on your finger in upgaze for 1 minute. Observe whether the eyelid droops more than expected.
3. Test for double vision in upgaze (hold the eyelid back so each eye can see your finger.)
4. Assess orbicularis strength by asking the patient to squeeze the eyelids shut while you attempt to force them open.
5. Test pupillary function.
6. Blood test for acetylcholine-receptor antibodies (positive in 60% to 88% of patients with myasthenia).

7. In adults, edrophonium chloride (e.g., Tensilon) test will often confirm the diagnosis. Test is performed as follows:
   a. Identify one prominent feature (e.g., ptosis, diplopia) to observe during test. Have cardiac monitor and injectable atropine readily available.
   b. Inject Tensilon, 0.2 ml i.v. Observe for 1 minute. If an improvement in the selected feature is noted, the test is positive and may be stopped at this point. If no improvement or untoward reaction to the medication develops, continue.
   c. Tensilon, 0.4 ml i.v. Observe for 30 seconds for a response or side effect. If neither develops, proceed.
   d. Tensilon, 0.4 ml i.v. If no improvement is noted within 2 additional minutes, the test is negative.

❖ **Note** *Cholinergic crisis, syncopal episode, and respiratory arrest, although rare, may be precipitated by a Tensilon test. Treatment includes atropine, 0.4 mg, i.v., while monitoring vital signs.*

Improvement within the stated time period is diagnostic of myasthenia gravis (rarely a patient with CPEO, an intracavernous tumor, or some other rare disorder will have a false-positive result). A negative test does not exclude myasthenia.
8. In children, observation for improvement immediately after a 1- to 2-hour nap (sleep test) is a safe alternative.
9. Check swallowing function and proximal limb muscle strength to rule out systemic involvement.
10. Thyroid function tests (T_3, T_4, TSH).
11. CT scan of the chest to rule out thymoma.
12 Consider anti-nuclear antibody (ANA), rheumatoid factor, and other tests to rule out other autoimmune disease.
13. Order single-fiber electromyography (EMG) of orbicularis muscle if Tensilon test is negative or contraindicated.

Treatment
Consider collaborating with a neurologist familiar with this disease.

1. If the patient is having difficulty swallowing or breathing, urgent hospitalization with consideration for plasmapheresis or ventilatory support or both may be indicated.
2. If the condition is mild and not disturbing to the patient, therapy need not be instituted (the patient may patch one eye as needed).
3. If the condition is disturbing or more than mild, an oral anticholinesterase agent such as pyridostigmine (e.g., Mestinon, 60 mg, p.o., q.i.d., for an adult) should be given. The dosage must be adjusted according to the response. (Patients rarely benefit from greater than 120

mg, p.o., q3h of pyridostigmine.) Overdosage may produce cholinergic crisis.

4. If symptoms persist, consider systemic steroids. (There is no uniform agreement concerning the dosage. One way is to start with prednisone, 20 mg, p.o., daily, increasing the dose slowly until the patient is receiving 100 mg/day. These patients are monitored in the hospital for several days when the steroids are started if they have systemic myasthenia.)
5. Azathioprine (e.g., Imuran, 1 to 2 mg/kg/day) may be helpful in older patients.
6. Treat any underlying thyroid disease or infection.
7. Surgical removal of a thymoma is usually performed. Thymectomy on patients without a thymoma occasionally helps.

Follow-up

If systemic symptoms are present, patients need to be monitored closely at first (every 1 to 4 days) until improvement is demonstrated. Patients who have had their isolated ocular abnormality for an extended time (e.g., months) need not be seen again for weeks (assuming no worsening of the condition develops). Patients should always be warned to return immediately if swallowing or breathing difficulties arise. After isolated ocular myasthenia has been present for about 2 years, progression to systemic involvement is unlikely.

❖ **Note** *Newborn infants of myasthenic mothers should be observed carefully for signs of myasthenia. Poor sucking reflex, ptosis, or decreased muscle tone may be seen.*

11.11 CHRONIC PROGRESSIVE EXTERNAL OPHTHALMOPLEGIA (CPEO)

Symptoms

Gradual onset of a droopy eyelid, ocular misalignment, and other muscle weakness may or may not be present; ocular involvement is usually bilateral; there is no diurnal variation; there may be a family history.

Critical Signs

Ptosis, limitation of ocular motility (sometimes complete limitation), normal pupils.

Other Signs

Weak orbicularis oculi muscles, weakness of limb and facial muscles, exposure keratopathy.

Differential Diagnosis

See Myasthenia Gravis, Section 11.10, for a complete list. The following are four syndromes that must be ruled out when CPEO is diagnosed. All of them may have CPEO as part of their clinical picture:

- Kearns–Sayre syndrome (Onset before age 20 years, retinal pigmentary degeneration with a salt-and-pepper appearance, heart block that generally occurs years after the ocular signs and may cause sudden death. There is usually no double vision. Other signs may include hearing loss, mental retardation, cerebellar signs, short stature, delayed puberty, nephropathy, vestibular abnormalities, increased cerebrospinal fluid protein, and characteristic findings on muscle biopsy. Inheritance pattern is maternal via mitochondrial DNA.)
- Abetalipoproteinemia (Bassen–Kornzweig syndrome) (Retinal pigmentary degeneration similar to retinitis pigmentosa, diarrhea, ataxia, and other neurologic signs, acanthocytosis of red blood cells seen on peripheral blood smear, increased cerebrospinal fluid protein. See Retinitis Pigmentosa, Section 12.24, for treatment.)
- Refsum's disease (Retinitis pigmentosa and increased blood phytanic acid level. May have polyneuropathy, ataxia, hearing loss, anosmia, others. See Retinitis Pigmentosa, Section 12.24, for treatment.)
- Ocular pharyngeal dystrophy (Difficulty swallowing, sometimes leading to aspiration of food; may have autosomal dominant inheritance.)

Workup

1. Careful history: determine the rate of onset (gradual vs. sudden, as in cranial nerve disease).
2. Family history.
3. Examine the pupils and ocular motility carefully.
4. Test orbicularis oculi strength.
5. Fundus examination: Look for diffuse pigmentary changes.
6. Check swallowing function.
7. Edrophonium chloride (e.g., Tensilon) test to rule out myasthenia gravis (see Section 11.10, Myasthenia Gravis).

❖ **Note** *Sometimes patients with CPEO are supersensitive to Tensilon.*

8. Consider a lumbar puncture if Kearns–Sayre syndrome is a possibility.
9. Yearly electrocardiograms (ECGs) by a cardiologist if Kearns–Sayre syndrome is a possibility.

10. Lipoprotein electrophoresis and peripheral blood smear if abeta-lipoproteinemia is suspected.
11. Serum phytanic acid level if Refsum's disease is suspected.

Treatment

There is no cure for CPEO, but associated abnormalities are managed as follows:

1. Treat exposure keratopathy with lubricants at night (e.g., Refresh PM ointment) and artificial tears during the day (e.g., Refresh tears 4 to 8 times per day). (See Exposure Keratopathy, Section 4.4.)
2. Base-down prisms within reading glasses may help reading when downward gaze is restricted.
3. In Kearns–Sayre syndrome, a pacemaker may be required.
4. In ocular pharyngeal dystrophy, dysphagia and aspirations may require cricopharyngeal surgery.
5. In severe ptosis, consider surgical repair, but watch for worsening exposure keratopathy.
6. Genetic counseling.

Follow-up

Depends on ocular and systemic findings.

11.12 INTERNUCLEAR OPHTHALMOPLEGIA (INO)

Symptoms

Blurry vision or double vision that disappears when one eye is occluded.

Critical Signs

Weakness or paralysis of inward (nasal) eye movement, with horizontal jerk nystagmus of the opposite eye when it attempts to look outward temporally.

Other Signs

A skew deviation (either eye is turned upward, but the three-step test cannot isolate a specific muscle; see Isolated Fourth-Nerve Palsy, Section 11.6), and upbeat nystagmus in upgaze when INO is bilateral. The involved eye can sometimes turn in when attempting to read (intact convergence). Unilateral or bilateral. Bilateral disease can give an exotropia.

Etiology
- Multiple sclerosis (more common in young patients)
- Ischemic vascular disease of the brainstem (more common in elderly patients)
- Brainstem mass lesion (e.g., tumor)

Differential Diagnosis
Other entities that may cause weakness of inward eye movement.

- Myasthenia gravis [May closely mimic INO; however, ptosis and orbicularis oculi weakness are common. Nystagmus of INO is faster; myasthenia gravis is more gaze paretic. Symptoms worsen toward the end of the day when the patient is fatigued. An edrophonium chloride (e.g., Tensilon) test is usually positive. See Section 11.10, Myasthenia Gravis.]
- Orbital disease (e.g., tumor, thyroid disease, inflammatory pseudotumor) (Proptosis, globe displacement, or pain may be present additionally. Nystagmus is usually not present. Orbital CT scan is abnormal. See Section 7.1, Orbital Disease.)

Workup
1. History: Age? Are symptoms always present or do they occur only toward the end of the day with fatigue? Previous episode of optic neuritis, urinary incontinence, numbness or paralysis of an extremity, or another unexplained neurologic event (multiple sclerosis)?
2. Complete ocular examination, including a careful evaluation of eye movement.

❖ **Note** *Ocular motility can appear full, but a muscle weakness can be detected by observing slower saccadic eye movement in the involved eye compared with the contralateral eye. The ability of the right eye to look medially is assessed by holding one of the fingers of the examiner's left hand lateral to the patient's right eye. The patient is asked to first look at the examiner's finger and then at the examiner's nose. If a right INO is present, the right eye will show slower eye movement from the finger to the nose than the left eye. The left eye may be tested in a similar fashion, by holding a finger from the examiner's right hand lateral to the patient's left eye.*

3. Edrophonium chloride (e.g., Tensilon) test when the diagnosis of myasthenia gravis cannot be ruled out (see Section 11.10, Myasthenia Gravis.).
4. MRI of the brainstem and midbrain.

Treatment/Follow-up
- Patients with the diagnosis of a stroke within 72 hours of the acute onset of symptoms are admitted to the hospital for neurologic evaluation and observation.
- Otherwise, patients are managed by physicians familiar with the underlying disease.

11.13 PAPILLEDEMA

Definition
Optic disc swelling produced by increased intracranial pressure.

Symptoms
Episodes of transient, often bilateral, visual loss (lasting seconds) often precipitated by changes in posture; headache; double vision; nausea; vomiting; and rarely, a decrease in visual acuity (a mild decrease in visual acuity can occur in the acute setting if associated with a macular disturbance). Visual-field defects and severe loss of central visual acuity can occur with chronic papilledema.

Critical Signs
Bilaterally swollen, hyperemic discs (in early papilledema, disc swelling may be asymmetric) with blurring of the disc margin, often obscuring the blood vessels. The nerve-fiber layer also usually is involved.

Other Signs
Papillary or peripapillary retinal hemorrhages (often flame-shaped); loss of venous pulsations (note that 20% of the normal population do not have venous pulsations); dilated, tortuous retinal veins; normal pupillary response and color vision; an enlarged physiologic blind spot by formal visual field testing.

As chronic papilledema progresses to optic atrophy, the hemorrhages and cotton-wool spots resolve, peripapillary gliosis and narrowing of the peripapillary retinal vessels occur, and optociliary shunt vessels may develop on the disc. Loss of color vision, central visual acuity, and peripheral visual field, especially inferonasally, also occur.

❖ **Note** *A unilateral or bilateral sixth-nerve palsy also may result from increased intracranial pressure.*

Etiology
- Primary and metastatic intracranial tumors
- Aqueductal stenosis producing hydrocephalus
- Pseudotumor cerebri (Often occurs in young, overweight females. See Section 11.14, Pseudotumor Cerebri.)
- Subdural and epidural hematomas (From trauma.)
- Subarachnoid hemorrhage [Severe headache, may have preretinal hemorrhages (Terson's syndrome).]
- Arteriovenous malformation
- Brain abscess (Often produces high fever.)
- Meningitis [Fever, stiff neck, headache (e.g., syphilis, tuberculosis, Lyme disease, bacterial).]
- Encephalitis (Often produces mental status abnormalities.)
- Sagittal sinus thrombosis

Differential Diagnosis
Other causes of disc swelling.

- Pseudopapilledema (e.g., optic disc drusen or congenitally anomalous disc) (Not true disc swelling. Vessels overlying the disc are not obscured, the disc is not hyperemic, and the surrounding nerve-fiber layer is normal. Spontaneous venous pulsations are often present. Buried drusen may be seen, especially with B-scan ultrasound.)
- Papillitis (An afferent pupillary defect and decreased color vision are often present, white blood cells are seen in the posterior vitreous, pain occurs with eye movement, and decreased visual acuity occurs in most cases, usually unilateral. See Optic Neuritis, Section 11.15.)
- Malignant hypertensive retinopathy (Blood pressure extremely high, narrowed arterioles. May have arteriovenous crossing changes. Hemorrhages with or without cotton-wool spots extend to the peripheral retina. See Section 12.5, Hypertensive Retinopathy.)
- Central retinal vein occlusion (Hemorrhages extend far beyond the peripapillary area, dilated and tortuous veins, generally unilateral, acute loss of vision in most cases. See Section 12.3, Central Retinal Vein Occlusion.)
- Ischemic optic neuropathy (Disc swelling is pale, not hyperemic; initially unilateral with sudden, sometimes severe, visual loss. See Sections 11.16, Giant Cell Arteritis, and 11.17, Nonarteritic Ischemic Optic Neuropathy.)
- Optic-disc vasculitis (Unilateral disc swelling in a young patient. There may be flame-shaped hemorrhages in the periphery.)
- Infiltration of the optic disc (e.g., sarcoid or tuberculous granuloma, leukemia, metastasis, other inflammatory disease or tumor) (Other ocu-

lar or systemic abnormalities may be present. The disc may have an irregular outline. Usually unilateral.)

- Leber's optic neuropathy (Usually occurs in men in the second to third decades of life; initially unilateral but rapidly bilateral; rapid, progressive visual loss; disc swelling associated with peripapillary telangiectasias. Optic atrophy later develops. See Section 11.18, Miscellaneous Optic Neuropathies.)
- Orbital optic-nerve tumors (Unilateral disc swelling, may or may not have proptosis. See Section 11.18, Miscellaneous Optic Neuropathies.)
- Diabetic papillitis (Disc edema in a young, type 1 diabetic; usually bilateral. May have moderate-to-severe retinopathy. See Section 14.6, Diabetes Mellitus.)
- Graves' ophthalmopathy (May have a history of thyroid dysfunction. May have lid lag or retraction, ocular misalignment, proptosis, increased intraocular pressure, and resistance to retropulsion. See Section 7.2, Thyroid Eye Disease.)
- Uveitis (e.g., syphilis or sarcoidosis) (May produce pain or photophobia. May have injection, keratic precipitates, anterior chamber cell and flare, posterior synechiae and vitreous cells. See Section 13.2, Posterior Uveitis.)

❖ **Note** *Optic-disc swelling in a patient with a history of leukemia is often a visually threatening sign of leukemic infiltration of the optic nerve. Immediate radiation therapy is usually required to preserve vision.*

Workup
1. History and physical examination, including blood pressure measurement.
2. Ocular examination, including a pupillary and color vision (using color plates) assessment, posterior vitreous evaluation to check for white blood cells, and a dilated fundus examination by using indirect ophthalmoscopy. The optic disc is best examined with a slit lamp and Hruby, fundus contact, or 60-diopter lens.
3. Emergency CT scan (axial and coronal views) or MRI of the head and orbit or both.
4. Lumbar puncture if the CT or MRI or both do not reveal the cause of the papilledema. Consider blood tests for thyroid disease, diabetes, and anemia.

Treatment
Treatment should be directed at the underlying cause of the increased intracranial pressure.

11.14 PSEUDOTUMOR CEREBRI
(Idiopathic Intracranial Hypertension)

Symptoms

Headache (usually worse in the morning), transient episodes of visual loss (typically lasting seconds) often precipitated by changes in posture, double vision (objects appear side by side; the double vision resolves when one eye is covered), tinnitus, dizziness, nausea, or vomiting. Occurs predominantly in women.

Critical Signs

By definition, a patient with pseudotumor cerebri will display the following findings:

1. Increased intracranial pressure with papilledema.
2. Normal MRI of the brain.
3. Normal cerebrospinal fluid composition.

Other Signs

See Papilledema, Section 11.13. As with other causes of papilledema, may have a unilateral or bilateral sixth-nerve palsy.

Etiology

Associated factors include obesity, pregnancy, and various medications, including oral contraceptives, tetracycline, nalidixic acid, and vitamin A. Systemic steroid withdrawal may also be causative.

Differential Diagnosis

See Papilledema, Section 11.13.

Workup

1. History: Inquire specifically about medications.
2. Ocular examination, including pupillary and intraocular pressure assessment, color vision test (color plates), and optic-nerve evaluation.
3. Systemic examination, including blood pressure and temperature.
4. MRI of the orbit and brain. Any patient with papilledema needs to be imaged immediately. If normal, the patient should have a thorough neuro-ophthalmologic evaluation, including a lumbar puncture, to rule out other causes of papilledema and to determine the opening pressure (see Section 11.13, Papilledema).
5. Visual field test (e.g., Octopus, Humphrey, Goldmann, or other).

Treatment

Pseudotumor cerebri may be a self-limited process. Treatment is indicated in the following situations:

- Severe intractable headache
- Evidence of progressive decrease in visual acuity or visual field loss.

Methods of treatment include the following.

1. Weight loss if overweight.
2. Acetazolamide (e.g., Diamox) 250 mg, p.o., q.i.d. initially, building up to 500 mg, q.i.d., if tolerated. Other diuretics (e.g., furosemide) have no proven efficacy.
3. Discontinuation of any causative medication.

If treatment by these methods is unsuccessful, one of the following may be tried.

4. Systemic steroids (controversial).
5. Optic-nerve sheath decompression surgery is often effective if vision is threatened (our choice).
6. Lumboperitoneal shunt if intractable headache is primary problem.

❖ **Note** *Any increase in intraocular pressure needs to be treated aggressively to avoid further injury to the optic nerve.*

Follow-up

Every 2 to 3 weeks initially, monitor for visual loss, especially visual field loss, and then every 4 to 6 weeks, depending on the response to treatment.

11.15 OPTIC NEURITIS

Symptoms

Loss of vision deteriorating over hours (rarely) to days (most commonly), with the nadir about 1 week after onset. Visual loss may be subtle or profound.

- Usually unilateral, but may be bilateral.
- Age typically 18 to 45 years.
- Orbital pain, especially with eye movement.
- Acquired loss of color vision.
- Reduced perception of light intensity.
- May have other focal neurologic symptoms (e.g., weakness, numbness, tingling in extremities).

- May have antecedent flu-like viral syndrome.
- Occasionally altered perception of moving objects (Pulfrich phenomenon), or a worsening of symptoms with exercise or increase in body temperature (Uhtoff's sign).

Critical Signs

Relative afferent pupillary defect (RAPD) in unilateral or asymmetric cases; decreased color vision; central, cecocentral, arcuate, or altitudinal visual-field defects.

Other Signs

Swollen disc with or without peripapillary flame-shaped hemorrhages (papillitis most commonly seen in children and young adults) or a normal disc (retrobulbar optic neuritis more common in adults). Posterior vitreous cells may be observed.

Etiology

- Idiopathic
- Multiple sclerosis (MS) (frequently optic neuritis is the initial manifestation of MS.)
- Childhood infections (e.g., measles, mumps, chickenpox)
- Other viral infections (e.g., mononucleosis, herpes zoster, encephalitis)
- Contiguous inflammation of the meninges, orbit, or sinuses
- Granulomatous inflammations (e.g., tuberculosis, syphilis, sarcoidosis, cryptococcus)
- Intraocular inflammations

Differential Diagnosis

- Ischemic optic neuropathy (ION) (Visual loss is sudden, no pain with ocular motility, optic nerve swelling tends to be pale. Visual-field defects are most commonly inferior altitudinal. In ION caused by giant cell arteritis (GCA), patients are older than 50 years. In nonarteritic ION, patients are typically 40 to 60 years of age. See Sections 11.16, Giant Cell Arteritis, and 11.17, Nonarteritic Ischemic Optic Neuropathy.)
- Acute papilledema (Bilateral disc edema, no decreased color vision, no decreased visual acuity, no pain with ocular motility, no vitreous cells. Spontaneous venous pulsations are almost always absent. An enlarged blind spot is often noted on visual field testing. See Section 11.13, Papilledema.)
- Severe systemic hypertension (Bilateral disc edema, increased blood pressure, flame-shaped retinal hemorrhages, and cotton-wool spots. See Section 12.5, Hypertensive Retinopathy.)
- Orbital tumor compressing the optic nerve (Unilateral, often proptosis or restriction of extraocular motility is evident; there are no vitreous

cells even when disc swelling is present. See Section 7.1, Orbital Tumor.)

- Intracranial mass compressing the afferent visual pathway (Normal disc, positive afferent pupillary defect, decreased color vision, mass evident on CT scan or MRI of the brain.)
- Leber's optic neuropathy (Usually occurs in men in the second or third decade of life, may or may not have family history, rapid visual loss of one and then the other eye within days to months, may have peripapillary telangiectasias. Disc swelling is followed by optic atrophy. See Section 11.18, Miscellaneous Optic Neuropathies.)
- Toxic or metabolic optic neuropathy [Progressive painless bilateral visual loss, may be secondary to alcohol, malnutrition, various toxins (e.g., ethambutol, chloroquine, isoniazid, chlorpropamide, heavy metals), anemia, and others. See Section 11.18, Miscellaneous Optic Neuropathies.]

Workup

1. History: Determine the patient's age and the rapidity of onset of the visual loss. Previous episode? Pain with eye movement?
2. Complete ophthalmic and neurologic examinations, including pupillary assessment, color vision evaluation with color plates, evaluation of the vitreous for cells, and dilated retinal examination with optic nerve assessment.
3. Check blood pressure.
4. Visual-field test, preferably automated (e.g., Octopus, Humphrey).
5. For atypical cases (e.g., out of typical age range, no pain with eye movement), consider the following: complete blood count (CBC), rapid plasma reagin (RPR), fluorescent treponemal antibody, absorbed (FTA-ABS), anti-nuclear antibody (ANA), erythrocyte sedimentation rate (ESR).
6. For first episode or atypical case, MRI of the brain and orbits with gadolinium.

Treatment

A. If patient seen acutely with no prior history of MS or optic neuritis:
1. If MRI reveals at least one area of demyelination, offer pulsed i.v. steroid in the following regimen: Methylprednisolone, 250 mg, i.v., over 30 minutes q6h for 12 doses, followed by prednisone, 1 mg/kg/day, p.o., for 11 days, and then taper off over 5 to 7 days. This treatment decreases recurrence of optic neuritis and shortens the duration of visual impairment. However, the long-term visual outcome is no different from observation alone, because spontaneous recovery is the natural course in most cases.
2. With a normal MRI, the risk of MS is low regardless of treatment, but pulsed i.v. steroid may still be used to hasten visual recovery.

3. Do not use oral prednisone as a primary treatment because of increased risk of recurrences.

B. In patient with diagnosis of prior MS or optic neuritis, observation.

❖ **Notes**

- *See Drug Glossary for systemic steroid evaluation.*
- *An antiulcer medication (e.g., ranitidine, 150 mg, p.o., b.i.d.) is given along with systemic steroids.*

Follow-up

In general, examine the patient every 1 to 3 months. Patients being treated with steroids must be followed more closely because of the risk of intraocular pressure increase. Patients with CNS demyelination on MRI or an abnormal neurologic examination should be referred to a neurologist for evaluation and management of possible MS.

REFERENCES

Beck R, Cleary PA, Anderson MM, et al. A randomized controlled trial of corticosteroids in the treatment of acute optic neuritis. *N Engl J Med* 1992;326:581–588.

Beck RW, Cleary PA, Trobe JD, et al., and the Optic Neuritis Study Group. The effect of corticosteroids for acute optic neuritis on the subsequent development of multiple sclerosis. *N Engl J Med* 1993;329:1764–1769.

Wray SH. Optic neuritis: guidelines. *Curr Opin Neurol* 1995;8:72–76.

11.16 ARTERITIC ISCHEMIC OPTIC NEUROPATHY
[Giant Cell Arteritis (GCA)]

Symptoms

Sudden, painless, nonprogressive visual loss; initially unilateral, but may rapidly become bilateral; occurs in patients older than 50 years; antecedent or simultaneous headache, jaw claudication (pain with chewing), scalp tenderness (tenderness with hair combing), proximal muscle and joint aches (polymyalgia rheumatica), anorexia, weight loss, or fever may occur.

Critical Signs

Afferent pupillary defect; devastating visual loss (often counting fingers or worse); pale, swollen disc, often with flame-shaped hemorrhages. Later, optic atrophy occurs as the edema resolves. The erythrocyte sedimentation rate (ESR) may be markedly increased.

Other Signs
Visual-field defect (commonly altitudinal or involving the central field); a palpable, tender, and often nonpulsatile temporal artery; a central retinal artery occlusion or a cranial nerve palsy (especially a sixth-nerve palsy) may occur.

Differential Diagnosis
- Nonarteritic ischemic optic neuropathy (Patients may be younger, usually have less severe visual loss, do not have the accompanying symptoms of giant cell arteritis (GCA) listed previously, and usually have a normal ESR. See Section 11.17.)
- Inflammatory optic neuritis (papillitis) (Affects a younger age group, typically less severe and less sudden onset of visual loss, pain with eye movements, optic-disc swelling is more hemorrhagic, posterior vitreous cells are often present, no symptoms of GCA. See Section 11.15, Optic Neuritis.)
- Compressive optic nerve tumor (Slowly progressive visual loss, few-to-no symptoms in common with GCA. See Section 11.18, Miscellaneous Optic Neuropathies)
- Central retinal vein occlusion (Severe visual loss may be accompanied by an afferent pupillary defect and disc swelling, but the retina shows diffuse retinal hemorrhages extending out to the periphery. See Section 12.3, Central Retinal Vein Occlusion.)
- Central retinal artery occlusion (Sudden, painless, severe visual loss with an afferent pupillary defect, but the disc is not swollen, and retinal edema with a cherry-red spot is frequently observed. See Section 12.1, Central Retinal Artery Occlusion.)

Workup
1. History: Attempt to elicit the symptoms. Age is critical.
2. Complete ocular examination, particularly pupillary assessment, color plates, dilated retinal examination to rule out retinal causes of severe visual loss, and optic nerve evaluation.
3. Immediate ESR (Westergren is the most reliable method) and C-reactive protein. A guideline for top normal ESR: men, age/2; women, (age + 10)/2.

4. Perform a temporal artery biopsy if GCA is suspected from the symptoms, signs, or ESR. The ESR may not be increased.

❖ **Note** *The biopsy should be performed within 1 week after starting systemic steroids, but a positive result may be seen up to 1 month later. Biopsy is especially important in patients in whom steroids are relatively contraindicated (e.g., diabetics).*

5. Consider ocular pneumoplethysmography (OPG) to look for reduced ocular blood flow as an aid in diagnosis.

Treatment

Systemic steroids should be given immediately once GCA is suspected. We give methylprednisolone, 250 mg i.v., q6h, for 12 doses in the hospital, and then switch to prednisone, 80 to 100 mg, p.o., daily. A temporal artery biopsy specimen is obtained while the patient is in the hospital.

- If the temporal artery biopsy is positive for GCA, then the patient must be maintained on prednisone, 80 to 100 mg, p.o., daily.
- If the biopsy is negative on an adequate (2-cm) section, then the likelihood of GCA is small. However, in highly suggestive cases, biopsy of the contralateral artery is performed. Steroids are usually discontinued when the disease is not found in adequate biopsy specimens, unless the clinical presentation is classic and a response to treatment has occurred.

❖ **Note**
- *Without steroids (and occasionally on adequate steroids), the contralateral eye can become involved within 24 hours.*
- *A histamine$_2$-blocker (e.g., ranitidine, 150 mg, p.o., b.i.d.) or another antiulcer medication is given along with systemic steroids.*
- *See Medical Glossary for systemic steroid workup.*

Follow-up

Patients suspected of having GCA must be evaluated and treated immediately. After the diagnosis is confirmed by biopsy, the initial oral steroid dosage is maintained for 2 to 4 weeks until the symptoms resolve and ESR normalizes. The dosage is then tapered slowly, repeating the ESR with each dosage change or monthly to ensure that the new steroid dosage is enough to suppress the disease. If the ESR increases or symptoms return, the dosage must be increased. Treatment should last at least 3 to 6 months and sometimes for 1 year or more. The smallest dose that suppresses the disease is used.

11.17 NONARTERITIC ISCHEMIC OPTIC NEUROPATHY (NAION)

Symptoms

Sudden, painless, nonprogressive visual loss of moderate degree, initially unilateral, but may become bilateral. Typically occurs in patients aged 40 to 60 years.

Critical Signs

Afferent pupillary defect, pale disc swelling often involving only a segment of the disc, flame-shaped hemorrhages, normal erythrocyte sedimentation rate (ESR).

1. Nonprogressive NAION: Sudden initial decrease in visual acuity and visual field, which stabilizes.
2. Progressive NAION: Sudden initial decrease in visual acuity and visual field followed by a second decrease in acuity or visual field days to weeks later.

Other Signs

Reduced color vision, altitudinal or central visual-field defect, optic atrophy (segmental or diffuse) after the edema resolves.

Etiology

Idiopathic. (Arteriosclerosis, diabetes, hypertension, and hyperlipidemia are associated risk factors, but causation has never been proven. Also, relative nocturnal hypotension is thought by some to play a role, especially in patients taking antihypertensive medication.)

Differential Diagnosis

See Arteritic Ischemic Optic Neuropathy, Section 11.16.

Workup

Same as Arteritic Ischemic Optic Neuropathy, Section 11.16. A medical evaluation by an internist is obtained to rule out cardiovascular disease, diabetes, and hypertension.

Treatment

1. Observation.
2. Consider aspirin, 80 to 325 mg, p.o., daily in conjunction with patient's primary medical doctor, although benefit in NAION has not been proven.

3. Patients should avoid taking blood pressure medication at bedtime if possible to help avoid nocturnal hypotension.

Follow-up

One month. Up to 40% of patients have shown mild improvement in vision over 3 to 6 months in some studies.

11.18 MISCELLANEOUS OPTIC NEUROPATHIES

Toxic/Metabolic Optic Neuropathy

Symptoms

Painless, progressive, bilateral loss of vision.

Critical Signs

Bilateral cecocentral or central visual field defects, signs of alcoholism or poor nutrition.

Other Signs

Visual acuity of 20/50 to 20/200, reduced color vision, temporal disc pallor, optic atrophy, or normal-appearing disc.

Etiology

- Tobacco/alcohol abuse
- Severe malnutrition with thiamine (vitamin B_1) deficiency
- Pernicious anemia (Usually due to a problem with vitamin B_{12} absorption.)
- Toxic [Often from chloramphenicol, ethambutol, isoniazid, digitalis, chloroquine, streptomycin, chlorpropamide, ethchlorvynol (e.g., Placidyl), disulfiram (e.g., Antabuse), and lead.]

Workup

1. History: Drug or substance abuse? Medications? Diet?
2. Complete ocular examination, including pupillary evaluation, color testing with color plates, and optic nerve examination.
3. Formal visual-field test (e.g., Goldmann).
4. Complete blood count (CBC).
5. Serum vitamin B_1, B_{12}, and folate levels (consider a gastrointestinal consult for possible Schilling's test if the vitamin B_{12} level is low).
6. Consider a heavy metal (i.e., lead, thallium) screen.

7. Consider blood test for Leber's hereditary optic neuropathy (clinical presentation of Leber's neuropathy may mimic toxic/metabolic optic neuropathy).

Treatment
1. Thiamine, 100 mg, p.o., b.i.d.
2. Folate, 1.0 mg, p.o., daily.
3. Multivitamin tablet daily.
4. Eliminate any causative agent (e.g., alcohol, medication).
5. Vitamin B_{12}, 1,000 μg, i.m. every month for pernicious anemia (usually coordinated by the patient's internist).

Follow-up
Every month at first, and then every 6 to 12 months.

Compressive Optic Neuropathy

Symptoms
Slowly progressive visual loss, although occasionally acute or noticed acutely.

Critical Signs
Central visual-field defect, relative afferent pupillary defect.

Other Signs
The optic nerve can be normal, pale, or occasionally, swollen; proptosis; optociliary shunt vessels (small vessels around the disc that shunt blood from the retinal to the choroidal venous circulation).

Etiology
- Optic nerve glioma (Patients usually younger than 20 years, often associated with neurofibromatosis.)
- Optic nerve meningioma [Usually affects adult women. Orbital imaging may show an optic nerve mass, diffuse optic nerve thickening, or a railroad-track sign (increased contrast of the periphery of the nerve).]
- Any intraorbital mass (e.g., hemangioma, schwannoma)

Workup
All patients with progressive visual loss and optic nerve dysfunction should have CT scan (coronal and axial views) or MRI of the orbit and brain.

Treatment/Follow-up
Depends on the etiology. Treatments of optic nerve glioma and meningioma are controversial. These lesions are often monitored unless there is evidence of intracranial involvement, at which point, surgical excision may be indicated.

Leber's Optic Neuropathy

Symptoms
Rapidly progressive visual loss of one and then the other eye within days to months of each other, painless.

Critical Signs
Mild swelling of optic disc progressing over weeks to optic atrophy; small telangiectatic blood vessels near the disc that do not leak on i.v. fluorescein angiography, usually occurs in young men aged 15 to 30 years, and less commonly in women in their second to third decade of life.

Other Signs
Visual acuity 20/200 to counting fingers, cecocentral visual-field defect.

Transmission
By mitochondrial DNA, so it is transmitted by women to all of offspring. However, 50% to 70% of sons and 10% to 15% of daughters manifest the disease. All daughters are carriers, and none of the sons can transmit the disease.

Workup
Send blood for known Leber's mutations.

Treatment
No effective treatment is available. Genetic counseling should be offered. A cardiology consult may be indicated, as patients have a higher incidence of cardiac conduction defects.

Dominant Optic Neuropathy

Mid-to-moderate bilateral visual loss (20/40 to 20/200) usually presenting about age 4 to 8 years, slow progression, temporal disc pallor, cecocentral visual-field defect, tritanopic (blue–yellow) color defect on Farnsworth–Munsell 100-hue test, strong family history, no nystagmus.

Complicated Hereditary Optic Atrophy

Bilateral optic atrophy with spinocerebellar degenerations (e.g., Friedreich's, Marie's, Behr's), polyneuropathy (e.g., Charcot–Marie–Tooth), or inborn errors of metabolism.

Radiation Optic Neuropathy

Delayed effect (usually 1 to 5 years) after radiation therapy to the eye, orbit, sinus, nasopharynx, and occasionally brain with acute or gradual step-wise visual loss, often severe. Disc swelling, radiation retinopathy, or both may or may not be present.

11.19 NYSTAGMUS

Nystagmus is divided into congenital or acquired forms.

Symptoms
Asymptomatic unless acquired after 8 years of age, at which point the environment may be noted to oscillate horizontally, vertically, or torsionally, or vision may seem blurred or unstable.

Critical Signs
Repetitive oscillations of the eye horizontally, vertically, or torsionally.

Jerk nystagmus: The eye slowly drifts in one direction (slow phase) and then abruptly returns to its original position (fast phase), only to drift again and repeat the cycle.

Pendular nystagmus: Drift occurs in two phases of equal speed, giving a smooth back-and-forth movement of the eye.

Congenital Forms of Nystagmus

A. Infantile Nystagmus

Onset at age 2 to 3 months, with wide, swinging eye movements. At age 4 to 6 months, small pendular eye movements are added, and at age 6 to 12 months, jerk nystagmus and a null point (a position of gaze where the nystagmus is minimized) develop. Compensatory head nodding develops at any point up to age 20 years. Infantile nystagmus is usually horizontal and typically dampens with convergence. May have a latent component.

Etiology
- Idiopathic
- Albinism (Iris transillumination defects and foveal hypoplasia are common. See Section 14.7, Albinism.)
- Aniridia (Bilateral, near-total absence of iris from birth. See Section 9.11, Developmental Anterior Segment and Lens Anomalies.)
- Leber's congenital amaurosis (Markedly abnormal or flat electroretinogram.)

- Others (e.g., bilateral optic nerve hypoplasia, bilateral congenital cataracts, rod monochromatism, optic nerve or macular disease.)

Differential Diagnosis
- Opsoclonus (Repetitive, irregular, multidirectional eye movements associated with cerebellar or brainstem disease, postviral encephalitis, visceral carcinoma, or neuroblastoma.)
- Spasmus nutans (Head nodding and head turn with vertical, horizontal, or torsional nystagmus appearing between 6 months and 3 years of age and resolving between 2 and 8 years of age. Unilateral or bilateral. Glioma of the optic chiasm may produce an identical clinical picture and needs to be ruled out with MRI.)
- Latent nystagmus (See the following.)
- Nystagmus blockage syndrome (See the following.)

Workup
1. History: Age of onset? Head nodding? Known ocular or systemic abnormalities? Medications? Family history?
2. Complete ocular examination: Carefully observe the eye movements, check for iris transillumination, and inspect the optic disc and macula for disease.
3. Consider obtaining an eye-movement recording if the diagnosis of infantile nystagmus is uncertain.
4. When opsoclonus cannot be ruled out, obtain a urinary vanillylmandelic acid and consider an abdominal CT scan to rule out neuroblastoma and visceral carcinoma.
5. In selected cases and in all cases of suspected spasmus nutans, a CT scan or MRI of the brain (axial and coronal views) may be obtained to rule out organic pathology.

Treatment
1. Maximize vision by refraction.
2. Treat amblyopia if indicated.
3. If small face turn: Prescribe prism in glasses with base in direction of face turn.
4. If large face turn: Consider muscle surgery.

B. Latent Nystagmus

Occurs only when one eye is viewing. Fast phase of nystagmus beats toward viewing eye.

Manifest latent nystagmus: occurs in children with strabismus or decreased vision in one eye, in whom the nonfixating or poorly seeing eye behaves as an occluded eye.

❖ **Note** *When testing visual acuity in one eye, fog (i.e., add plus lenses in front of) rather than occluding the opposite eye to minimize induction of latent nystagmus.*

Treatment
1. Maximize vision by refraction.
2. Treat amblyopia if indicated.
3. Consider muscle surgery if symptomatic strabismus exists.

C. Nystagmus Blockage Syndrome (NBS)

Any nystagmus that decreases when the fixating eye is in adduction and demonstrates an esotropia to dampen the nystagmus.

Treatment
For large face turn, consider muscle surgery.

Acquired Forms of Nystagmus

Etiology
- Visual loss (e.g., dense cataract, trauma, cone dystrophy) (Usually monocular and vertical nystagmus.)
- Toxic/metabolic (e.g., alcohol intoxication, lithium, barbiturates, phenytoin, salicylates, benzodiazepines, phencyclidine, other anticonvulsants or sedatives, Wernicke's encephalopathy, thiamine deficiency)
- CNS disorders [e.g., thalamic hemorrhage, tumor, stroke, trauma, multiple sclerosis (MS)]
- Nonphysiologic (Voluntary, rapid, horizontal, small oscillatory movements of the eyes that usually cannot be sustained more than 30 seconds without fatigue.)

Types of Nystagmus with Localizing Neuroanatomic Significance

- See-saw (One eye rises and intorts while the other descends and extorts. Most commonly, the lesion involves the chiasm or third ventricle or both. May have a bitemporal hemianopia resulting from a parasellar mass. Rarely congenital.)
- Convergence retraction (Convergence-like eye movements are accompanied by retraction of the globe into the orbit when the patient attempts to look up. There is limitation of upward gaze, eyelid retraction, and large, unreactive pupils. Papilledema may be present. Usually, a pineal gland tumor or other midbrain abnormality is responsible.)
- Upbeat (The fast phase of the nystagmus is up. Most commonly, the lesion involves the brainstem or vermis of the cerebellum when the nys-

tagmus is present in primary position. If the nystagmus is present only in upgaze, the most likely etiology is drug effect.)

- Rebound (Triggered by changing directions of gaze. The fast phase is in the direction of gaze, but fatigue occurs with sustained gaze, and the fast phase then changes direction. When gaze is returned to primary position, the fast phase increases in the direction the eye takes in returning to the primary position. Most commonly, the lesion involves the cerebellum.)
- Gaze-evoked (Not present when the individual looks straight, but appears as the eyes look to the side. Nystagmus increases when looking in direction of fast phase. Slow frequency. Most commonly the result of alcohol intoxication, sedatives, cerebellar or brainstem disease.)
- Downbeat [The fast phase of nystagmus is down. Most commonly, the lesion is at the cervicomedullary junction (e.g., Arnold–Chiari malformation).]
- Periodic alternating [Fast eye movements are in one direction (with head turn) for 60 to 90 seconds, and then reverse direction for 60 to 90 seconds. The cycle repeats continuously. May be congenital, or rarely, the result of blindness. Acquired forms not caused by blindness are most commonly the result of lesions of the cervicomedullary junction.]
- Vestibular [Horizontal or horizontal rotary nystagmus. May be accompanied by vertigo, tinnitus, or deafness. May be due to dysfunction of vestibular end organ (inner-ear disease), eighth cranial nerve, or eighth-nerve nucleus in brainstem. Destructive lesions produce fast phases opposite to affected end organ or nerve. Irritative lesions produce fast phase in the same direction as the affected end organ. Vestibular nystagmus associated with interstitial keratitis is called Cogan's syndrome.]

Differential Diagnosis
- Superior oblique myokymia (Small, unilateral, vertical, and torsional movements of one eye can be seen with a slit lamp or ophthalmoscope. Symptoms and signs are more pronounced when the involved eye looks inferonasally. Usually benign, resolving spontaneously. Can be treated with carbamazepine, 200 mg, p.o., t.i.d. A medical consult for hematologic evaluation before carbamazepine use and periodic evaluation during therapy are recommended.)
- Opsoclonus (Rapid, chaotic conjugate saccades. Etiology in children is neuroblastoma or encephalitis. In adults, it can be seen with drug intoxication or following infarction.)
- Myoclonus [Pendular oscillation associated with contraction of nonocular muscles (e.g., palate, tongue, facial muscles). Involves olive nucleus in medulla.]

Workup
1. History: Nystagmus, strabismus, or amblyopia in infancy? Oscillopsia? Drug or alcohol use? Vertigo? Episodes of weakness, numbness, or decreased vision in the past (MS)?
2. Family history: Nystagmus? Albinism? Eye disorder?
3. Complete ocular examination: Pay close attention to the eye movements. Slit-lamp or optic-disc observation may be helpful in subtle cases. Iris transillumination should be performed to rule out albinism.
4. Obtain an eye-movement recording when congenital nystagmus is being considered.
5. Visual field examination, particularly with see-saw nystagmus.
6. Consider a drug/toxin/dietary screen of the urine, serum, or both.
7. CT scan or MRI as needed. (Make sure the scan carefully evaluates the area that most commonly causes the particular nystagmus.)

❖ **Note** *The cervicomedullary junction and cerebellum are best evaluated with MRI.*

Treatment
1. The underlying etiology must be treated.
2. The nystagmus of periodic alternating nystagmus may respond to baclofen. (Baclofen is given in three divided doses, starting with a total daily dose of 15 mg, p.o., and increasing by 15 mg every 3 days until a desired therapeutic effect is obtained. Do not exceed 80 mg/day. If there is no improvement with the maximal tolerated dose, the dosage should be tapered slowly. Baclofen is not recommended for use in children.)
2. Severe disabling nystagmus can be treated with retrobulbar injections of botulinum toxin.

Follow-up
A workup should be instituted as soon as possible to rule out a CNS abnormality.

11.20 VERTEBROBASILAR ARTERY INSUFFICIENCY

Symptoms
Transient bilateral blurred vision lasting from a few seconds to a few minutes, sometimes accompanied by flashing lights. Ataxia, vertigo, dysarthria or dysphasia, and hemiparesis or hemisensory loss may accompany

the visual symptoms. History of drop attacks (the patient suddenly falls to the ground without warning or loss of consciousness). Recurrent attacks are common.

Signs
Normal ocular examination.

Differential Diagnosis
Causes of transient visual loss.

- Papilledema (Bilateral visual loss lasts 5 to 15 seconds. See Section 11.13, Papilledema.)
- Migraine (Visual loss from 10 to 45 minutes, often with history of migraine headache or car-sickness, or a family history of migraine. May or may not be followed by a headache. See Section 15.4, Migraine.)
- Amaurosis fugax (Monocular, usually lasts minutes, appears as if a curtain drops down in front of the eye. See Section 12.6, Amaurosis fugax.)
- Giant cell arteritis (GCA) (Can cause transient visual loss in patients older than 50 years. Usually associated with temporal headache, scalp tenderness, pain with chewing, weight loss, fever, and anorexia. See Section 11.16, Giant Cell Arteritis.)
- Vertebral artery dissection (After trauma or resulting from atherosclerotic disease.)

Workup
1. History: Associated symptoms of vertebrobasilar insufficiency? History of car-sickness or migraine? Symptoms of GCA?
2. Dilated fundus examination: Look for retinal emboli or papilledema.
3. Blood pressure in each arm: Look for the subclavian steal syndrome.
4. Cardiac auscultation to rule out arrhythmia.
5. ECG and Holter monitor for 24 hours: Look for sick sinus syndrome, ventricular ectopy.
6. Consider carotid noninvasive flow studies.
7. Magnetic resonance angiography (MRA) or transcranial/vertebral artery Doppler ultrasound to evaluate posterior cerebral blood flow.
8. CBC to rule out anemia and polycythemia, with immediate ESR if GCA is possible.
9. Consider cervical spine radiographs to rule out compressive cervical spine disease if arthritis of the neck is present.

Treatment
1. Aspirin, 80 mg, p.o., daily.
2. Control hypertension, diabetes, and hyperlipidemia if present, as per medical internist.

3. Reduce fat and cholesterol intake; stop smoking.
4. Correct any underlying problem revealed by the workup.

Follow-up
One week to check test results.

11.21 CORTICAL BLINDNESS

Symptoms
Bilateral complete or severe loss of vision. Patients may deny they are blind (Anton's syndrome).

Critical Signs
Markedly decreased vision and visual field in both eyes (sometimes no light perception) with normal pupillary responses.

Etiology
Most common Bilateral occipital lobe infarctions.
Rare Neoplasm (e.g., metastasis, meningioma).

Workup
1. Test vision with a near card (sometimes patients with bilateral occipital lobe infarcts appear completely blind, but actually have a very small residual visual field and are unable to locate a distant eye chart.)
2. Complete ocular and neurologic examinations.
3. Rule out functional visual loss by appropriate testing (see Nonphysiologic Visual Loss, Section 11.22).
4. Cardiac auscultation to rule out arrhythmia.
5. Check blood pressure.
6. MRI of the brain.
7. CBC to rule out polycythemia in cases of stroke.
8. Refer to a neurologist or internist for evaluation of stroke risk factors.

Treatment
1. Patients diagnosed with a stroke within 72 hours of the onset of symptoms are admitted to the hospital for neurologic evaluation and observation.
2. If possible, treat the underlying condition.
3. Arrange for services to help the patient function at home and in the environment.

Follow-up
As per the internist or neurologist.

11.22 NONPHYSIOLOGIC VISUAL LOSS

Symptoms

Loss of vision. Malingerers frequently are involved with an insurance claim or are looking for some other form of financial gain. Hysterics truly believe they have lost vision.

Critical Signs

No ocular or neuro-ophthalmic findings that would account for the decreased vision. Normal pupillary light reaction.

Differential Diagnosis

The following must be considered in anyone with a normal neuro-ophthalmic examination:

- Amblyopia [Poor vision in one eye since childhood, rarely both eyes. Patient often has strabismus (eye misalignment best seen with a cover test) or anisometropia (one eye is usually more far-sighted, astigmatic, or very near-sighted). May have a history of eye patching as a child. Vision is no worse than counting fingers, especially in the temporal periphery of an amblyopic eye. See Section 9.6, Amblyopia.]
- Cortical blindness (Bilateral complete or severe visual loss with normal pupils. MRI of the brain shows bilateral occipital lobe infarcts in most cases. See Section 11.21, Cortical Blindness.)
- Retrobulbar optic neuritis (Afferent pupillary defect may be present. See Section 11.15, Optic Neuritis.)
- Cone–rod dystrophy [Positive family history, decreased color vision, abnormal dark adaptation studies and electroretinogram (ERG). See Section 12.27, Cone Dystrophies.]
- Chiasmal tumor (Visual loss may precede optic atrophy. Pupils usually react sluggishly to light, and an afferent pupillary defect is usually present. Visual fields are abnormal.)

Workup

The following tests may be used to deceive a patient with nonphysiologic visual loss (i.e., to fool the malingerer or hysteric into seeing better than he or she admits to seeing).

Two codes are used in the list below:

U: this test may be used in patients feigning unilateral decreased vision;
B: this test may be used in patients feigning bilateral vision loss.

PATIENTS CLAIMING NO LIGHT PERCEPTION

Determine whether each pupil reacts to light (U): When one eye has no light perception, its pupil will not react to light. The pupil should not appear dilated unless the patient has bilateral no light perception or third-nerve involvement.

PATIENTS CLAIMING HAND-MOTION TO NO LIGHT PERCEPTION

1. Test for an afferent pupillary defect (U): A defect should be present in unilateral visual loss to this degree. If not, the diagnosis of nonphysiologic visual loss is made.
2. Mirror test (U or B): If the patient claims unilateral visual loss, cover the better-seeing eye with a patch; otherwise leave both uncovered. Ask the patient to hold eyes still and slowly tilt a large mirror from side to side in front of the eyes, holding it beyond the patient's range of hand-motion vision. If the eyes move, the patient can see better than hand motion.
3. Optokinetic test (U or B): Patch the uninvolved eye when unilateral visual loss is claimed. Ask the patient to look straight ahead, and slowly move an optokinetic tape in front of the eyes (or rotate an optokinetic drum). If nystagmus can be elicited, vision is better than hand motion.
4. Worth four-dot test (U): Place red–green glasses on patient, and quickly turn on four-dot pattern and ask patient how many dots are seen. If patient closes one eye (cheating), try reversing the glasses and repeating test. If all four dots are seen, vision is better than hand-motion.

PATIENTS CLAIMING 20/40 TO 20/400 VISION

1. Visual acuity testing (U or B): Start with the 20/10 line and ask the patient to read it. When the patient claims incompetence, look amazed and then offer reassurance. Inform the patient you will go to a larger line and show the 20/15 line. Again, force the patient to work to see this line. Slowly proceed up the chart, asking the patient to read each line as you pass it (including the three or four 20/20 lines). Make the patient feel incompetent. By the time the 20/30 or 20/40 lines are reached, the patient may in fact read one or two letters correctly. The visual acuity can then be recorded.
2. Fog test (U): For example, in a patient feigning visual loss on the right. If patient wears glasses, dial patient's correction into phoropter, if not dial in plano. Add +4.00 to the left. Put patient in phoropter with both eyes open. Tell patient to use both eyes to read each line, starting at the 20/15 line and working up the chart slowly, as described previously. Record visual acuity (this should be visual acuity of the right eye). Close phoropter over the right eye. Ask patient to read the same line as before; work up the chart until patient is able to read line. Record visual acuity (this should be visual acuity of the left eye with +4.00 fog).

3. Retest visual acuity in the supposedly "poorly seeing eye" at 10 feet from the chart (U or B): Vision should be twice as good (e.g., a patient with 20/100 vision at 20 feet should read 20/50 at 10 feet). If it is better than expected, record the better vision. If it worse, the patient has nonphysiologic visual loss.
4. Test near vision (U or B): If normal near vision can be documented, nonphysiologic visual loss or myopia has been documented.
5. Visual-field testing (U or B): Goldmann visual-field tests often reveal inconsistent responses and nonphysiologic field losses.

CHILDREN

1. Tell the child that there is an eye abnormality, but the strong drops about to be administered will cure it. Dilate the child's eyes (e.g., tropicamide, 1%), and retest the visual acuity in 40 minutes. Children, as well as adults, sometimes need a "way out."
2. Test as above.

Treatment
Patients are usually told that no ocular abnormality can be found that accounts for their decreased vision. Hysterical patients often benefit from being told that everything is going to be all right and that their vision can be expected to return to normal by their next visit. Psychiatric referral is sometimes indicated.

Follow-up
If nonphysiologic visual loss is highly suspected but cannot be proven, reexamine in 1 to 2 weeks. Consider obtaining an electroretinogram (ERG), a fluorescein angiogram, or a CT scan or MRI of the brain, or a combination of these. If functional visual loss can be documented, have the patient return as needed.

❖ **Note** *Always try to determine the patient's actual visual acuity if possible, and carefully document your findings.*

RETINA

12.1 CENTRAL RETINAL ARTERY OCCLUSION (CRAO)

Symptoms

Unilateral, painless, acute vision loss (counting fingers to light perception in 94% of eyes) occurring over seconds; may have a history of amaurosis fugax.

Critical Signs

Superficial opacification or whitening of the retina in the posterior pole and a cherry-red spot in the center of the macula.

Other Signs

A marked afferent pupillary defect; narrowed retinal arterioles; box-carring or segmentation of the blood column in the arterioles. Occasionally, retinal arteriolar emboli or cilioretinal artery sparing of the foveola is evident. If visual acuity is light perception or worse, strongly suspect ophthalmic artery occlusion.

Etiology

- Embolus (especially carotid or cardiac)
- Thrombosis
- Giant cell arteritis (GCA) (May produce CRAO or an ischemic optic neuropathy. See later for concomitant symptoms.)
- Collagen–vascular disease other than GCA (e.g., systemic lupus erythematosus, polyarteritis nodosa)

- Hypercoagulation disorders (e.g., oral contraceptives, polycythemia, antiphospholipid syndrome)
- Rare causes (e.g., migraine, Behçet's disease, syphilis, sickle-cell disease)
- Trauma

Differential Diagnosis
- Acute ophthalmic artery occlusion. (Usually no cherry-red spot in the foveola; the entire retina appears whitened. The treatment is the same as for CRAO.)
- Inadvertent intraocular injection of gentamicin.
- Arteritic ischemic optic neuropathy [Age older than 50 years, acute severe visual loss, history of temporal headache with scalp tenderness, jaw claudication, muscle pains, weakness, weight loss, a significant afferent pupillary defect, pale optic disc swelling, and a markedly increased erythrocyte sedimentation rate (ESR) are typical. See Section 11.16, Anterior Ischemic Optic Neuropathy.]
- Other causes of a cherry-red spot (e.g., Tay–Sachs or other storage diseases) (Present in early life, other systemic manifestations, usually bilateral.)

Treatment
To be instituted immediately after the diagnosis is made, before the workup, if the CRAO has been present >24 hours.

1. Immediate ocular massage (fundus contact lens or digital massage).
2. Anterior-chamber paracentesis (Fig. 12-1): Place a drop of topical anesthetic (e.g., cocaine 2% to 4%) in the eye and anesthetize the base of the medial rectus muscle by holding a cotton-tipped applicator dipped in the topical anesthetic against the muscle for 1 minute. Retract the eyelid with an eyelid speculum, and with an operating microscope or slit lamp (a microscope is easier), grasp the base of the medial rectus muscle with fixation forceps at the anesthetized site. With a 30-gauge short needle on a tuberculin syringe, enter the eye temporally at the limbus with the bevel of the needle pointing up and away from the eye. Be sure to keep the tip of the needle over the iris (not the lens) when entering the anterior chamber. Withdraw fluid until the chamber shallows slightly (usually 0.1 to 0.2 ml). Withdraw the needle and place a drop of antibiotic on the eye [e.g., ofloxacin (Ocuflox), or ciprofloxacin (Ciloxan)].
3. Acetazolamide, 500 mg i.v., or two 250-mg tablets, p.o., and/or a topical β-blocker (e.g., timolol, or levobunolol, 0.5% b.i.d.) is used to reduce the intraocular pressure.

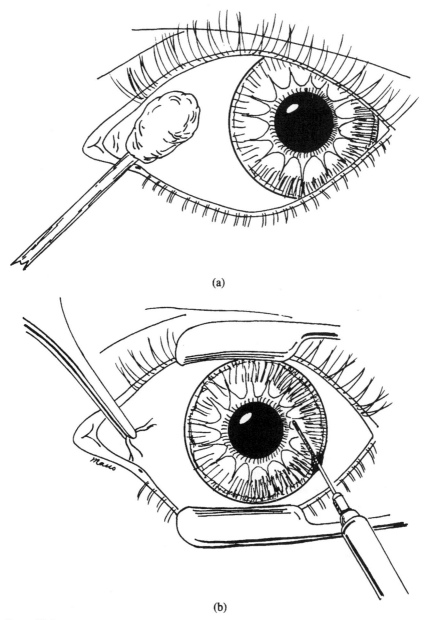

(a)

(b)

Figure 12-1

Anterior-chamber paracentesis. (a) The base of the medial rectus muscle is anesthetized with a cotton-tipped applicator dipped in cocaine, 2% to 4%. **(b)** While the globe is fixated with forceps, a 30-gauge needle is passed through the cornea into the anterior chamber. The needle should stay over the iris.

Comment: *Although there was no significant improvement in outcomes with either anterior-chamber paracentesis or carbogen inhalation in one study, we often do perform paracentesis. There are anecdotal reports of patients experiencing visual improvement after paracentesis.*

Workup

1. Immediate ESR to rule out GCA if the patient is 50 years or older. This is obtained immediately after the paracentesis. If the patient's history or ESR or both are consistent with GCA, high-dose systemic steroids are started. See Section 11.16, Arteritic Ischemic Optic Neuropathy, for additional details.
2. Check blood pressure.
3. Other blood tests: Fasting blood sugar (FBS), glycosylated hemoglobin, complete blood count (CBC) with differential, prothrombin time/activated partial thromboplastin time (PT/PTT). In patients younger than 50 years or with appropriate risk factors or positive review of systems, consider lipid profile, antinuclear antibody (ANA), rheumatoid factor, fluorescence treponemal antibody, absorbed (FTA-ABS), serum protein electrophoresis, hemoglobin electrophoresis, and antiphospholipid antibodies.
4. Carotid artery evaluation (Duplex Doppler ultrasound of the carotid arteries).
5. Cardiac evaluation (ECG, echocardiogram, and possibly Holter monitor).
6. Consider intravenous fluorescein angiography, electroretinogram (ERG), or both to confirm the diagnosis.

Comment: *Recently it was suggested that only patients with high-risk characteristics for cardioembolic disease merit echocardiography. These high-risk characteristics include the following: a history of subacute bacterial endocarditis, rheumatic heart disease, mitral valve prolapse, recent myocardial infarction, prosthetic valve, i.v. drug abuse, congenital heart disease, valvular heart disease, any detectable heart murmur, and ECG changes (atrial fibrillation, acute ST elevation or Q waves).*

Follow-up

The patient is referred to an internist for a complete workup. A repeated eye examination is performed in 1 to 4 weeks, checking for neovascularization of the iris/disc, which develops in up to 20% of patients, at a mean of 4 weeks after onset. If neovascularization develops, panretinal photocoagulation should be performed.

---

*Sharma S, Naqvi A, Sharma SM, Cruess AF, Brown GC. Transthoracic echocardiographic findings in patients with acute retinal artery obstruction: a retrospective review. *Arch Ophthalmol* 1996; 114:1189–1192.

12.2 BRANCH RETINAL ARTERY OCCLUSION (BRAO)

Symptoms

Unilateral, painless, abrupt loss of partial visual field; a history of transient visual loss (amaurosis fugax) may be elicited.

Critical Sign

Superficial opacification or whitening along the distribution of a branch retinal artery. The affected retina becomes edematous.

Other Signs

Narrowed branch retinal artery; box-carring, segmentation of the blood column, or emboli are sometimes seen in the affected branch retinal artery. Cotton-wool spots may appear in the involved area.

Etiology

See Central Retinal Artery Occlusion, Section 12.1.

Workup

See Central Retinal Artery Occlusion, Section 12.1. An electroretinogram (ERG), however, is not helpful.

❖ **Note:** *When a BRAO is accompanied by optic nerve edema or retinitis, obtain appropriate serologic testing to rule out cat-scratch disease* [Bartonella (Rochalimaea) henselae], *syphilis, Lyme disease, and toxoplasmosis.*

Treatment

1. No ocular therapy of proven value is available. Ocular massage (and rarely, anterior-chamber paracentesis) may dislodge a cholesterol embolus (cholesterol emboli appear as bright, reflective crystals, generally at a vessel bifurcation).
2. Treat any underlying medical problem.

Follow-up

Patients need to be evaluated immediately to treat any underlying disorders (especially giant cell arteritis). Reevaluate every 3 to 6 months initially to monitor progression. Ocular neovascularization after BRAO is rare.

12.3 CENTRAL RETINAL VEIN OCCLUSION (CRVO)

Symptoms
Painless loss of vision, usually unilateral.

Critical Signs
Diffuse retinal hemorrhages in all four quadrants of the retina; dilated, tortuous retinal veins.

Other Signs
Cotton-wool spots; disc edema and hemorrhages; retinal edema; optociliary shunt vessels on the disc; neovascularization of the optic disc, retina, or iris.

Types
Ischemic CRVO   Multiple cotton-wool spots (usually >10), extensive retinal hemorrhage, and widespread capillary nonperfusion on intravenous fluorescein angiogram (IVFA). Often a relative afferent pupillary defect is present, and acuity is 20/400 or worse.
Nonischemic CRVO   Mild fundus changes. No afferent pupillary defect is present, and often acuity is better than 20/400.

Etiology
- Atherosclerosis of the adjacent central retinal artery. (The artery compresses the central retinal vein in the region of the lamina cribrosa, secondarily inducing thrombosis in the lumen of the vein.)
- Hypertension
- Optic-disc edema
- Glaucoma (The ocular disease most commonly associated with CRVO.)
- Optic-disc drusen
- Hypercoagulable state (e.g., polycythemia, lymphoma, leukemia, sickle-cell disease, multiple myeloma, cryoglobulinemia, Waldenström's macroglobulinemia, antiphospholipid syndrome, activated protein C resistance, hyperhomocysteinemia)
- Vasculitis (e.g., sarcoid, syphilis, systemic lupus erythematosus)
- Drugs (e.g., oral contraceptives, diuretics)
- Abnormal platelet function
- Retrobulbar external compression (e.g., thyroid disease, orbital tumor)
- Migraine (Rare)

Differential Diagnosis
- Ocular ischemic syndrome (carotid occlusive disease) [Veins are usually dilated and irregular (but not tortuous). Although neovasculariza-

tion of the disc is present in one third of cases, disc edema and hemorrhages are not characteristic. Retinal hemorrhages tend to be in the midperiphery. Patients may have a history of amaurosis fugax, transient ischemic attacks, or orbital pain. Intraocular pressure (IOP) is often low. Central retinal artery perfusion pressure is low in this entity. See Section 12.7, Ocular Ischemic Syndrome.)

- Diabetic retinopathy (Hemorrhages and microaneurysms are usually concentrated in the posterior pole, exudate is more prominent, and the condition is typically bilateral. IVFA may be required to distinguish this condition from CRVO. See Section 14.6, Diabetes mellitus.)
- Papilledema (Bilateral disc swelling with flame-shaped hemorrhages surrounding the disc but not extending to the peripheral retina; results from increased intracranial pressure. See Section 11.13, Papilledema.)
- Radiation retinopathy (History of irradiation is critical in diagnosis. Disc swelling with radiation papillopathy, and retinal neovascularization may be present. Generally, cotton-wool spots are a more prominent feature than hemorrhages.)

Workup

OCULAR

1. Complete ocular examination, including IOP measurement, careful slit-lamp biomicroscopy and gonioscopy to rule out neovascularization of the iris or angle, and dilated fundus examination.
2. IVFA. The more the retinal capillary nonperfusion noted on IVFA, the greater the risk of neovascularization.
3. If the diagnosis of CRVO is uncertain, oculopneumoplethysmography (OPG) or ophthalmodynamometry may help to distinguish CRVO from carotid disease. Ophthalmic artery pressure is low in carotid disease but is normal to increased in CRVO.

Comment: *It is important to distinguish ischemic from nonischemic CRVO. Reportedly the presence of a relative afferent pupillary defect, decreased b-wave amplitude on electroretinography, visual-field constriction, and visual acuity 20/400 or worse are the most reliable signs of an ischemic CRVO.* *

SYSTEMIC

1. History: Medical problems, medications, eye diseases?
2. Check blood pressure.
3. Blood tests: fasting blood sugar, glycosylated hemoglobin, complete blood count (CBC) with differential, platelets, serum protein elec-

*Hayreh SS, Klugman MR, Beri M, Kimura AE, Podhajsky P. Differentiation of ischemic from non-ischemic central retinal vein occlusion during the early acute phase. *Graefe's Arch Clin Exp Ophthalmol* 228; 1990:201–217.

trophoresis, lipid profile, fluorescent treponemal antibody, absorbed (FTA-ABS), and anti-nuclear antibody (ANA).

4. If clinically indicated, consider hemoglobin electrophoresis, prothrombin time/activated partial thromboplastin time (PT/PTT), erythrocyte sedimentation rate (ESR), Veneral Disase Research Laboratories test (VDRL), cryoglobulins, antiphospholipid antibodies, and chest radiograph.

5. Complete medical evaluation, with careful attention to the possibility of cardiovascular disease.

Treatment

1. Discontinue oral contraceptives; change diuretics to other antihypertensive medications if possible.

2. Reduce IOP if increased (e.g., >20 mm Hg) in either eye (see Primary Open-Angle Glaucoma, Section 10.1).

3. Treat underlying medical disorders.

4. If neovascularization of the iris, retina, or optic nerve is present, panretinal photocoagulation (PRP) is performed. In a large, multicenter trial, prophylactic PRP was not shown to have an advantage over PRP performed once neovascularization had occurred. Nonetheless, if timely follow-up cannot be assured, prophylactic PRP is a reasonable consideration for ischemic CRVO.

5. Aspirin, 80 to 325 mg, p.o., daily is often recommended. Although in theory this treatment seems logical, no clinical trials demonstrated efficacy to date.

Follow-up

Nonischemic Every 4 weeks for the first 6 months; if the fundus picture worsens and can be categorized as ischemic, treat as ischemic.

Ischemic Every 3 to 4 weeks after treatment for the first 6 months; watch for neovascularization of the iris or the angle. Check gonioscopy each visit. If neovascularization occurs, PRP is appropriate.

12.4 BRANCH RETINAL VEIN OCCLUSION (BRVO)

Symptoms

Blind spot in the visual field or loss of vision, generally unilateral.

Critical Signs

Superficial hemorrhages in a sector of the retina along a retinal vein. The hemorrhages almost never cross the horizontal raphé (midline).

Other Signs

Cotton-wool spots, retinal edema, a dilated and tortuous retinal vein, narrowing and sheathing of the adjacent artery, retinal neovascularization, vitreous hemorrhage.

Etiology

Disease of the adjacent arterial wall (usually the result of hypertension, arteriosclerosis, or diabetes) compresses the venous wall at a crossing point.

Differential Diagnosis

- Diabetic retinopathy (Dot-and-blot hemorrhages and microaneurysms extend across the horizontal raphe. Nearly always bilateral. See Section 14.6, Diabetes Mellitus.)
- Hypertensive retinopathy (Narrowed retinal arterioles. Hemorrhages are not confined to a sector of the retina and usually cross the horizontal raphe. Bilateral in most. See Section 12.15, Hypertensive Retinopathy.)

Workup

1. History: Systemic disease, particularly hypertension or diabetes?
2. Complete ocular examination, including dilated retinal examination with indirect ophthalmoscopy to look for retinal neovascularization and a macular examination with a slit lamp and a Hruby, 60- or 90-diopter, or fundus contact lens to detect macular edema.
3. Check blood pressure.
4. Consider obtaining fasting blood sugar, complete blood count (CBC) with differential and platelets, prothrombin time (PT), activated partial thromboplastin time (PTT), erythrocyte sedimentation rate (ESR), antinuclear antibody (ANA), rheumatoid factor, and chest radiograph.
5. Medical examination (usually performed by an internist to check for cardiovascular disease).
6. An intravenous fluorescein angiogram (IVFA) is obtained after the hemorrhages have cleared or sooner if neovascularization is suspected.

Treatment

1. Retinal laser photocoagulation is indicated for:
   a. Chronic macular edema (3 to 6 months' duration) reducing vision below 20/40 in the absence of macular capillary nonperfusion. Grid treatment to the area of macular edema is used.
   b. Retinal neovascularization. Sector panretinal photocoagulation to the ischemic area, as delineated by IVFA evidence of capillary nonperfusion, is performed.
2. Underlying medical problems are treated appropriately.

Follow-up

Every 1 to 2 months at first, and then every 3 to 12 months, checking for neovascularization and macular edema.

12.5 HYPERTENSIVE RETINOPATHY

Symptoms
Usually asymptomatic, although may have decreased vision.

Critical Sign
Generalized or localized retinal arteriolar narrowing, almost always bilateral.

Other Signs
- Chronic hypertension: Arteriovenous crossing changes, retinal arteriolar sclerosis ("copper" or "silver" wiring), cotton-wool spots, flame-shaped hemorrhages, arterial macroaneurysms, central or branch occlusion of an artery or vein. Rarely, neovascular complications can develop.
- Acute ("malignant") hypertension: Hard exudates often in a "macular star" configuration, retinal edema, cotton-wool spots, flame-shaped hemorrhages, swelling of the optic-nerve head (disc edema). Rarely, retinal detachment (RD), vitreous hemorrhage. Focal chorioretinal atrophy (Elschnig spots of choroidal nonperfusion) are a sign of past episodes of acute hypertension.

❖ **Note**: *When hypertensive changes are only found in one eye, suspect carotid artery obstruction on the side of the normal-appearing eye, sparing the retina from the effects of the hypertension.*

Etiology
- Primary hypertension (No known underlying cause.)
- Secondary hypertension (Typically the result of preeclampsia/eclampsia, pheochromocytoma, kidney disease, adrenal disease, or coarctation of the aorta.)

Differential Diagnosis
- Diabetic retinopathy (Hemorrhages are generally dot and blot, microaneurysms are common, vessel attenuation is less common. See Section 14.6, Diabetes Mellitus.)
- Collagen–vascular disease (May show multiple cotton-wool spots, but few-to-no other fundus findings characteristic of hypertension.)
- Anemia (Hemorrhage predominates without marked arterial changes.)
- Radiation retinopathy (Can appear similar to hypertension. A history of irradiation to the eye or an adnexal structure such as the brain, sinus, or nasopharynx can usually be elicited. It may develop any time

after the radiation therapy, but it most commonly occurs within a few years.)

- Central retinal vein occlusion (CRVO) or branch retinal vein occlusion (BRVO) (Unilateral, multiple hemorrhages, venous dilatation and tortuosity, no arteriolar narrowing. May be the result of hypertension. See Sections 12.3, Central Retinal Vein Occlusion, or 12.4, Branch Retinal Vein Occlusion.)

Workup
1. History: Known hypertension, diabetes, or adnexal radiation?
2. Complete ocular examination, particularly dilated fundus examination.
3. Check blood pressure.
4. Refer patient to a medical internist or the emergency room of a hospital. The urgency generally depends on the blood pressure reading and whether the patient is symptomatic. As a general rule, a diastolic blood pressure of 110 to 120 mm Hg or the presence of chest pain, difficulty breathing, headache, change in mental status, or blurred vision with optic disc swelling requires immediate medical attention.

Treatment
Control the hypertension (as per the internist).

Follow-up
Every 2 to 3 months at first, and then every 6 to 12 months.

12.6 AMAUROSIS FUGAX

Symptoms
Monocular visual loss that usually lasts seconds to minutes, but may last up to 1-2 hours. Vision returns to normal.

Critical Signs
May see an embolus within an arteriole or the ocular examination may be normal.

Other Signs
Signs of the ocular ischemic syndrome (dilated veins; midperipheral dot and blot hemorrhages; neovascularization of the iris, disc, or retina), an old branch retinal artery occlusion (BRAO) (sheathed arteriole), or neurologic signs caused by ischemia of a cerebral hemisphere [transient ischemic attacks (TIA)] (e.g., contralateral arm or leg weakness).

Etiology

Embolus from the carotid artery (most common), heart, or aorta; vascular insufficiency as a result of arteriosclerotic disease of vessels anywhere along the path from the aorta to the globe causing hypoperfusion precipitated by a postural change or cardiac arrhythmia; hypercoagulable/hyperviscosity state. Rarely, an intraorbital tumor may compress the optic nerve or a nourishing vessel in certain gaze positions, causing transient visual loss.

Differential Diagnosis

All of the following conditions may produce transient visual loss:

- Papilledema (Optic-disc swelling is evident. Visual loss lasts seconds, is usually bilateral and is often associated with postural change or Valsalva's maneuver. See Section 11.13, Papilledema.)
- Giant cell arteritis (GCA) (Patients are typically more than 50 years of age and have an elevated erythrocyte sedimentation rate (ESR), temporal headache, scalp tenderness, jaw claudication, or muscle pains. Transient visual loss may precede an ischemic optic neuropathy or central retinal artery occlusion. See Section 11.16.)
- Impending central retinal vein occlusion (CRVO) (Dilated, tortuous retinal veins are observed on funduscopic examination. See Section 12.3, Central Retinal Vein Occlusion.)
- Glaucoma (Characteristicc optic-nerve changes and visual field loss. See Chapter 10.)
- Retinal migraine (Usually a diagnosis of exclusion. Typically occurs in patients less than 40 years of age. May have recurrent episodes. Focal retinal arteriolar narrowing is sometimes observed. See Section 15.4.)
- Intermittent intraocular hemorrhage (e.g., vitreous hemorrhage)
- Others (e.g., optic nerve head drusen)

Work-up

1. *Immediate ESR when GCA is suspected.*
2. History: Monocular visual loss or homonymous hemianopsia? (Did the patient cover one eye to test vision?) Duration of visual loss? Previous episodes of amaurosis fugax or TIA? Cardiovascular disease factors? Use of oral contraceptives? Heart disease or operations?
3. Ocular examination, including a confrontational visual field examination and a dilated retinal evaluation: Look for an embolus or signs of other disorders mentioned previously.
4. Medical examination (cardiac and carotid auscultation).
5. Consider an intravenous fluorescein angiogram (focal arterial staining at the site of the embolus may be seen).

6. Ophthalmic color Doppler ultrasound may reveal a retrolaminar central retinal artery stenosis or embolus proximal to the lamina cribrosa.
7. Complete blood count (CBC) with differential and platelet count, fasting blood sugar, glycosylated hemoglobin, and lipid profile (to rule out polycythemia, thrombocytosis, diabetes, and hyperlipidemia).
8. Noninvasive carotid artery evaluation (e.g., Duplex Doppler ultrasound).
9. Cardiac evaluation (including an echocardiogram).

Treatment
A. Carotid disease
   1. Consider aspirin 325 mg po daily.
   2. Consider referral for carotid endarterectomy in the presence of a surgically accessible, high-grade carotid stenosis or occlusion if the potential benefit of the procedure outweighs the risks.
   3. Control hypertension and diabetes (follow-up with a medical internist).
   4. Stop smoking.
B. Cardiac disease
   1. Consider aspirin 325 mg po daily (e.g., for mitral valve prolapse).
   2. Consider hospitalization and anticoagulation (e.g., heparin therapy) in the presence of a mural thrombus.
   3. Consider referral for cardiac surgery as needed.
   4. Control arteriosclerotic risk factors as described previously (follow-up with medical internist).
C. If carotid and cardiac disease are ruled out, a vasospastic etiology can be considered. Treatment with a calcium channel blocker is at least theoretically beneficial.

Follow-up
Patients with recurrent episodes of amaurosis fugax (especially if accompanied by signs of cerebral TIA) require immediate diagnostic and sometimes therapeutic attention.

12.7 OCULAR ISCHEMIC SYNDROME (OIS)
(CAROTID OCCLUSIVE DISEASE)

Symptoms
Decreased vision, ocular or periorbital pain, afterimages or prolonged recovery of vision after exposure to bright light, may have a history of transient monocular visual loss (amaurosis fugax). Usually unilateral. Typi-

cally occurs in patients who are aged 50 to 80 years. Men outnumber women, 2:1.

Critical Signs

Although retinal veins are dilated and irregular in caliber, they are typically not tortuous. The retinal arterioles are narrowed. Associated findings include midperipheral retinal hemorrhages (80% prevalence), iris neovascularization (66%), and posterior segment neovascularization (37%).

Other Signs

Episcleral injection, corneal edema, mild anterior uveitis, neovascular glaucoma, iris atrophy, cataract, retinal microaneurysms, cotton-wool spots, spontaneous pulsations of the central retinal artery, and cherry-red spot. Central retinal artery occlusion may occur.

Etiology

- Carotid disease (Usually >90% stenosis)
- Ophthalmic artery disease (Less common)

Differential Diagnosis

- Central retinal vein occlusion (CRVO). (Similar signs, but may have optociliary shunt vessels or edema of the disc and dilated retinal veins that are tortuous and regular in caliber. Decreased vision after exposure to light and orbital pain are not typically found. Ophthalmodynamometry may distinguish this condition from ocular ischemic syndrome. See Section 12.3, Central Retinal Vein Occlusion.)
- Diabetes (Bilateral, usually symmetric. Retinal hemorrhages usually concentrate in the posterior pole, and hard exudates are often present. See Section 14.6, Diabetes Mellitus.)
- Aortic arch disease (Caused by atherosclerosis, syphilis, or Takayasu's arteritis. Produces a clinical picture identical to OIS, which is generally bilateral. Examination reveals absent arm and neck pulses, cold hands, and spasm of the arm muscles with exercise.)

Workup

1. History: Previous episodes of transient monocular visual loss? Cold hands or spasm of arm muscles with exercise?
2. Complete ocular examination: Search carefully for neovascularization of the iris, disc, or retina.
3. Medical examination (arm pulses, cardiac and carotid auscultation). Evaluate for hypertension, diabetes, and atherosclerotic disease.
4. Consider fluorescein angiography (FA) for diagnostic or therapeutic purposes.

5. Noninvasive carotid artery evaluation (e.g., Duplex Doppler ultrasound, oculoplethysmography, magnetic resonance angiography).
6. Consider orbital color Doppler ultrasound.
7. Consider ophthalmodynamometry if the diagnosis of CRVO cannot be excluded (ophthalmic artery pressure is low in carotid disease but is normal to increased in CRVO).
8. Carotid arteriography is reserved for patients in whom surgery is to be performed.
9. Consider a cardiology consultation, given the high association with cardiac disease.

Treatment
Often unsuccessful.

1. Carotid endarterectomy for significant stenosis (refer to neurovascular surgeon).
2. Consider panretinal photocoagulation (PRP) in the presence of neovascularization.
3. Manage glaucoma if present (see Neovascular Glaucoma, Section 10.13).
4. Control hypertension and diabetes, and reduce cholesterol level (refer to internist).
5. Stop smoking.

Follow-up
Depends on the age and general health of the patient and the symptoms and signs of disease. Surgical candidates should be evaluated urgently.

12.8 CENTRAL SEROUS CHORIORETINOPATHY (CSCR)

Symptoms
Blurred or dim vision, objects appear distorted and miniature in size, colors appear washed-out, central scotoma. Usually unilateral, sometimes asymptomatic.

Critical Signs
Localized serous detachment of the neurosensory retina in the region of the macula without subretinal blood or lipid exudates. The margins of the detachment are sloping and merge gradually into the attached retina. It is best seen with a fundus contact lens by using a slit lamp.

Other Signs

Visual acuity generally ranges from 20/20 to 20/80, Amsler's grid testing reveals distortion of straight lines often with scotoma; a small afferent pupillary defect or a concomitant retinal pigment epithelial detachment may be present. Focal pigment epithelial irregularity may mark sites of previous episodes.

Etiology

Idiopathic. Generally occurs in men aged 25 to 50 years. Patients with lupus have an increased incidence of CSCR. In women, CSCR typically occurs at a slightly older age. There is also an association with pregnancy. Increased endogenous cortisol levels may play a role in the pathogenesis of CSCR. (This helps explain a putative association with psychologic or physiologic stress.) Exogenous cortisol (i.e., corticosteroid use) also has been postulated as a cause of CSCR.

Differential Diagnosis

These entities may produce a serous detachment of the sensory retina in the macular area.

- Age-related macular degeneration (ARMD) [Patient generally older than 50 years, drusen, pigment epithelial alterations, may have a choroidal (subretinal) neovascular membrane, often bilateral. See Section 12.10, Age-Related Macular Degeneration.]
- Optic pit (The optic disc has a small defect, a pit, in the nerve tissue. A serous retinal detachment may be present contiguous with the optic disc. See Section 12.9, Optic Pit.)
- Macular detachment as a result of a rhegmatogenous RD (A hole in the retina can be found. See Section 12.19, Retinal Detachment.)
- Choroidal tumor (A mass is visible by indirect ophthalmoscopy. See Section 8.3, Malignant Melanoma of the Choroid.)
- Pigment epithelial detachment (PED) (The margins of a PED are more distinct than those of CSCR. Occasionally, PED may accompany CSCR or ARMD.)
- Others (e.g., idiopathic choroidal effusion, inflammatory choroidal disorders.)

Workup

1. Optional Amsler's grid test to document the area of field involved (see Appendix 3).
2. Slit-lamp examination of the macula with a fundus contact, Hruby, or 60- or 90-diopter lens to rule out a concomitant choroidal neovascular membrane. Additionally, search for an optic pit of the disc.
3. Dilated fundus examination by using indirect ophthalmoscopy to rule out a choroidal tumor or rhegmatogenous RD.

4. Consider an intravenous fluorescein angiography (FA) if the diagnosis is uncertain or presentation atypical, a choroidal neovascular membrane is suspected, or laser treatment is to be instituted.

Treatment/Follow-up

The prognosis for spontaneous recovery of visual acuity to ≥20/30 is excellent. The prognosis is worse for patients with recurrent disease, multiple areas of detachment, or prolonged course. Recovery of maximal visual acuity is hastened by laser therapy and recurrences after laser are less likely; nonetheless, laser treatment prolongs recovery of contrast sensitivity and may ultimately reduce contrast sensitivity. Because of these issues, the following recommendations have been made:

1. Examine most patients every 6 to 8 weeks until the condition spontaneously resolves or, if no resolution occurs, for 4 to 6 months.
2. Laser photocoagulation may be considered under the following circumstances:
   a. Persistence of a serous detachment beyond 4 to 6 months.
   b. Recurrence of the condition in an eye that sustained a permanent visual deficit from a previous episode.
   c. Occurrence in the contralateral eye after a permanent visual deficit resulted from a previous episode.
   d. Patient absolutely requires prompt restoration of vision (e.g., occupational necessity).

12.9 OPTIC PIT

Symptoms

Asymptomatic if isolated. May notice distortion of straight lines or edges, blurred vision, a blind spot, or micropsia if a serous macular detachment develops.

Critical Sign

Small round depression (usually hypopigmented or gray in appearance) in the nerve tissue of the optic disc. The majority are temporal, but approximately one third are central.

Other Signs

May develop a localized detachment of the sensory retina extending from the disc to the macula, usually unilateral.

Differential Diagnosis
- Acquired pit (pseudopit) (Sometimes seen in patients with low-tension glaucoma or primary open-angle glaucoma. May be accompanied by flame hemorrhages at the disc margin. See Sections 10.1, Primary Open-Angle Glaucoma, and 10.2, Low-Tension Glaucoma)
- Other causes of a serous macular detachment (e.g., central serous chorioretinopathy. See Section 12.8, Central Serous Chorioretinopathy).

Workup
1. Optic-disc evaluation to detect the pit.
2. Slit-lamp examination of the macula with a fundus contact lens or 60- or 90-diopter lens to evaluate for a serous macular detachment and to rule out a choroidal (subretinal) neovascular membrane.
3. Measure intraocular pressure (IOP).
4. Consider an intravenous fluorescein angiogram (IVFA) to help detect a pit and rule out a choroidal neovascular membrane in patients with a serous macular detachment.

Treatment
Isolated optic pit   No treatment required.

Optic pit with a serous macular detachment   Laser photocoagulation to the temporal margin of the optic disc is used in most cases. Surgery (vitrectomy) may be used in refractory cases.

Follow-up
Isolated optic pits   Yearly examination; sooner if symptomatic.

Optic pits with serous macular detachment   Reexamine every few weeks after treatment to check for resorption of subretinal fluid. Watch for amblyopia in children.

12.10 AGE-RELATED MACULAR DEGENERATION (ARMD)

Two types: Nonexudative (dry form) and exudative (wet form). Both forms almost always occur in patients older than 50 years.

A. Nonexudative ("Dry") ARMD

Symptoms
Gradual loss of central vision, Amsler's grid defects; may be asymptomatic.

Critical Signs

Macular drusen, clumps of pigment in the outer retina, and retinal pigment epithelial (RPE) atrophy, almost always in both eyes.

Other Signs

Confluent retinal and choriocapillaris atrophy (e.g., geographic atrophy), dystrophic calcification.

Differential Diagnosis

- Peripheral drusen (Drusen are located outside of the macular area, not within it.)
- Myopic degeneration (Typically, high myopia with characteristic peripapillary changes in addition to the macular degeneration. Drusen are not seen. See Section 12.12, High Myopia.)
- Central serous chorioretinopathy (Parafoveal serous retinal elevation, RPE detachments, and mottled RPE atrophy, without drusen, usually in patients younger than 50 years of age. See Section 12.8, Central Serous Chorioretinopathy.)
- Inherited central retinal dystrophies (e.g., Stargardt's disease, pattern dystrophy, Best's disease, others) (Variable macular pigmentary changes, atrophy, or accumulation of lipofuscin or a combination of these. Usually younger than 50 years, without drusen, familial occurrence. See specific entity.)
- Toxic retinopathies (e.g., chloroquine toxicity) [Mottled hypopigmentation with ring of hyperpigmentation ("bull's eye" maculopathy) without drusen. History of drug ingestion.]
- Inflammatory maculopathies (e.g., multifocal choroiditis, rubella, serpiginous choroidopathy) (Variable chorioretinal atrophy, often with vitreous cells and without drusen. See specific entity.)

Workup

1. Amsler's grid to document or detect a central or paracentral scotoma (see Appendix 3).
2. Macular examination with a 60- or 90-diopter or a fundus contact lens: Look for signs of the exudative form.
3. Fluorescein angiogram (FA) when exudative ARMD cannot be ruled out clinically, when RPE detachment is present, or when visual acuity has declined rapidly to rule out choroidal neovascularization (see part B later). Drusen and RPE atrophy are often more visible on FA.

Treatment

No proven treatment is available. Some physicians advocate the use of oral nutrition supplements containing antioxidant vitamins (e.g., vitamins A, C, E), and trace minerals (e.g., selenium, zinc). Whereas not likely harmful at standard dosages, this treatment has not been scientifically confirmed to be beneficial. Low-vision aids may benefit some patients with bilateral loss of macular function.

Follow-up

Every 6 to 12 months, watching for signs of the exudative form. Patients are given an Amsler's grid to take home and use on a daily basis. They are instructed to return immediately if a change is noted on Amsler's grid.

B. Exudative ("Wet") ARMD

Symptoms

Distortion of straight lines or edges, rapid onset of visual loss, blind spot in the central or paracentral visual field.

Critical Signs

Drusen accompanied by a choroidal (subretinal) neovascular membrane (CNVM; grayish green membrane beneath the retina).

Other Signs

Subretinal hemorrhages, subretinal exudates, subretinal pigment ring, subretinal fibrosis (disciform scar), retinal or vitreous hemorrhage. Nonexudative signs may be present.

Risk Factors for Loss of Vision

Advanced age, hyperopia, family history, soft (larger ill-defined) drusen, focal pigment clumping, RPE detachments, systemic hypertension, smoking.

❖ **Note:** *In patients with wet ARMD in one eye, the risk of a CNVM in the contralateral eye is 10% to 12% per year. Eyes at highest risk are those with multiple or confluent soft drusen with RPE clumping.*

Differential Diagnosis

All of the following are associated with a CNVM:

- Ocular histoplasmosis syndrome (Small white–yellow chorioretinal scars are seen in the midperiphery and posterior pole along with chorioretinal scarring adjacent to the optic disc. See Section 12.11, Ocular Histoplasmosis Syndrome.)
- Angioid streaks (Bilateral subretinal red–brown or gray bands of irregular contour that radiate from the optic disc. See Section 12.13, Angioid Streaks.)
- High myopia (Significant myopic refractive error, lacquer cracks in the posterior pole, myopic disc changes. See Section 12.12, High Myopia.)

- Traumatic choroidal rupture (History of trauma, usually unilateral; a choroidal tear concentric to the optic disc is often noted. See Section 3.9, Traumatic Choroidal Rupture.)
- Others conditions disrupting Bruch's membrane (Drusen of the optic nerve, choroidal tumors, photocoagulation scars, inflammatory chorioretinal lesions, and idiopathic.)

Workup
1. Amsler's grid testing to detect and document the degree of central field involved (see Appendix 3).
2. Macular slit-lamp examination with a 60- or 90-diopter, Hruby, or fundus contact lens to detect a CNVM. Must examine both eyes.
3. Blood pressure measurement. The presence of systemic hypertension in patients with a CNVM appears to have a negative effect on the response to laser therapy.
4. IVFA is performed as soon as possible if a CNVM is suspected on clinical examination. IVFA classically shows an area of lacy, fine capillaries at the outer retinal level or beneath the RPE in early transit phase, with leakage obscuring the boundaries of these vessels in the middle and late phases.
5. Indocyanine green (ICG) angiography may be a helpful adjuvant test in delineating the borders of some CNVM, especially in the presence of subretinal blood or exudate.

❖ **Note:** *Neither IVFA nor ICG angiography are indicated when there is no hope of preserving central vision, such as in advanced stages of macular scarring (despite the presence of choroidal neovascularization).*

Treatment
Laser photocoagulation should be applied within 72 hours of the IVFA to reduce the risk of severe visual loss in patients with treatable macular CNVM as outlined by the Macular Photocoagulation Study (MPS) Group. Argon blue–green or green is used to treat CNVM located greater than 200 μm from the center of the foveal avascular zone (FAZ).* Krypton red may be considered for juxtafoveal CNVM (i.e., membrane or associated blood or pigment extending within 200 μm from the FAZ center), but studies comparing outcome to Argon green are equivocal. Treatment of well-demarcated subfoveal CNVM less than 3.5 disc-areas with Argon green or Krypton red laser, although usually causing an immediate decrease in visual acuity, has been shown to lessen incidence of severe vision loss at 24 months after treatment.

*The FAZ is an avascular area about 500 microns in diameter in the center of the fovea. It is easily observed with IVFA.

Follow-up

PATIENTS TEATED FOR CNVM WITH LASER PHOTOCOAGULATION

Because of the high rate of neovascular activity after treatment (persistent and new CNVM), patients need to be monitored closely, especially during the first posttreatment year:

1. Amsler's grid to be used at home daily. The patient is instructed to return immediately if a change is noted.
2. Scheduled examinations at 2 weeks, 6 weeks, 3 months, and 6 months after treatment, and then every 6 months. Careful macular examination is performed as described previously.
3. IVFA is repeated 2 weeks after treatment and again when renewed neovascular activity is suspected.
4. Retreatment with laser photocoagulation should be considered when renewed neovascular activity is identified.

Risk Factors

1. Persistence: Incomplete treatment of CNVM.
2. Recurrence: Hypertension, cigarette smoking, contralateral eye with CNVM or disciform scar, and/or high-risk fundus features (soft drusen and pigment clumping).

REFERENCES

Macular Photocoagulation Study Group. Laser photocoagulation for juxtafoveal choroidal neovascularization: five-year results from randomized clinical trials. *Arch Ophthalmol* 1994;112:500.

Zimmer-Galler IE, Bressler NM, Bressler SB. Treatment of choroidal neovascularization. Updated information from recent macular photocoagulation study group reports. *Int Ophthalmol Clin* 1995;35:37.

12.11 OCULAR HISTOPLASMOSIS SYNDROME

Symptoms

May be asymptomatic or have decreased or distorted vision. Patients often have lived in or visited the Ohio–Mississippi River Valley area and are usually in the 20- to 50-year age range.

Critical Signs

Classic triad. Need two of the three to make the diagnosis.

1. Yellow–white punched-out round spots usually <1 mm in diameter, deep to the retina in any fundus location ("histo-spots").

2. A macular choroidal neovascular membrane (CNVM) appearing as a gray–green patch beneath the retina, associated with detachment of the sensory retina, subretinal blood or exudate, or a pigment ring evolving into a disciform scar.
3. Atrophy or scarring adjacent to the optic disc, sometimes with nodules or hemorrhage. There may be a rim of pigment separating the disc from the area of atrophy or scarring.

Other Signs

Linear streaks of chorioretinal atrophy in the peripheral fundus. The eye is uninflamed with minimal to no vitreous cells and no aqueous cells or flare.

Differential Diagnosis

- High myopia [May have atrophic spots in the posterior pole and a myopic crescent on the temporal side of the disc. A CNVM may develop. The atrophic spots are whiter than histo-spots and are not seen beyond the posterior pole. The myopic crescent has a rim of pigment on the outer (not inner) edge, separating the crescent from the retina. May have lacquer cracks. The disc is often tilted. See Section 12.12, High Myopia.]
- Age-related macular degeneration (The macular changes may appear similar, but typically, there are macular drusen and patients are older than 50 years. There are no atrophic round spots similar to histoplasmosis and no scarring or atrophy around the disc. See Section 12.8, Age-Related Macular Degeneration.)
- Toxoplasmosis (White chorioretinal lesion associated with vitreous and sometimes aqueous cells. See Section 13.3, Toxoplasmosis.)
- Angioid streaks (Histo-like spots may be seen in the midperiphery, and macular degeneration may occur. Jagged red, brown, or gray lines appearing deep to the retinal vessels and radiating from the optic disc are typically seen. Often associated with pseudoxanthoma elasticum, sickle-cell anemia, Paget's disease, and other rarer systemic diseases. See Section 12.13, Angioid Streaks.)
- Multifocal choroiditis with panuveitis (Similar clinical findings, except anterior or vitreous inflammatory cells or both are also present. See Section 13.2, Posterior Uveitis.)

Workup

1. History: Time spent in the Ohio–Mississippi River Valley area? Prior exposure to fowl?
2. Amsler's grid test (see Appendix 3) to evaluate the central visual field of each eye.
3. Slit-lamp examination: Anterior-chamber cells and flare should not be present.

4. Dilated fundus examination: Concentrate on the macular area with a slit lamp and fundus contact, Hruby, or 60- or 90-diopter lens. Look for signs of CNVM and vitreous cells.
5. Fluorescein angiogram (FA) (to help detect or treat a CNVM).

Treatment
Focal laser photocoagulation is indicated for well-defined CNVM. Surgical removal of CNVM can also be considered when laser is likely to cause visual loss. Antifungal treatment is not helpful.

Follow-up
Treatment should be instituted within 72 hours of confirming the presence of CNVM by FA. All patients (whether they will be, will not be, or have been treated) are to use an Amsler's grid daily. Patients are instructed to return immediately if any sudden visual change is noted. Treated patients are seen at 2 to 3 weeks, 4 to 6 weeks, 3 months, and 6 months after treatment and then every 6 months. A careful macular examination is performed at each visit. FA is repeated at the 2- to 3-week posttreatment visit and whenever renewed neovascular activity is suspected. Patients without CNVM are seen every 6 months when macular changes are present in one or both eyes and yearly when no macular pathology is present in either eye.

12.12 HIGH MYOPIA

Symptoms
Decreased vision. (Patients are usually beyond the fifth decade of life before progressive decrease in visual acuity occurs.)

Critical Signs
Myopic crescent (a crescent-shaped area of white sclera or choroidal vessels adjacent to the disc, separated from the normal-appearing fundus by a hyperpigmented line; this crescent may enlarge with time); an oblique (tilted) insertion of the optic disc; macular pigmentary abnormalities, a hyperpigmented spot in the macula (Fuchs' spot); typically, but not always, a refractive correction of more than 6.00 to 8.00 diopters. Axial length greater than 26 to 27 mm.

Other Signs
Temporal optic-disc pallor, posterior staphyloma, entrance of the retinal vessels into the nasal part of the cup, the retina and choroid may be seen to

extend over the nasal border of the disc, well-circumscribed areas of atrophy, spots of subretinal hemorrhage, choroidal sclerosis, yellow subretinal streaks (lacquer cracks), peripheral retinal thinning, lattice degeneration. A choroidal neovascular membrane (CNVM) or retinal detachment (RD) may develop. Visual-field defects may be present. Increased intraocular pressure (IOP) with other evidence for primary open-angle glaucoma may be seen.

Differential Diagnosis
- Age-related macular degeneration (ARMD) (May develop CNVM and a similar macular appearance, but typically, drusen are present, and the myopic features of the optic disc described previously are absent. See Section 12.10, Age-Related Macular Degeneration.)
- Ocular histoplasmosis [May develop CNVM and exhibit a peripapillary scar. A pigmented ring may separate the disc from the peripapillary atrophy, as opposed to pigmented ring separating the atrophic area from the adjacent retina. Round choroidal scars (punched-out lesions) are often seen scattered throughout the fundus. See Section 12.11, Ocular Histoplasmosis Syndrome.]
- Tilted discs [Anomalous discs with a scleral crescent, most often infer-onasally, an irregular vascular pattern as the vessels emerge from the disc (situs inversus), and an area of fundus ectasia in the direction of the tilt (inferonasally). Many patients have myopia and astigmatism. They do not have chorioretinal degeneration or lacquer cracks. Visual-field defects corresponding to the areas of fundus ectasia are often seen. Most cases are bilateral.]
- Gyrate atrophy (Rare. Multiple, sharply defined areas of chorioretinal atrophy beginning in the midperiphery in childhood and then coalescing to involve a large portion of the fundus. Body fluid levels of ornithine are markedly increased. Patients are often highly myopic. Autosomal recessive. See Section 12.26, Gyrate Atrophy.)
- Toxoplasmosis (Well-circumscribed chorioretinal scar that does not typically develop CNVM; active disease shows retinitis and vitritis. See Section 13.3, Toxoplasmosis.)

Workup
1. Manifest or cycloplegic refraction or both.
2. IOP measurement by applanation tonometry (Schiötz tonometry may underestimate IOP in highly myopic eyes.)
3. Dilated retinal examination, by using indirect ophthalmoscopy to search for retinal breaks or detachment. Scleral depression helps to reveal the far peripheral retina, but should not be performed over a staphyloma.
4. Slit-lamp and fundus contact, Hruby, or 60- or 90-diopter lens examination of the macula, searching for CNVM (dirty-gray or green lesion beneath the retina, subretinal blood or exudate, or subretinal fluid).

5. Fluorescein angiogram (FA) when a CNVM is suspected.
6. Formal visual-field examinations (e.g., Humphrey, Octopus) to document field stability or change when glaucoma is suspected.

Treatment

1. Symptomatic retinal breaks are treated with laser photocoagulation, cryotherapy, or scleral-buckling surgery. Treatment of asymptomatic retinal breaks should be considered when there is no surrounding pigmentation or demarcation line.
2. Extrafoveal or juxtafoveal CNVM may be considered for laser photocoagulation therapy within several days of obtaining an FA (see Age-Related Macular Degeneration, Section 12.10).
3. For glaucoma suspects, a single visual field often cannot distinguish myopic visual field loss from early glaucoma. Progression of visual-field loss in the absence of progressive myopia, however, suggests the presence of glaucoma and the need for therapy (see Primary Open-Angle Glaucoma, Section 10.1).
4. Recommend wearing polycarbonate safety glasses for sports because there is an increased risk of choroidal rupture from minor trauma.

Follow-up

In the absence of complications, reexamine every 6 to 12 months, watching for the related disorders discussed earlier. See Primary Open-Angle Glaucoma, Section 10.1; Age-Related Macular Degeneration, Section 12.10 (for treatment of choroidal neovascularization); Retinal Break, Section 12.18; and Retinal Detachment, Section 12.19 for further information on these conditions.

12.13 ANGIOID STREAKS

Symptoms

Usually asymptomatic; decreased vision may result from choroidal (subretinal) neovascularization (CNVM).

Critical Signs

Bilateral reddish brown or gray bands located deep to the retina, radiating in an irregular or spoke-like pattern from the optic disc. Choroidal neovascular membranes leading to macular degeneration may occur.

Other Signs

Mottled-background fundus appearance ("peau d'orange"); subretinal hemorrhages after mild blunt trauma; reticular pigmentary changes in the macula; small, white, pinpoint chorioretinal scars ("histo-like spots") in the midperiphery; drusen of the optic disc (especially with pseudoxanthoma elasticum); granular pattern of hyperfluorescent on intavenous fluorescein angiography (IVFA).

Etiology

(Fifty percent of cases are associated with systemic diseases; the remainder are idiopathic.)

- Pseudoxanthoma elasticum [Most common. Loose skin folds in the neck and on flexor aspects of joints, cardiovascular complications, increased risk of gastrointestinal (GI) bleeds.]
- Paget's disease (Enlarged skull, bone pain, history of bone fractures, hearing loss, possible cardiovascular complications. May be asymptomatic. Increased serum alkaline phosphatase and urine calcium.)
- Sickle-cell disease [May be asymptomatic; may have decreased vision from fundus abnormalities (see Sickle-Cell Disease, Section 12.23), or may have a history of recurrent infections or painless or painful crises. Positive sickle-cell preparation and abnormal hemoglobin (Hgb) electrophoresis.]
- Ehlers–Danlos syndrome (Hyperelasticity of skin, loose joints.)
- Less common (Acromegaly, senile elastosis, lead poisoning, Marfan's syndrome.)

Differential Diagnosis

- Myopic chorioretinal degeneration (lacquer cracks) (High myopia, often with a tilted disc and peripapillary atrophy; may have macular degeneration. See Section 12.12, High Myopia.)
- Choroidal rupture (Subretinal streaks are usually concentric to the optic disc, yellow–white in color, and result from ocular trauma. See Section 3.9, Traumatic Choroidal Rupture.)

Workup

1. History: Any known systemic disorders? Previous ocular trauma?
2. Complete ocular examination: Look carefully at the macula with a slit lamp and a Hruby, 60- or 90-diopter, or a fundus contact lens to detect choroidal neovascularization.
3. Intravenous fluorescein angiogram (IVFA) if uncertain of the diagnosis or if choroidal neovascularization is suspected.
4. Physical examination: Look for clinical signs of etiologic diseases.

5. Serum alkaline phosphatase and urine calcium levels if Paget's disease is suspected.
6. Sickle-cell preparation and Hgb electrophoresis in African-American patients.
7. Skin biopsy if pseudoxanthoma elasticum is suspected.

Treatment
1. Focal laser photocoagulation for treatable choroidal neovascularization (see Age-Related Macular Degeneration, Section 12.10).
2. Management of any underlying systemic disease, if present, by a medical internist.
3. Recommend wearing polycarbonate safety glasses for sports because there is an increased risk of choroidal rupture from minor trauma.

Follow-up
Fundus examination every 6 months, observing for choroidal neovascularization. Amsler's grid (see Appendix 3) is to be used at home on a daily basis. Patients are instructed to return immediately if a change is noted on Amsler's grid. (See Age-Related Macular Degeneration, Section 12.10, for management of choroidal neovascularization.)

12.14 CYSTOID MACULAR EDEMA (CME)

Symptoms
Decreased vision.

Critical Signs
Irregularity and blurring of the foveal light reflex, thickening with or without small intraretinal cysts in the foveal region.

Other Signs
Loss of the choroidal vascular pattern underlying the macula. Vitreous cells, optic-nerve swelling, and dot hemorrhage can appear in severe cases. A lamella macular hole causing permanent visual loss can develop.

Etiology
- After any type of ocular surgery (including laser photocoagulation and cryotherapy) (The peak incidence after cataract surgery is about 6 to 10 weeks; the incidence increases with surgical complications including vitreous to the wound, iris prolapse, and vitreous loss.)
- Diabetic retinopathy

- Central retinal vein occlusions (CRVOs) and branch retinal vein occlusions (BRVOs)
- Uveitis (particularly pars planitis; see Section 13.5, Pars Planitis)
- Retinitis pigmentosa
- Topical drops (e.g., epinephrine, dipivefrin, and latanoprost) drops, especially in postoperative cataract patients (Often reversed by discontinuing the drops.)
- Retinal vasculitis (e.g., Eales' disease, Behçet's syndrome, sarcoidosis, necrotizing angiitis, multiple sclerosis, cytomegalovirus retinitis)
- Retinal telangiectasias (e.g., Coats' disease)
- Age-related macular degeneration (ARMD) [Commonly over long-standing choroidal neovascular membrane (CNVM)]
- Associated with other conditions (occult inferior rhegmatogenous retinal detachment or occult foveal CNVM)
- Others (Intraocular tumors, systemic hypertension, collagen–vascular disease, surface-wrinkling retinopathy, autosomal dominant CME, others.)
- Pseudocystoid macular edema (No leakage on fluorescein angiogram [FA] [e.g., nicotinic acid maculopathy (relatively high doses of nicotinic acid are used to treat hypercholesterolemia)], X-linked retinoschisis, Goldmann–Favre disease, pseudohole from an epiretinal membrane)

Workup

1. History: Recent intraocular surgery? Diabetes? Previous uveitis or eye inflammation? Night blindness or family history of eye disease? Medications, including topical epinephrine, dipivefrin, or latanoprost?
2. Complete ocular examination, including a peripheral fundus evaluation (scleral depression inferiorly may be required to detect pars planitis). A macular examination is best performed with a slit lamp and a fundus contact lens, a Hruby lens, or a 60- or 90-diopter lens.
3. FA often shows early leakage of dye out of perifoveal capillaries and late macular staining, classically in a flower-petal or spoke-wheel pattern. Optic nerve head leakage is sometimes observed. Fluorescein leakage does not occur in nicotinic acid maculopathy.
4. Other diagnostic tests when indicated (e.g., fasting blood sugar or glucose tolerance test, electroretinogram)

❖ **Note**: *Subclinical CME commonly develops after cataract extraction and is noted on FA. These cases are not treated.*

Treatment

Most of these cases resolve spontaneously within 6 months.

1. Treat the underlying disorder if possible.
2. Topical nonsteroidal antiinflammatory drug (NSAID; e.g., ketorolac, q.i.d.) for 6 weeks (other topical NSAIDs not yet approved for CME)

3. Discontinue topical epinephrine, dipivefrin, or xalatan drops and medications containing nicotinic acid.
4. Consider acetazolamide, 500 mg p.o., daily, especially for postoperative patients, but also for those with retinitis pigmentosa and uveitis.
5. Other forms of therapy that have unproven efficacy but are occasionally used:
   a. Systemic NSAIDs (e.g., indomethacin, 25 mg p.o., t.i.d., for 6 weeks).
   b. Topical steroids (e.g., prednisolone acetate, 1%, q.i.d., for 3 weeks, and then taper over 3 weeks).
   c. Systemic steroids (e.g., prednisone, 40 mg p.o., daily for 5 days, and then taper over 2 weeks).
   d. Subtenon's steroid (e.g., methylprednisolone 80 mg/ml, in 0.5 ml).
   • Diabetic macular edema may benefit from focal laser treatment (see Diabetes Mellitus, Section 14.6).
   • Macular edema persisting for 3 to 6 months after a BRVO and reducing vision below 20/40 may improve with laser photocoagulation (see Branch Retinal Vein Occlusion, Section 12.4).
   • Macular edema with or without vitreous incarceration in a surgical wound may be improved by vitrectomy or YAG-laser lysis of the vitreous strand.
   • Macular edema from pars planitis is often treated with steroids when vision is reduced below 20/40 (see Pars Planitis, Section 13.5).

Follow-up

Postsurgical CME is not an emergency condition. Other forms of macular edema may require an etiologic workup and may benefit from early treatment (e.g., elimination of nicotinic acid–containing medications).

REFERENCES

Cox SN, Hay E, Bird AC. Treatment of chronic macular edema with acetazolamide. *Arch Ophthalmol* 1988;106:1190–1195.

12.15 MACULAR HOLE

Symptoms

Decreased vision, typically around the 20/200 level for a full-thickness hole, better for a partial-thickness hole; sometimes distortion of vision. More commonly, middle-aged to elderly women are affected.

Critical Signs
A round, red spot in the center of the macula, usually from one third to two thirds of a disc diameter in size, surrounded by a gray halo (marginal retinal detachment). A stage 1 idiopathic macular hole demonstrates loss of the normal foveolar depression and often a yellow spot or ring in the center of the macula.

Other Signs
Small, yellow precipitates within the hole, deep to the retina; retinal cysts at the margin of the hole or a small operculum above the hole, anterior to the retina (stage 4) or both.

❖ **Note**: *A partial-thickness (lamellar) hole is not so red and the surrounding gray halo is usually not present.*

Etiology
May be caused by vitreous or epiretinal membrane traction on the macula, trauma, or cystoid macular edema (CME).

Differential Diagnosis
- Macular pucker with a pseudohole [An epiretinal membrane (surface wrinkling) on the surface of the retina may simulate a macular hole.]
- Solar retinopathy (Small, round, red or yellow lesion at the center of the fovea, with surrounding fine gray pigment in a sun-gazer or eclipse watcher.)
- Intraretinal cysts (e.g., chronic CME with prominent central cyst.)

Workup
1. History: Previous trauma? Previous eye surgery? Sun-gazer?
2. Complete ocular examination, including a macular examination with a slit-lamp and 60- or 90-diopter, Hruby, or fundus contact lens. Because many macular hole patients have a posterior vitreous detachment, examination of the peripheral fundus to rule out peripheral breaks is important.
3. A true macular hole can be differentiated from a pseudohole by directing a thin, vertical slit beam across the area in question by using a 60- or 90-diopter lens with the slit-lamp biomicroscope. The patient with a true hole will report a break in the line. A pseudohole may cause distortion of the line, but it should not be broken (Watzke–Allen test).

Treatment
In selected cases of macular hole or impending macular hole, vitrectomy may be beneficial. It is preferable to operate within the first 12 months of onset with the possibility of regaining half of the visual angle. The risk of RD is very small. However, symptoms of an RD (e.g., sudden increase in

flashes and floaters, abundant "cobwebs" in the vision, or a curtain coming across the field of vision) are explained to patients, particularly those with high myopia. It is in this latter group that the macular hole sometimes leads to an RD, which requires surgical repair.

Follow-up

Patients with high myopia are seen every 6 months; other patients may be seen yearly. All patients are seen sooner if RD symptoms develop. Because there is a small risk that the condition may develop in the contralateral eye, patients are given an Amsler's grid for periodic home monitoring.

12.16 EPIRETINAL MEMBRANE
(MACULAR PUCKER, SURFACE-WRINKLING RETINOPATHY)

Symptoms

Decreased or distorted vision or both. Occasionally bilateral. Typically occurs in middle-aged or elderly patients.

Critical Signs

Spectrum ranges from a fine, glistening membrane (cellophane maculopathy) to a thick, gray–white membrane (macular pucker) present on the surface of the retina in the macular area.

❖ **Note:***When the epiretinal membrane is thin, it is often best appreciated with a 60- or 90-diopter lens. A glistening sparkle, much like cellophane, may be observed in the macular area.*

Other Signs

Retinal folds radiating out from the membrane, displacement or straightening of the macular retinal vessels, macular edema or detachment, signs of other ocular disease. A round, dark condensation of the epiretinal membrane in the macula may simulate a macular hole (termed pseudohole).

Etiology

Idiopathic, retinal break, rhegmatogenous retinal detachment, after retinal cryotherapy or photocoagulation, after intraocular surgery, trauma, uveitis, diabetic retinopathy, and other retinal vascular disease.

Differential Diagnosis

- Diabetic retinopathy (May produce preretinal fibrovascular tissue, which may displace retinal vessels or detach the macula. Macular edema may be present. Hemorrhages and microaneurysms are usually found in addition, and the changes are commonly bilateral.)

Workup

1. History: Previous eye surgery or eye disease? Diabetes?
2. Complete ocular examination, particularly a thorough dilated fundus evaluation. The macula is often best seen with a slit lamp and a 60- or 90-diopter, Hruby, or fundus contact lens.

Treatment

Treat the underlying disorder. Surgical peeling of the membrane can be considered when it significantly reduces the vision.

Follow-up

This is not an emergency condition, and treatment may be instituted at any time. Infrequently, membranes separate from the retina, resulting in spontaneously improved vision. A small percentage of epiretinal membranes recur after surgical removal.

12.17 POSTERIOR VITREOUS DETACHMENT (PVD)

Symptoms

Floaters ("cobwebs," "bugs," "tadpole," or comma-shaped objects that change position with eye movement), blurred vision, flashes of light, which are more common in dim illumination and are temporally located.

Critical Signs

One or more discrete light gray to black vitreous opacities, often in the shape of a ring (termed Weiss ring), suspended over the optic disc. The opacities float within the vitreous as the eye moves from side to side.

Other Signs

Vitreous hemorrhage, peripheral retinal and disc-margin hemorrhages, pigmented cells in the anterior vitreous, retinal break or detachment.

❖ **Note:** *The presence of pigmented cells (released retinal pigment epithelial cells) in the anterior vitreous or vitreous hemorrhage in association with acute PVD indicates a high probability of a coexisting retinal break (see Section 12.18, Retinal Break).*

Differential Diagnosis
- Vitritis (It may be difficult to distinguish PVD with pigmented anterior vitreous cells from vitreous inflammatory cells. In vitritis, the vitreous cells may be found in both the posterior and anterior vitreous, the condition may be bilateral, and the cells are not typically pigmented. A history of uveitis may be elicited. See Section 13.2, Posterior Uveitis.)
- Migraine (Patients complain of flashing lights in a zig-zag pattern that obstruct vision, last approximately 20 minutes, and are sometimes multicolored. A headache may or may not follow. No vitreous or retinal abnormalities are found on examination. See Section 15.3, Headache.)

The following may occur with or without PVD, producing similar symptoms:

- Retinal break
- Vitreous hemorrhage
- Retinal detachment (RD)

Workup
1. History: Distinguish between the visual distortion of migraine, from the light sparks of PVD, which are commonly accompanied by new floaters. Determine the duration of the symptoms.
2. Complete ocular examination, particularly a dilated retinal examination by using indirect ophthalmoscopy and scleral depression to rule out a retinal break and detachment. A slit-lamp examination of the anterior vitreous, looking for pigmented cells, should be performed (see Appendix 8).
3. PVD may be visualized by focusing in the vitreous, anterior to the disc, by using
   a. Indirect ophthalmoscopy.
   b. Direct ophthalmoscopy. (The ophthalmoscope is initially focused on the cornea, and the lens wheel is moved from higher toward lower plus lenses while the patient is asked to move his or her eye from left to right. The Weiss ring is seen to float by.)
   c. A slit-lamp and a 60- or 90-diopter, Hruby, or contact lens examination. (Pull the slit lamp back once focus on the disc is obtained. A gray-to-black strand may be seen suspended in the vitreous.)

Treatment
No treatment is indicated for PVD. If an acute retinal break is found, the patient should receive laser or cryotherapy within 24 to 72 hours to avoid the development of an RD (see Section 12.18, Retinal Break).

❖ **Note:** *A retinal break surrounded by pigment is old and usually does not require treatment.*

Follow-up

The patient should be given a list of retinal-detachment symptoms (an increase in floaters or flashing lights, or the appearance of a persistent curtain or shadow anywhere in the field of vision) and told to return immediately if these symptoms develop.

- If no retinal break or hemorrhage is found, the patient should be scheduled for repeated examination with scleral depression in 2 to 4 weeks, 2 to 3 months, and 6 months after the symptoms first develop.
- If no retinal break is found, but mild vitreous hemorrhage or peripheral punctate retinal hemorrhages are present, repeated examinations are performed 1 to 2 weeks, 4 weeks, 3 months, and 6 months after the event.
- If a vitreous hemorrhage dense enough to obscure visualization of the retina is found, ultrasonography is indicated to rule out an RD, tumor, or hemorrhagic macular degeneration. Occasionally the flap of a tear can be identified. Bed rest, with the head of the bed elevated, may be used for 24 to 48 hours to hasten settling of the blood (see Section 12.22, Vitreous Hemorrhage).

12.18 RETINAL BREAK

Symptoms

Acute retinal break Flashes of light, floaters ("cobwebs" or "flies" that move with eye movement), and sometimes blurred vision.
Chronic retinal break or an atrophic retinal hole Usually asymptomatic.

Critical Sign

A full-thickness retinal defect.

Other Signs

Acute retinal break Pigmented cells in the anterior vitreous, vitreous hemorrhage, posterior vitreous detachment, retinal flap, an operculum (a free-floating piece of retina) suspended in the vitreous cavity above the retinal hole.
Chronic retinal break A ring of pigmentation surrounding the break, demarcation line between attached and detached retina, signs (but not symptoms) of an acute retinal break.

Predisposing Lesions

Lattice degeneration, high myopia, aphakia, pseudophakia, age-related retinoschisis, vitreoretinal tufts, meridional folds, history of previous retinal break or detachment in the fellow eye.

Workup

Complete ocular examination, particularly a dilated fundus examination of both eyes by using indirect ophthalmoscopy and scleral depression. Scleral depression is generally not performed until 2 to 4 weeks after a traumatic hyphema or microhyphema. A slit-lamp examination with a fundus contact lens is often quite helpful in evaluating retinal breaks.

Treatment

In general, laser therapy, cryotherapy, or scleral-buckling surgery is required within 24 to 72 hours for acute retinal breaks, and only rarely for chronic breaks. Each case must be individualized; however, we follow these general guidelines:

A. Treatment recommended
   1. Acute symptomatic break (e.g., a horseshoe or operculated tear).
   2. Acute traumatic break (including a dialysis).
B. Treatment to be considered
   1. Asymptomatic retinal break that is large (e.g., >1.5 mm) or above the horizontal meridian or both, particularly if there is no posterior vitreous detachment.
   2. Asymptomatic retinal break in an aphakic or pseudophakic eye, an eye in which the involved or the contralateral eye has had a retinal detachment (RD), or in a highly myopic eye.

Follow-up

Patients with predisposing lesions or retinal breaks that do not require treatment are followed up every 6 to 12 months. Patients treated for a retinal break are reexamined in 1 week, 1 month, 3 months, and then every 6 to 12 months. RD symptoms (an increase in floaters or flashing lights or the appearance of a curtain, shadow, or bubble anywhere in the field of vision) are explained to all patients, and patients are told to return immediately if these symptoms develop.

12.19 RETINAL DETACHMENT

There are three distinct types of retinal detachment (RD). All three forms show an elevation of the retina.

A. Rhegmatogenous (RRD)

Symptoms

Flashes of light, floaters, a curtain or shadow moving over the field of vision, peripheral or central visual loss or both.

Critical Sign

Elevation of the retina with an accompanying retinal break(s) (See Section 12.18, Retinal Break).

Other Signs

Pigmented cells in the anterior vitreous, vitreous hemorrhage, posterior vitreous detachment, usually lower intraocular pressure (IOP) in the affected eye than the contralateral eye, clear subretinal fluid that does not shift with body position, sometimes fixed retinal folds. The detached retina is often corrugated in appearance. An afferent pupillary defect (APD) may be present.

❖ **Note:** *A chronic RRD often shows a pigmented demarcation line at the posterior extent of the RD, intraretinal cysts, fixed folds, or white dots underneath the retina (subretinal precipitates) or a combination of these. It should be differentiated from retinoschisis, which produces an absolute visual-field defect.*

B. Exudative (ERD)

Symptoms

Minimal-to-severe visual loss or a visual-field defect.

Critical Sign

Serous elevation of the retina with shifting subretinal fluid (SRF). (The area of detached retina changes when the patient changes position: while sitting, the SRF accumulates inferiorly, detaching the retina inferiorly; while in the supine position, the fluid accumulates in the posterior pole, detaching the macula.) There is no retinal break.

Other Signs

The detached retina is smooth and may become quite bullous. A mild APD may be present.

Etiology
- Neoplastic (e.g., choroidal malignant melanoma, metastasis, choroidal hemangioma, multiple myeloma, capillary retinal hemangioma) (Fluorescein angiogram and ultrasound may be helpful in making a differential diagnosis.)
- Inflammatory disease [e.g., Vogt–Koyanagi–Harada (VKH) syndrome, posterior scleritis, other chronic inflammatory processes]

- Congenital abnormalities (e.g., optic pit, morning-glory syndrome, choroidal coloboma, Coats' disease)
- Nanophthalmos (Small eyes with a small cornea and a shallow anterior chamber but a large lens and a thick sclera.)
- Idiopathic central serous chorioretinopathy (May be seen with bullous RD from multiple, large retinal pigment epithelial detachments.)
- Uveal effusion syndrome (Bilateral detachments of the peripheral choroid, ciliary body, and retina; leopard-spot retinal pigment epithelial changes (when retina is reattached); cells in the vitreous; dilated episcleral vessels.)

C. Tractional (TRD)

Symptoms

Visual loss or visual-field defect; may be asymptomatic.

Critical Signs

The detached retina appears concave with a smooth surface; vitreous membranes exerting traction on the retina are present. (Detachment may become a convex RRD if a tractional retinal tear develops.)

Other Signs

The retina is immobile, and the detachment rarely extends to the ora serrata. A mild APD may be present.

Etiology

Fibrous bands in the vitreous (e.g., resulting from proliferative diabetic retinopathy, sickle-cell retinopathy, retinopathy of prematurity, toxocariasis, trauma, previous giant retinal tear) contract and detach the retina.

Differential Diagnosis for All Three Types of RD
- Acquired/Age-related degenerative retinoschisis (Commonly bilateral, usually inferotemporal, no pigmented cells or hemorrhage are present in the vitreous, the retinal vessels in the inner retinal layers are often sheathed peripherally, white "snowflakes" are often seen on the inner retinal layers; the patient is asymptomatic. An absolute scotoma, as opposed to a relative scotoma as seen with a RRD, is found on visual-field testing. A demarcation line is generally not present. When a demarcation line is present, we must look for a retinal break because long-standing detachments may simulate schisis and may even demonstrate an absolute field defect.)
- Juvenile retinoschisis (Petaloid foveal changes are present when the schisis is posterior to the equator, X-linked recessive, bilateral, the retinoschisis does not extend to the ora serrata.)

- Choroidal detachment (Orange–brown, more solid in appearance than an RD, the ora serrata can usually be seen without scleral depression, the detachment often extends 360 degrees around the globe. Hypotony is generally present.)

Treatment/Follow-up
1. Patients with acute RRD or TRD that threatens the fovea should be placed on bed rest until surgical repair is performed urgently.
2. All RRDs that do not threaten fixation or with macula-off detachments or TRDs that involve the macula are repaired at the earliest convenience, preferably within a few days.
3. Chronic RDs are treated within 1 week.
4. For ERD, successful treatment of the underlying condition often leads to resolution of the detachment.

12.20 RETINOSCHISIS

Retinoschisis, a splitting of the retina, occurs in X-linked (juvenile) and age-related degenerative forms.

A. X-Linked (Juvenile) Retinoschisis

Symptoms
Decreased vision (often due to vitreous hemorrhage) or asymptomatic. The condition is congenital, but may not be detected at birth if an examination is not performed. A family history may or may not be elicited.

Critical Signs
Cystoid foveal changes with retinal folds that radiate from the center of the foveal configuration (petaloid pattern). Unlike the cysts of cystoid macular edema, they do not stain on fluorescein angiogram.

Other Signs
Separation of the nerve-fiber layer from the outer retinal layers in the retinal periphery with the development of nerve-fiber layer breaks; this peripheral retinoschisis occurs most commonly in the inferotemporal quadrant of the fundus and is bilateral. The retinoschisis does not extend to the ora serrata. Retinal detachment (RD), vitreous hemorrhage, and pigmentary changes also may occur. Pigmented demarcation lines may be seen even though the retina is not detached. This is not the case for acquired age-related degeneration.

Inheritance
X-linked recessive.

Differential Diagnosis
- Age-related degenerative retinoschisis (see the following)
- Rhegmatogenous RD (Usually unilateral and acquired. It extends to the ora serrata and lacks the foveal changes described previously. Anterior-chamber cells and flare and pigment in the vitreous are often seen. See Section 12.19, Retinal Detachment.)

Workup
1. Family history.
2. Dilated retinal examination with scleral depression to rule out an outer-layer retinal break or detachment.

Treatment
Surgical repair of an RD should be performed. Superimposed amblyopia should always be considered in children younger than 9 to 11 years when one eye is more severely affected, and a trial of patching should be considered (see Section 9.6, Amblyopia).

Follow-up
Every 6 months; sooner if treating amblyopia.

B. Age-Related Degenerative Retinoschisis

Symptoms
Usually none, may have decreased vision.

Critical Signs
The retinal split is usually bilateral and may show sheathing of retinal vessels and "snowflakes," or "frosting" on the elevated inner wall of the schisis cavity. (In contrast to X-linked juvenile retinoschisis, splitting usually occurs at the level of the outer plexiform layer.) The schisis cavity is dome-shaped with a smooth surface and is usually located temporally, especially inferotemporally.

Other Signs
Prominent cystoid degeneration near the ora serrata, an absolute scotoma is found on visual-field testing, hyperopia is common, and there are no pigment cells or hemorrhage in the vitreous. A rhegmatogenous RD may occasionally develop.

Differential Diagnosis

- Rhegmatogenous RD (The surface is not smooth but corrugated in appearance and can be seen to move more with eye movements. Schisis does not; retinal vessels are not sheathed, and no "snowflakes" or "frosting" can be seen on the retinal elevation; one or more full-thickness holes are present, and pigmented cells or hemorrhage may be present in the vitreous. A long-standing RD may resemble retinoschisis, but intraretinal cysts, demarcation lines between attached and detached retina, and white retroretinal dots may be seen. A relative scotoma is found on visual-field testing. See Section 12.19, Retinal Detachment.)
- X-linked juvenile retinoschisis (see previous)

Workup

1. Slit-lamp evaluation to rule out the presence of anterior-chamber inflammation or pigmented anterior-vitreous cells, both of which should not be present in isolated retinoschisis.
2. Dilated retinal examination with scleral depression to rule out a concomitant RD or an outer-layer retinal hole, which may lead to an RD.
3. A fundus contact lens evaluation of the retina as needed to aid in recognizing outer-layer retinal breaks.

Treatment

Surgery is indicated when a clinically significant RD develops. A small RD walled off by a demarcation line is generally not treated. This may take the form of pigmentation at the posterior border of outer-layer breaks.

Follow-up

Every 6 months. RD symptoms (an increase in floaters or flashing lights or the appearance of a curtain or shadow anywhere in the field of vision) are explained to all patients, and patients are told to return immediately if these symptoms develop.

12.21 CHOROIDAL DETACHMENT

Symptoms

Decreased vision or asymptomatic in a serous choroidal detachment. Moderate to severe pain, decreased vision may occur if the choroidal detachments are touching ("kissing choroidals"), and red eye may occur with a hemorrhagic choroidal detachment.

Critical Signs

Smooth, bullous, orange–brown elevation of the retina and choroid that usually extends 360 degrees around the periphery in a lobular configuration. The ora serrata can be seen without scleral depression.

Other Signs

Serous choroidal detachment Low intraocular pressure (IOP) (often <6 mm Hg), shallow anterior chamber with mild cell and flare, positive transillumination.

Hemorrhagic choroidal detachment High IOP (if detachment is large), shallow anterior chamber with mild cell and flare, no transillumination.

Etiology

SEROUS

- Intra- or postoperative (Wound leak, perforation of the sclera from a superior rectus bridle suture, iritis, cyclodialysis cleft, leakage or excess filtration from a filtering bleb, or after laser photocoagulation or cryotherapy. May occur days to weeks after the surgery.)
- Traumatic (Often associated with a ruptured globe.)
- Rhegmatogenous retinal detachment (RRD) or after scleral buckling repair of a detachment
- Rare [Nanophthalmos, uveal effusion syndrome, carotid–cavernous fistula, primary or metastatic tumor, scleritis, Vogt-Koyanagi-Harada (VKH) syndrome.]

HEMORRHAGIC

- Intra- or postoperative (From anterior displacement of the ocular contents and rupture of the short posterior ciliary arteries.)
- Spontaneous (e.g., after perforation of a corneal ulcer)
- Rupture of a choroidal neovascular membrane (CNVM) in a patient taking anticoagulants

Differential Diagnosis

- Melanoma of the ciliary body (Not typically multilobular or symmetrical in each quadrant of the globe. Pigmented melanomas do not transilluminate. B-scan ultrasound may help to differentiate between the two. See Section 8.3, Malignant Melanoma of the Choroid.)
- RRD (Appears white and undulates with eye movements. A break usually seen in the retina, and pigment cells are present in the vitreous. See Section 12.19, Retinal Detachment.)

Workup

1. History: Recent ocular surgery or trauma? Known eye or medical problem?

2. Slit-lamp examination: Check for the presence of a filtering bleb and perform Seidel's test to rule out a wound leak (see Appendix 4).
3. Gonioscopy of the anterior-chamber angle: Look for a cyclodialysis cleft.
4. Dilated retinal examination: Determine whether there is subretinal fluid, indicating a concomitant retinal detachment (RD), and whether an underlying choroidal disease or tumor is present. Examination of the contralateral eye may be helpful in diagnosis.
5. In cases suggestive of melanoma, B-scan ultrasonography and transillumination of the globe are helpful in making a diagnosis.
6. Check the skin for vitiligo and the head for alopecia (VKH).

Treatment
  A. General treatment
    1. Cycloplegic (e.g., atropine, 1%, t.i.d.).
    2. Topical steroid (e.g., prednisolone acetate, 1%, 4 to 6 times per day).
    3. Surgical drainage of the suprachoroidal fluid may be indicated for a flat or progressively shallow anterior chamber, particularly in the presence of inflammation (because of the risk of peripheral anterior synechiae), corneal decompensation resulting from lens–cornea touch, or "kissing" choroidals (apposition of two lobules of detached choroid).
  B. Specific treatment: Repair the underlying problem.

SEROUS

- Wound leak or leaky filtering bleb: Patch for 24 hours, suture the site, use cyanoacrylate glue, or place a bandage contact lens on the eye, or a combination of these.
- Cyclodialysis cleft: Laser therapy, diathermy, cryotherapy, or suture the cleft to close it.
- Uveitis: Topical cycloplegic and steroid as discussed previously.
- Inflammatory disease: See the specific entity.
- RD: Surgical repair. Proliferative vitreoretinopathy (PVR) after repair is common.

HEMORRHAGIC

An anterior vitrectomy and drainage of the choroidal detachment is performed for severe cases with retina or vitreous to the wound. Otherwise use general treatment.

Follow-up
In accordance with the underlying problem.

12.22 VITREOUS HEMORRHAGE

Symptoms

Sudden painless loss of vision or sudden appearance of black spots with flashing lights.

Critical Signs

In a severe vitreous hemorrhage, the red fundus reflex may be absent, and there may be no fundus view on ophthalmoscopy. Red blood cells can sometimes be appreciated when a slit lamp is focused posterior to the lens. In a mild vitreous hemorrhage, blood may be seen to obscure part of the retina and retinal vessels. Chronic vitreous hemorrhage has a yellow ochre appearance resulting from the breakdown of hemoglobin.

Other Signs

A mild afferent pupillary defect is possible. Depending on the etiology, there may be other fundus abnormalities.

Etiology

- Diabetic retinopathy (Almost always have a known history of diabetes and usually one of diabetic retinopathy. Diabetic retinopathy is usually evident in the contralateral eye. See Section 14.6, Diabetes Mellitus.)
- Retinal break (Commonly superior in cases of dense vitreous hemorrhage. This may be demonstrated by ultrasonography and scleral depression. See Section 12.18, Retinal Break.)
- Retinal detachment (RD) (May be diagnosed by ultrasound if the retina cannot be viewed on clinical examination. See Section 12.19, Retinal Detachment.)
- Retinal vein occlusion (usually a branch retinal vein occlusion) (Commonly occurs in older patients with a history of high blood pressure. May have a history of a vein occlusion or sudden visual loss in the eye months to years previously. See Section 12.4, Branch Retinal Vein Occlusion.)
- Posterior vitreous detachment (Common in middle-aged or elderly patients. Usually, patients note floaters and flashing lights. See Section 12.17, Posterior Vitreous Detachment.)
- Age-related macular degeneration (ARMD) (Patients often acknowledge poor vision before the vitreous hemorrhage as a result of their underlying disease. Macular drusen or other findings of ARMD or both are found in the contralateral eye. May use B-scan ultrasound to aid in the diagnosis. See Section 12.10, Age-Related Macular Degeneration.)
- Sickle-cell disease (particularly SC disease) African-American patients. May have peripheral retinal neovascularization in the contralateral eye,

typically in a "sea-fan" configuration and salmon color. See Section 12.23, Sickle-Cell Disease.)
- Trauma (by history)
- Intraocular tumor (May be visible on ophthalmoscopy or B-scan ultrasonography. See Sections 8.2, Malignant Melanoma of the Iris, and 8.3, Malignant Melanoma of the Choroid.)
- Subarachnoid or subdural hemorrhage (Terson's syndrome) (Frequently bilateral preretinal or vitreous hemorrhages may occur. A severe headache usually precedes the fundus findings. Coma may occur.)
- Eales' disease (Usually occurs in men aged 20 to 30 years with peripheral retinal ischemia and neovascularization of unknown etiology. Decreased vision as a result of vitreous hemorrhage is frequently the presenting sign. The disease is often bilateral and is a diagnosis of exclusion.)
- Others (Coats' disease, retinopathy of prematurity, retinal capillary angiomas of von Hippel–Lindau syndrome, congenital prepapillary vascular loop, hypertension, radiation retinopathy, anterior-segment hemorrhage because of an intraocular lens (IOL), bleeding diathesis, others.)

❖ **Note:** *In infancy and childhood consider birth trauma, shaken baby syndrome, traumatic child abuse, juvenile X-linked retinoschisis.*

Differential Diagnosis
- Vitritis (white blood cells in the vitreous) (The onset is rarely as sudden as in vitreous hemorrhage; anterior or posterior uveitis may also be present. No red blood cells and no hemorrhage in the vitreous are present. See Section 13.2, Posterior Uveitis.)
- RD (May occur without a vitreous hemorrhage, yet the symptoms may be identical. The fundus view may be difficult in a highly elevated detachment; however, the retina can usually be viewed with an indirect ophthalmoscope. In cases of highly elevated detachments, slit-lamp examination may show the retina behind the lens. See Section 12.19, Retinal Detachment.)

Workup
1. History: Any ocular or systemic diseases, specifically the ones mentioned previously? Trauma?
2. Complete ocular examination, including a slit-lamp examination to check for iris neovascularization, intraocular presure (IOP) measurement, and a dilated fundus examination of both eyes by using indirect ophthalmoscopy. In cases of spontaneous vitreous hemorrhage, scleral depression is performed if a retinal view can be obtained (we do not generally depress eyes until 3 to 4 weeks after traumatic hemorrhages.)

3. When no retinal view can be obtained, a B-scan ultrasound is performed to detect an associated RD or intraocular tumor. Flap retinal tears may be detected with scleral depression and sometimes seen on B-scan.
4. A fluorescein angiogram may aid in defining the etiology, although the quality of the angiogram may depend on the density of the hemorrhage.

Treatment

1. If the etiology of the vitreous hemorrhage is not known and a retinal break or a RD or both cannot be ruled out (e.g., there is no known history of one of the diseases mentioned previously, there are no changes in the contralateral eye, and the fundus is obscured by a total vitreous hemorrhage), the patient is admitted to the hospital or monitored closely as an outpatient.
2. Bed rest with the head of the bed elevated (and sometimes bilateral patching) for 2 to 3 days (this reduces the chance of recurrent bleeding and allows the blood to settle inferiorly, permitting a view of the superior peripheral fundus, a common site for responsible retinal breaks).
3. Eliminate aspirin, nonsteroidal antiinflammatory drugs, and other anticlotting agents unless they are medically necessary.
4. The underlying etiology is treated as soon as possible (e.g., retinal breaks are sealed with cryotherapy or laser photocoagulation, detached retinas are repaired, and proliferative retinal vascular diseases are treated with laser photocoagulation or cryotherapy when there is no retinal view).
5. Surgical removal of the blood (vitrectomy) is usually performed for:
   a. Vitreous hemorrhage accompanied by RD or break seen on B-scan.
   b. Chronic vitreous hemorrhage (>6 months in duration).
   c. Vitreous hemorrhage with neovascularization of the iris.
   d. Hemolytic or ghost cell glaucoma.

❖ **Note:** *Vitrectomy for isolated vitreous hemorrhage (e.g., without RD) may be considered earlier than 6 months for diabetics or patients with bilateral vitreous hemorrhage.*

Follow-up

The patient is evaluated daily for the first 2 to 3 days. If a total vitreous hemorrhage persists, and the etiology remains unknown, the patient is followed up with a B-scan ultrasound every 1 to 3 weeks to rule out an RD.

12.23 SICKLE-CELL DISEASE
(SICKLE-CELL HEMOGLOBIN C DISEASE, SICKLE-CELL THALASSEMIA, SICKLE-CELL ANEMIA, AND SICKLE-CELL TRAIT)

Symptoms
Usually without ocular symptoms. May have floaters, flashing lights, or loss of vision with advanced disease. Systemically, patients with sickle-cell anemia often have painful crises with severe abdominal or musculoskeletal discomfort. Patients are of African or Mediterranean extraction in most cases.

Critical Signs
Peripheral retinal neovascularization in the shape of a fan ("sea-fan" sign), sclerosed peripheral retinal vessels, or an abnormal dull gray peripheral fundus background color (as a result of peripheral arteriolar occlusions and ischemia).

Other Signs
Tortuosity of retinal veins, black midperipheral fundus lesions with spiculated borders (black sunbursts), intraretinal and subretinal hemorrhages (salmon patch), refractile (iridescent) intraretinal deposits, angioid streaks, comma-shaped capillaries of the conjunctiva (especially along the inferior fornix). Vitreous hemorrhage and traction bands, retinal detachment (RD), central retinal artery occlusion (CRAO), and macular arteriolar occlusions may develop.

❖ **Note:** *Proliferative sickle-cell retinopathy is thought to progress from peripheral arteriolar occlusions (stage 1) to peripheral arteriovenous anastomoses (stage 2) to retinal neovascularization (stage 3). The retinal neovascularization may spontaneously regress or may produce vitreous hemorrhage (stage 4) or traction RD (stage 5).*

Differential Diagnosis
(Other causes of peripheral retinal neovascularization.)

- Sarcoidosis (May also produce peripheral sea-fan neovascularization in young black individuals. However, granulomatous uveitis, vitritis with vitreous opacities, and sheathing of retinal veins are often present. See Section 13.4, Sarcoidosis.)
- Diabetes (Tends to have a more posterior retinal location, dot/blot hemorrhages, and increased blood sugar. See Section 14.6, Diabetes Mellitus.)

- Branch Retinal Vein Occlusion [Flame-shaped hemorrhages involving a sector or one half of the retina (the inferior or superior half); the hemorrhages do not cross the horizontal raphé. May see a sclerosed arteriole only in late stages. See Section 12.4, Branch Retinal Vein Occlusion.]
- Embolic (e.g., talc) retinopathy (History of intravenous drug abuse. May see refractile talc particles in the macular arterioles.)
- Eales' disease (Peripheral retinal vascular occlusion of unknown etiology; a diagnosis of exclusion.)
- Others (Retinopathy of prematurity, familial exudative vitreoretinopathy, chronic myelogenous leukemia, radiation retinopathy, pars planitis, carotid–cavernous fistula, ocular ischemic syndrome, collagen–vascular disease.)

Workup
1. Medical history and family history: Sickle-cell disease, diabetes, or known medical problems? Intravenous drug abuse?
2. Dilated fundus examination by using indirect ophthalmoscopy.
3. Sickle-cell preparation and hemoglobin electrophoresis (patients with sickle-cell trait, as well as hemoglobin C disease, may have a negative sickle-cell preparation).
4. Consider fluorescein angiogram to aid in diagnostic and therapeutic considerations.

Treatment
There are no well-established indications or guidelines for treatment. The presence of retinal neovascularization, vitreous hemorrhage, or RD, however, typically warrants treatment. Laser photocoagulation or retinal surgery is typically performed.

Follow-up
- No retinal pathology present: Repeat dilated fundus examination yearly.
- Retinal pathology present: Repeat dilated fundus examination every 1 to 6 months, depending on the degree of pathology.

12.24 RETINITIS PIGMENTOSA (RP)

Symptoms
Difficulty with night vision (often night blindness) and loss of peripheral vision are most common. Poor central vision or difficulty with color vision are late findings.

Critical Signs

Classically, clumps of pigment dispersed throughout the peripheral retina in a perivascular pattern, often assuming a "bone spicule" arrangement, areas of depigmentation or atrophy of the retinal pigment epithelium (RPE), narrowing of arterioles, vitreous cells, and later, optic-disc pallor. Patients have progressive visual-field loss, usually a ring scotoma, which progresses to a small central field. Electroretinography (ERG) is usually moderately to markedly reduced.

Other Signs

Focal or sectoral pigment clumping, cystoid macular edema (CME), epi-retinal membrane, posterior subcapsular cataract.

INHERITANCE PATTERNS

Autosomal recessive   Diminished vision and night blindness occur early in life.

Autosomal dominant   More gradual onset of RP, typically in adult life, late onset of cataract.

X-linked recessive   Onset similar to autosomal recessive. Female carriers often have salt-and-pepper fundus.

SYSTEMIC DISEASES ASSOCIATED WITH HEREDITARY RETINAL DEGENERATION

Many systemic diseases and syndromes are associated with RP. The following is a short list of those syndromes for which treatment may be beneficial.

Refsum's disease   (phytanoyl-CoA hydroxylase deficiency) Autosomal recessive RP with increased serum phytanic acid level. May have cerebellar ataxia, progressive weakness of distal extremities, deafness, dry skin, anosmia, or progressive restriction of ocular motility.
Treatment:
1. Give a low-phytanic acid, low-phytol diet (minimize the amount of milk products, animal fats, and green leafy vegetables in the patient's diet).
2. Examine serum phytanic acid levels every 6 months.

Hereditary abetalipoproteinemia   (Bassen-Kornzweig syndrome) RP with fat intolerance, diarrhea, crenated erythrocytes (acanthocytes), ataxia, progressive restriction of ocular motility, and other neurologic symptoms as a result of deficiency in lipoproteins and malabsorption of the fat-soluble vitamins A, D, E, and K. Diagnosis based on serum Apo-B deficiency.
Treatment:
1. Water-miscible vitamin A, 10,000 to 15,000 IU, p.o., daily.
2. Vitamin E, 200 to 300 IU/kg, p.o., daily.

3. Vitamin K, 5 mg, p.o., weekly.

4. Restrict dietary fat to 15% of caloric intake.

5. Biannual serum levels of vitamin A and E; yearly ERG, dark adaptometry, and prothrombin time (PT); periodic nerve-conduction studies.

6. Consider supplementing the patient's diet with zinc.

Kearns–Sayre syndrome Pigmentary degeneration of the retina, often salt-and-pepper in appearance, with normal arterioles, progressive limitation of ocular movement, ptosis, and later, heart block. Ocular signs generally appear before age 20 years. See Section 11.11, Chronic Progressive External Ophthalmoplegia. Transmitted by mitochondrial DNA.

Treatment:

Refer the patient to a cardiologist for yearly electrocardiograms. Patients may need a pacemaker.

PSEUDORETINITIS PIGMENTOSA

Disorders that produce a fundus picture similar to that of RP.

- Phenothiazine toxicity (Especially in patients taking >800 mg/day of thioridazine.)
- Syphilis (Positive FTA-ABS, asymmetric visual fields, abnormal fundus appearance, may have a history of recurrent uveitis, no family history of RP; the ERG is generally preserved to some degree.)
- Congenital rubella (A salt-and-pepper fundus appearance may be accompanied by microphthalmos, cataract, deafness, a congenital heart abnormality, or another systemic abnormality. The ERG is usually normal.)
- After resolution of a retinal detachment (RD) (e.g., toxemia of pregnancy or Harada's disease). The history is diagnostic.
- Pigmented paravenous retinochoroidal atrophy (Paravenous localization of RPE degeneration and pigment deposition. No definite hereditary pattern. Variable visual fields and ERG. May be nonprogressive, but long-term follow-up is not available.)
- After severe blunt trauma (Usually due to spontaneous resolution of RD)

❖ **Note:** *The pigment abnormalities are at the level of the RPE with phenothiazine toxicity, syphilis, and congenital rubella. With resolved RD, the pigment is intraretinal.*

OTHER CAUSES OF NYCTALOPIA (NIGHT BLINDNESS)

- Gyrate atrophy [The fundus shows well-demarcated, scalloped areas of full-thickness atrophy, white–yellow in appearance, with thin margins of pigment outlining the areas of atrophy; the changes extend from the periphery toward the macula. Patients have high levels of ornithine in their blood (often 10 times normal levels), urine, aqueous humor, and cerebrospinal fluid. Abnormal or nonrecordable ERG, visual-field defects, high myopia, and cataracts are common. Autosomal recessive. See Section 12.26, Gyrate Atrophy.]

- Choroideremia (Choroidal atrophy accompanies scattered, small pigment granules, sparing the macula. Bone spicules are not seen. X-linked recessive. See Section 12.25, Choroideremia.)
- Vitamin A deficiency [Usually acquired from malnutrition or surgical resection of the bowel, but may be inherited (familial carotinemia). Marked night blindness; numerous small, yellow–white, well-demarcated spots deep in the retina seen peripherally; dry eye and/or Bitot's spots (white lesions) on the conjunctiva. See Section 14.10, Vitamin A Deficiency.]
- Congenital stationary night blindness (Night blindness from birth, normal visual fields, may have a normal or abnormal fundus, not progressive. Paradoxic pupillary response.)

Workup
1. Medical and ocular history pertaining to the diseases discussed previously.
2. Drug history.
3. Family history (for diagnostic and counseling purposes).
4. Ophthalmoscopic examination.
5. Formal visual-field testing (e.g., Goldmann).
6. ERG (may help distinguish stationary rod–cone dysfunction from RP, a progressive disease) and dark adaptation studies.
7. Fundus photographs.
8. Fluorescent treponemal antibody, absorbed (FTA-ABS) if the diagnosis is uncertain.
9. If the patient is male and the type of inheritance is unknown, examine his mother and perform an ERG on her (women carriers of X-linked disease often have abnormal pigmentation in the midperiphery and have abnormal dark-adapted ERGs.)
10. If neurologic abnormalities such as ataxia, polyneuropathy, deafness, or anosmia are present, obtain a fasting (at least 14 hours) serum phytanic acid level to rule out Refsum's disease.
11. If hereditary abetalipoproteinemia is suspected, obtain serum cholesterol and triglyceride levels (levels are low), a serum protein and lipoprotein electrophoresis (lipoprotein deficiency is detected), and peripheral blood smears (acanthocytosis is seen).
12. If Kearns–Sayre syndrome is suspected, the patient must be examined by a cardiologist with sequential ECGs; patients can die of complete heart block.

Treatment/Follow-up

For the following conditions, consult

Choroideremia, Section 12.25
Gyrate Atrophy, Section 12.26
Acquired Syphilis, Section 14.2
Vitamin A Deficiency, Section 14.10

No definitive treatment for RP is currently known. However, vitamin A palmitate, 15,000 IU, was found in one study to slow ERG dysfunction. This is recommended only for nonpregnant patients older than 21 years. Watch liver-function tests (LFTs) and vitamin A levels.

Cataract surgery may improve central visual acuity. Oral acetazolamide is often effective for CME.

All patients will benefit from genetic counseling and instruction on how to deal with their visual handicaps. In advanced cases, low-vision aids and vocational rehabilitation are helpful.

REFERENCE

Berson EL, Rosner B, Sanberg MA, et al. A randomized trial of vitamin A and vitamin E supplementation for retinitis pigmentosa. *Arch Ophthalmol* 1993;111(6):761–772.

12.25 CHOROIDEREMIA

Symptoms

Night blindness in male patients aged 4 to 30 years, followed by insidious loss of peripheral vision. Decreased central vision occurs late in the disease. Women, who are asymptomatic carriers, often have a salt-and-pepper fundus.

Critical Signs

Males   Early: Dispersed pigment granules throughout, sparing the macula. Late: Total absence of retinal pigment epithelium (RPE) and choriocapillaris.

Females   Small, scattered, square intraretinal pigment granules overlying choroidal atrophy, most marked in the midperiphery.

Other Signs

Retinal arteriolar narrowing and optic atrophy can occur late in the process; constriction of visual fields, normal color vision, abnormal electro-retinogram (ERG). Late stages, near-total absence of choroid and RPE.

Inheritance

X-linked recessive.

Differential Diagnosis

- Retinitis pigmentosa (No choroidal atrophy, may see bone spicules of pigment. See Section 12.24, Retinitis Pigmentosa.)
- Gyrate atrophy (Scalloped RPE and choriocapillaris atrophy, posterior subcapsular cataract, high myopia with astigmatism, hyperornithinemia. Autosomal recessive. See Section 12.26, Gyrate Atrophy.)
- Albinism (Blond fundus without RPE clumping; the choroidal vasculature is easily seen. Iris transillumination defects are present, and the foveal reflex is absent. See Section 14.7, Albinism.)
- Thioridazine (e.g., Mellaril) retinopathy (Patients taking >800 mg/day of thioridazine. See Section 12.29, Phenothiazine Toxicity.)

Workup

1. History: Family history? Medications?
2. Dilated fundus examination of the patient's mother and other family members if possible.
3. Formal visual fields (e.g., Octopus, Humphrey).
4. ERG with or without dark-adaptation studies.
5. Fluorescein angiogram (FA) may be diagnostic.

Treatment

No effective treatment for this condition is currently available. The following may be helpful in management.

1. Darkly tinted sunglasses may ameliorate symptoms.
2. Genetic counseling.

12.26 GYRATE ATROPHY

Symptoms

Decreased vision, night blindness.

Critical Signs

Multiple sharply defined areas of chorioretinal atrophy separated from each other by thin margins of pigment. The lesions begin in the midperiphery in childhood and then coalesce to involve the entire fundus, sparing the fovea until late in the disease, usually in midlife. Ornithine levels are markedly increased in all body fluids.

Other Signs

Posterior subcapsular cataract, high myopia, and astigmatism; optic-disc pallor and narrowing of the retinal vessels appear later in the disease. Constriction of visual fields and abnormal-to-nonrecordable electroretinogram (ERG), electro-oculogram (EOG), and dark-adaptation studies occur. Color vision typically remains relatively intact until late in the course of the disease. Carriers have normal fundi, but may have mild increase of ornithine levels.

Inheritance

Autosomal recessive.

Differential Diagnosis

All of the following can be distinguished by the presence of normal ornithine levels.

- Thioridazine retinopathy (Patient taking >800 mg/day of thioridazine. See Section 12.29, Phenothiazine Toxicity.)
- Paving-stone degeneration (Patches of chorioretinal atrophy limited to the retinal periphery, usually inferiorly.)
- Choroideremia (Diffuse retinal pigment epithelial and choroidal atrophy spread throughout the fundus. X-linked recessive. See Section 12.25, Choroideremia.)
- High myopia (Chorioretinal atrophy, most marked in the posterior pole, often with a staphyloma. See Section 12.12, High Myopia.)

Workup

1. Family history: Check for night blindness or severely decreased vision.
2. Dilated fundus examination.
3. Plasma ornithine and amino acid levels (expect ornithine to be 6 to 10 times normal).
4. Consider ERG and fluorescein angiogram (FA) if the ornithine level is not markedly increased.

Treatment

1. Supplemental vitamin B_6 (pyridoxine). The dose is not currently established; can try 20 mg/day, p.o., initially and increase up to 500 mg/day, p.o., if there is no response.

❖ **Note:** *Only a small percentage of patients are vitamin B_6 responders.*

2. Reduce dietary protein consumption and substitute artificially flavored solutions of essential amino acids without arginine (i.e., arginine-restricted diet).

Follow-up
- Frequent serum ornithine levels are obtained initially to determine the amount of supplemental vitamin B_6 and the degree to which dietary protein needs to be restricted. Serum ornithine levels between 0.15 and 0.20 mM are optimal. The frequency of blood tests may be reduced after the ornithine levels stabilize in this range.
- Serum ammonia levels are monitored in patients restricting dietary arginine.

12.27 CONE DYSTROPHIES

Symptoms
Slowly progressive bilateral visual loss, photophobia, and poor color vision. Vision is worse during the day than at night.

Critical Signs
Early Essentially a normal fundus examination, even with poor visual acuity. Abnormal cone function on the electroretinogram (ERG) (i.e., a reduced single-flash photopic response and a reduced flicker response).
Late Bull's-eye macular appearance or central geographic atrophy of the retinal pigmental epithelium (RPE) and choriocapillaris.

Other Signs
Nystagmus, temporal pallor of the optic disc, spotty pigment clumping in the macular area, tapetal-like retinal sheen. Rarely rod degeneration may ensue, leading to a retinitis pigmentosa–like picture (i.e., a cone–rod degeneration, which may have an autosomal dominant inheritance pattern).

Inheritance
Usually sporadic. Hereditary forms are usually autosomal dominant, but autosomal recessive and X-linked also occur.

Differential Diagnosis
- Stargardt's disease (In early cases when the fundus flavimaculatus is absent. A normal ERG is usually present in the early stage. Primarily autosomal recessive. See Section 12.28, Stargardt's Disease.)
- Chloroquine retinopathy (May produce a bull's-eye macular appearance and poor color vision. History of chloroquine or hydroxychloroquine use, no family history of cone degeneration, no nystagmus. See Section 12.30, Chloroquine/Hydroxychloroquine Toxicity.)

- Central areolar choroidal dystrophy (Geographic atrophy of the retinal pigment epithelium with normal photopic ERG.)
- Age-related macular degeneration (ARMD) (Can have geographic atrophy of the RPE, but with normal color vision and photopic ERG. See Section 12.10, Age-Related Macular Degeneration).
- Congenital color blindness (Normal visual acuity, onset at birth, not progressive.)
- Retinitis pigmentosa (Night blindness and peripheral visual-field loss are the first symptoms. Often peripheral retinal bone spicules are seen. Can be distinguished by dark-adaptation testing and ERG. See Section 12.24, Retinitis Pigmentosa.)
- Optic neuropathy or atrophy (Decreased acuity, impaired color vision, temporal or diffuse optic-disc pallor or both. May have a family history. See Sections 11.16, Giant Cell Arteritis, 11.17, Nonarteritic Ischemic Optic Neuropathy, and 11.18, Miscellaneous Optic Neuropathies.)
- Nonphysiologic visual loss (Normal ophthalmoscopic examination, fluorescein angiogram (FA), ERG, and electro-oculogram (EOG). Patients can often be tricked into seeing better by special testing. See Section 11.22, Nonphysiologic Visual Loss.]

Workup
1. Family history.
2. Complete ophthalmic examination, including color plates and formal color testing (e.g., Farnsworth–Munsell 100-hue test, red test object for chloroquine).
3. Formal visual field test (e.g., Humphrey, Octopus).
4. ERG.
5. FA to help detect the bull's-eye macular pattern.

Treatment
There is no proven cure for this disease. The following measures may be palliative:

1. Heavily tinted glasses or contact lenses may help maximize vision.
2. Miotic drops (e.g., pilocarpine, 0.5% to 1%, q.i.d., during the day) are occasionally tried to improve vision and reduce photophobia.
3. Genetic counseling.
4. Low-vision aids as needed.

Follow-up
Yearly.

12.28 STARGARDT'S DISEASE
(FUNDUS FLAVIMACULATUS)

Symptoms
Usually bilateral decreased vision in childhood or young adulthood. In the early stages, the decrease in vision is often out of proportion to the clinical ophthalmoscopic appearance; therefore we must be careful not to label the child a malingerer.

Critical Signs
Any of the following may be present.

A. A relatively normal-appearing fundus except for a heavily pigmented retinal pigment epithelium (RPE).
B. Yellow or yellow–white fleck-like deposits at the level of the RPE, usually in a pisciform (fish-tail) configuration.
C. Atrophic macular degeneration: May have a bull's-eye appearance as a result of atrophy of the RPE around a normal central core of RPE, a "beaten-metal" appearance, pigment clumping, or marked geographic atrophy.

Other Signs
Atrophy of the RPE just outside of the macula or in the midperipheral fundus, normal peripheral visual fields in most cases, and rarely an accompanying cone or rod dystrophy. The electroretinogram (ERG) is typically normal in the early stages, but may become abnormal late in the disease. The electro-oculogram (EOG) is usually normal.

Inheritance
Usually autosomal recessive, but occasionally autosomal dominant.

Differential Diagnosis
- Fundus albipunctatus (Diffuse, small, white, discrete dots, most prominent in the midperipheral fundus and rarely present in the fovea; nonprogressive congenital night blindness; no atrophic macular degeneration or pigmentary changes. Visual acuity and visual fields remain normal.)
- Retinitis punctata albescens (Similar clinical appearance to fundus albipunctatus, but visual acuity, visual field, and night blindness progressively worsen. A markedly abnormal ERG develops.)

- Drusen [Small, yellow–white spots deep to the retina, sometimes calcified, usually developing later in life. Fluorescein angiogram (FA) helps distinguish: All drusen hyperfluoresce, whereas some lesions of fundus flavimaculatus do and some lesions do not hyperfluoresce, and some areas without flecks show hyperfluorescence.]
- Cone or cone–rod dystrophy (May have a bull's-eye macula, but have a significant color vision deficit and a characteristic ERG. See Section 12.27, Cone Dystrophies.)
- Batten's Disease and Spielmeyer–Vogt (May have bull's eye maculopathy, autosomal recessive lysosomal storage disease, progressive dementia, seizures; may have variable degree of optic atrophy, attenuation of retinal vasculature, and peripheral RPE changes. Shows characteristic curvilinear or fingerprint inclusions on electron microscopy of peripheral blood or conjunctival biopsy.)
- Chloroquine/hydroxychloroquine maculopathy (History of use of this medication. Dose related. See Section 12.30, Chloroquine/Hydroxychloroquine Toxicity.)
- Nonphysiologic visual loss (Normal ophthalmoscopic examination, FA, ERG, and EOG. Patients can often be tricked into seeing better by special testing. See Section 11.22, Nonphysiologic Visual Loss.)

Workup

Indicated when the diagnosis is uncertain or must be confirmed.

1. History: Age at onset, medications, family history?
2. Dilated retinal examination.
3. FA often shows blockage of choroidal fluorescence producing a "silent choroid" or "midnight fundus" as a result of increased lipofuscin in the RPE cells.
4. ERG and EOG.
5. Formal visual-field examination (e.g., Octopus, Humphrey).

Treatment

No known medical or surgical therapy is beneficial. The patient may benefit from low-vision aids, services dedicated to helping the visually handicapped, and genetic counseling.

12.29 PHENOTHIAZINE TOXICITY

A. Thioridazine (e.g., Mellaril)

Symptoms

Blurred vision, brownish vision, difficulty with night vision.

Signs

Pigment clumps between the posterior pole and the equator, areas of retinal depigmentation, retinal edema, visual-field abnormalities (central scotoma and general constriction), depressed or extinguished electroretinogram (ERG).

❖ **Note:** *Symptoms and signs may occur within weeks of starting phenothiazine therapy, particularly if very large doses (>2,000 mg/day) are taken.*

Dosage Generally Required to Produce Toxicity

800 mg/day chronically.

Differential Diagnosis

Pigment clumps in the retina.

- Retinitis pigmentosa (Family history, pale optic disc, narrowed arterioles. See Section 12.24, Retinitis Pigmentosa.)
- Old syphilitic chorioretinopathy (Positive fluorescent treponemal antibody, absorbed, may have a history of an acute visual problem.)
- Viral chorioretinitis (Often associated with an anterior-chamber reaction, vitreous cells, and other ocular signs.)
- Trauma (Usually unilateral, history of trauma.)

Treatment

Discontinue the medication.

Baseline Workup

For patients in whom long-term treatment is anticipated.

1. Visual acuity.
2. Complete ophthalmoscopic examination.
3. Fundus photographs.
4. Visual field, preferably automated (e.g., Humphrey, Octopus, with or without a red test object).
5. Consider ERG.
6. Color vision testing, preferably with a Farnsworth–Munsell 100-hue test.

Follow-up

Every 6 months.

B. Chlorpromazine (e.g., Thorazine)

Symptoms

Blurred vision or none.

Signs

Abnormal pigmentation of the eyelids, cornea, conjunctiva (especially within the palpebral fissure), and anterior-lens capsule; anterior and posterior subcapsular cataract; rarely, a pigmentary retinopathy within the visual field and ERG changes described for thioridazine.

Dosage Generally Required to Produce Toxicity

From 1,200 to 2,400 mg/day for longer than 12 months.

Treatment

Discontinue the medication if vision is affected.

Baseline Workup

Same as for thioridazine.

Follow-up

Every 6 months.

12.30 CHLOROQUINE/HYDROXYCHLOROQUINE TOXICITY

Symptoms

Decreased vision, abnormal color vision, difficulty adjusting to darkness.

Critical Signs

Bull's-eye macula (a ring of depigmentation surrounded by a ring of increased pigmentation), loss of the foveal reflex.

Other Signs

Increased pigmentation in the macula, arteriolar narrowing, vascular sheathing, peripheral pigmentation, decreased color vision, visual field abnormalities (central, paracentral, or peripheral scotoma), abnormal electroretinogram (ERG) and electro-oculogram (EOG), and normal dark adaptation. Whorl-like corneal changes also may be observed.

Dosage Generally Required to Produce Toxicity

Chloroquine: >300 g total cumulative dose.
Hydroxychloroquine: >750 mg/day taken over months to years.
(Some believe that retinopathy will not develop if the daily dose is kept <4.4 mg/kg/day of chloroquine and 7.7 mg/kg/day of hydroxychloroquine.)

Differential Diagnosis

The following can produce a bull's-eye macula.

- Cone dystrophy (Family history, generally <30 years old, severe photophobia, abnormal to nonrecordable photopic ERG. See Section 12.27, Cone Dystrophies.)
- Stargardt's disease/fundus flavimaculatus (Family history, generally younger than 25 years, may have white–yellow flecks in the posterior pole and midperiphery. See Section 12.28, Stargardt's Disease.)
- Age-related macular degeneration (ARMD) (Drusen; pigment clumping and atrophy and detachment of the retinal pigment epithelium or sensory retina may or may not occur. See Section 12.10, Age-Related Macular Degeneration.)
- Spielmeyer–Vogt syndrome (Retinitis pigmentosa, seizures, ataxia, and progressive dementia.)

Treatment

Discontinue the medication if signs of toxicity develop.

Baseline Workup

For patients in whom long-term treatment is anticipated.

1. Visual acuity.
2. Ophthalmoscopic examination.
3. Posterior-pole fundus photographs.
4. Visual field, preferably automated (e.g., Humphrey, Octopus, with or without red test object).
5. Color vision testing, preferably Farnsworth–Munsell 100-hue test.

Follow-up

Every 6 months.

❖ **Note**: *Once ocular toxicity develops, it usually does not regress even if the drug is withdrawn. In fact, new toxic effects may develop, and old ones may progress even after the chloroquine/hydroxychloroquine has been discontinued.*

12.31 BEST'S DISEASE
(VITELLIFORM MACULAR DYSTROPHY)

Symptoms

Decreased vision or asymptomatic. Onset at birth, but may not be detected until years later if examination is not performed.

Critical Signs

Yellow, round, subretinal lesion(s) likened to an egg yolk or in some cases to a pseudohypopyon. Typically bilateral and located in the fovea, measuring approximately one to two disc areas in size. Ten percent of lesions are multiple and extrafoveal. Normal electroretinogram (ERG), abnormal electro-oculogram (EOG).

Other Signs

The lesions may degenerate, and macular choroidal neovascularization, hemorrhage, and scarring may develop. In the scar stage, it may be indistinguishable from age-related macular degeneration. May be hyperopic and have esophoria or esotropia.

Inheritance

Autosomal dominant with variable penetrance and expression. Carriers may have normal fundi but an abnormal EOG.

Workup

1. Family history (often helpful to examine family members).
2. Complete ocular examination, including a dilated retinal examination, carefully inspecting the macula with a slit lamp and a fundus contact, Hruby, or 60- or 90-diopter lens.
3. EOG to confirm the diagnosis or to detect the carrier state of the disease.
4. Consider fluorescein angiography to confirm the presence of or delineate a choroidal neovascular membrane (CNVM).

Treatment

There is no effective treatment for the underlying disease. Laser should be considered for well-defined choroidal neovascularization outside the foveal center.

Follow-up

Patients with treatable CNVM should be attended to promptly. Otherwise, there is no urgency in seeing patients with this disease. Patients are given an Amsler's grid (see Appendix 3), instructed on its use, and told to return immediately if a change is noted.

❖ **Note**: *An adult form of vitelliform macular dystrophy (a "pattern dystrophy") has been described. The egg-yolk lesions usually appear from ages 30 to 50 years, the disease is dominantly inherited, and the EOG may or may not be abnormal. There also is no effective treatment for this entity.*

UVEITIS

13.1 ANTERIOR UVEITIS (IRITIS/IRIDOCYCLITIS)

Symptoms

Acute Pain, red eye, photophobia, mildly decreased vision, tearing. May have recurrent episodes.

Chronic May have periods of exacerbations and remissions, fewer or none of the acute symptoms.

Critical Signs

Cells and flare in the anterior chamber.

Differentiating Signs

Nongranulomatous Fine keratic precipitates (KP) (white cells on the corneal endothelium).

Granulomatous Large "mutton-fat" KP, Koeppe's nodules (clusters of cells on the pupillary border), Busacca's nodules (clusters of cells on the anterior iris surface).

Other Signs

Cells in the anterior vitreous (spillover), posterior synechiae (adhesions of the iris to the lens), miosis, low intraocular pressure (IOP) but occasionally increased (especially with herpes simplex and herpes zoster), injection of the perilimbal blood vessels ("ciliary flush"), fibrinous hypopyon (layering of white cells in the anterior chamber) if severe, cystoid macular edema if chronic, occasionally a cataract.

❖ **Note** *Patients will often complain of increased pain in the involved eye when light is shined in the uninvolved eye because of the consensual pupillary response.*

Etiology

ACUTE, NONGRANULOMATOUS

- Idiopathic
- Human leukocyte antigen (HLA)-B27–associated uveitis (without systemic disease).
- Trauma (see Traumatic Iritis, Section 3.6)
- Ankylosing spondylitis (Young adult men, often with low back pain, abnormal sacroiliac spine radiographs, increased erythrocyte sedimentation rate (ESR), positive HLA-B27.)
- Inflammatory bowel disease (Chronic intermittent diarrhea, often alternating with constipation.)
- Reiter's syndrome (Young adult men, conjunctivitis, urethritis, polyarthritis, occasionally keratitis, increased ESR, positive HLA-B27, may have recurrent episodes.)
- Psoriatic arthritis (Iritis is not associated with psoriasis without arthritis.)
- Glaucomatocyclitic crisis (Recurrent episodes of acute IOP increase, open angle on gonioscopy, corneal edema, fine KP, fixed middilated pupil, and mild iritis. See Section 10.12, Glaucomatocyclitic Crisis.)
- Lens-induced uveitis (Often after incomplete extracapsular cataract extraction or trauma damaging the lens capsule; also may be secondary to a hypermature cataract.)
- Postoperative iritis (An anterior-chamber reaction is expected after intraocular surgery. Severe reactions with excessive pain, however, must make the examiner consider endophthalmitis. See Postoperative Uveitis, Section 13.9.)
- UGH syndrome (uveitis–glaucoma–hyphema) [Usually secondary to irritation from an intraocular lens (especially a closed-loop anterior-chamber lens). See Postoperative Glaucoma, Section 10.15.]
- Behçet's disease (Young adults, acute hypopyon, iritis, aphthous mouth ulcers, genital ulcerations, erythema nodosum, positive Behçet's skin-puncture test if active systemic disease is present, often retinal vasculitis and hemorrhages, may have recurrent episodes.)
- Lyme disease (Often a history of a tick bite. May have a skin rash and/or arthritis. See Section 14.4, Lyme Disease.)
- Anterior-segment ischemia (Caused by carotid insufficiency, flare out of proportion to the cellular reaction, pain.)
- Mumps, influenza, adenovirus, measles, chlamydia (Rare causes of transient anterior uveitis.)

- Medication (Rifabutin, systemic sulfonamides, cidofovir, and topical optipranolol can all cause uveitis.)
- Tight contact lens (Red eye, corneal edema, epithelial defects, iritis ± hypopyon, no stromal infiltrates.)
- Other rare causes of anterior uveitis (Leptospirosis, Kawasaki's disease, rickettsial disease.)

CHRONIC, USUALLY NONGRANULOMATOUS

- Juvenile rheumatoid arthritis (JRA) [Usually young girls, eye may be white and without pain, often bilateral, iritis can occur before the arthritis, pauciarticular arthritis (fewer than five joints involved), positive antinuclear antibody (ANA), negative rheumatoid factor, increased ESR, glaucoma, cataracts, and occasionally fever and lymphadenopathy.]
- Chronic iridocyclitis of children (Usually young girls, same as JRA, except no arthritis.)
- Fuchs' heterochromic iridocyclitis (Usually unilateral, few symptoms, diffuse iris stromal atrophy often causing a lighter colored iris, iris transillumination defects, blunting of the iris architecture, fine KP over the entire corneal endothelium, mild anterior-chamber reaction, few if any posterior synechiae. Vitreous opacities, glaucoma, and cataracts are common.)

CHRONIC, USUALLY GRANULOMATOUS

- Sarcoidosis [Usually African-American, usually bilateral; may have dense posterior synechiae, conjunctival nodules, or signs of posterior uveitis (see Section 13.2, Posterior Uveitis). Mild-to-moderate anergy, an abnormal chest radiograph, positive gallium scan, and increased serum angiotensin-converting enzyme (ACE) are common. See Section 13.4, Sarcoidosis.]
- Herpes simplex/herpes zoster/varicella (Look for corneal scars, history of past unilateral recurrent red eye, occasionally history of skin vesicles, associated with increased IOP, followed by iris atrophy.)
- Syphilis [May have a maculopapular rash (often on the palms and soles), iris roseola (vascular papules on the iris), and interstitial keratitis with ghost vessels in late stages. Usually seen with uveitis in acquired syphilis versus interstitial keratitis in congenital syphilis. A positive VDRL or rapid plasma reagin (RPR) and positive fluorescent treponemal antibody, absorbed (FTA-ABS) are usually present. See Section 14.2, Acquired Syphilis.]
- Tuberculosis [Positive purified protein derivative (PPD), typical chest x-ray, occasionally phlyctenular keratitis, sometimes signs of posterior uveitis (see Section 13.2, Posterior Uveitis).]
- Others [Rare (e.g., leprosy, brucellosis).]

Differential Diagnosis

The following may be associated with an anterior-chamber reaction.

- Rhegmatogenous retinal detachment (RRD) (Elevated retina with a retinal break, pigment cells in the vitreous or anterior chamber. See Section 12.19, Retinal Detachment.)
- Posterior segment tumor (e.g., retinoblastoma or leukemia in children, malignant melanoma in adults. See Section 8.3, Malignant Melanoma of the Choroid.)
- Juvenile xanthogranuloma (Age younger than 15 years, often with a spontaneous hyphema, yellow–gray poorly demarcated iris nodule or nodules, and slightly raised orange skin lesions.)
- Intraocular foreign body
- Sclerouveitis (Uveitis secondary to scleritis.)
- Endophthalmitis (See Sections 13.9, Postoperative Uveitis, 13.10, Post-operative Endophthalmitis, 13.11, Traumatic Endophthalmitis, 13.12, Endogenous Bacterial Endophthalmitis.)

Workup

1. Obtain a history, attempting to define the etiology.
2. Complete ocular examination, including an IOP check and a dilated fundus examination. The vitreous should be evaluated for cells (see Appendix 8).

If a unilateral, nongranulomatous uveitis develops for the first time and the history and examination are unremarkable, then no further workup is pursued.

If the uveitis is bilateral, granulomatous, or recurrent, and the history and examination are unremarkable, then a nonspecific initial workup is conducted:

3. Complete blood count (CBC).
4. ESR.
5. HLA-B27.
6. ACE level, ANA.
7. RPR or VDRL.
8. FTA-ABS or MHA-TP.
9. PPD and anergy panel.
10. Chest radiograph, especially to rule out sarcoidosis and tuberculosis.
11. In endemic areas, a Lyme titer is recommended (see the following).

If the history, symptoms, or signs, or a combination of these point strongly to a certain etiology, then the workup should be tailored accordingly:

- Syphilis: RPR or VDRL, FTA-ABS or MHA-TP.
- Ankylosing spondylitis: Sacroiliac spine radiographs show sclerosis and narrowing of the joint spaces, ESR, HLA-B27.

- Inflammatory bowel disease: Medical or gastrointestinal consult, HLA-B27.
- Reiter's syndrome: Conjunctival, urethral, and prostatic cultures (for chlamydia) if indicated; joint radiographs if arthritis is present; a medical or rheumatology consult; consider an HLA-B27.
- Psoriatic arthritis: A rheumatology or dermatology consult, HLA-B27.
- Glaucomatocyclitic crisis: Diagnosed clinically.
- Lens-induced uveitis: Diagnosed clinically. See Phacolytic Glaucoma, Section 10.8; Lens-Particle Glaucoma, Section 10.9; and Phacoanaphylactic Endophthalmitis, Section 13.14.
- Herpes: Diagnosed clinically.
- UGH: Diagnosed clinically.
- Behçet's disease: Behçet's skin-puncture test (if a blister develops minutes to hours after puncturing the skin intradermally with a sterile 25- to 30-gauge needle, a positive test is noted), a medical or rheumatology consult, consider an HLA-B27 or HLA-B5.
- Lyme disease: Lyme immunofluorescent assay or enzyme-linked immunosorbent assay (ELISA).
- JRA: ANA, rheumatoid factor, radiographs of arthritic joints (if no arthritic symptoms are present, then radiographs of the knees are obtained), and a pediatric or rheumatology consult.
- Chronic iridocyclitis of children: Same as JRA.
- Fuchs' heterochromic iridocyclitis: Diagnosed clinically.
- Sarcoidosis: Chest x-ray, ACE, serum lysozyme, and a PPD and anergy panel, gallium scan of the head and neck; consider a biopsy of any skin or conjunctival nodule for pathologic diagnosis (see Sarcoidosis, Section 13.4).

❖ **Note** *ACE and gallium scans may give false-negative results if the patient is taking systemic steroids. ACE levels also may be low if the patient is taking ACE inhibitors for cardiac reasons.*

- Tuberculosis: PPD and anergy panel, chest radiograph, referral to a medical specialist.

Treatment
1. Cycloplegic (e.g., cyclopentolate, 1% to 2%, t.i.d., or scopolamine, 0.25%, b.i.d., for mild-to-moderate inflammation; scopolamine, 0.25%, t.i.d., for moderate inflammation, or atropine, 1%, t.i.d., for severe inflammation. Use atropine if a hypopyon is present).
2. Topical steroid (e.g., prednisolone acetate, 1%, q 1 to 6 hours, depending on the severity). Most cases of moderate-to-severe acute uveitis require q 1 to 2 hour dosing initially.
    If the anterior uveitis is severe and is not responding well to frequent topical steroids, then consider periocular repository steroids

(e.g., methylprednisolone, 40 to 80 mg subtenons). Before injecting depot steroids periocularly, it is wise to use topical steroids at full strength for 6 weeks to make certain that the patient is not a steroid responder (i.e., develops a significant IOP increase from taking steroids). See Appendix 7, which describes the technique of a subtenons injection.

If there is no improvement on maximal topical and repository steroids, then consider systemic steroids, or last, systemic immuno-suppressive agents. A medical or rheumatology consult is often advisable when systemic therapy is to be instituted. See Medical Glossary for a systemic steroid workup.

3. Treat secondary glaucoma with aqueous suppressants (not with pilocarpine or latanoprost). Glaucoma may result from:
   a. A severe inflammatory reaction with cellular blockage of the trabecular meshwork. See Inflammatory Open-Angle Glaucoma, Section 10.4.
   b. Synechiae formation giving rise to secondary angle closure. See Acute Angle-Closure Glaucoma, Section 10.10.
   c. Neovascularization of the iris, producing blockage of the trabecular meshwork or closure of the angle. See Neovascular Glaucoma, Section 10.13.
   d. A response to steroids. See Steroid-Response Glaucoma, Section 10.5.

4. If an exact etiology for the anterior uveitis is determined, then the specific management outlined later should be added to these treatments.

   Ankylosing spondylitis Often requires systemic antiinflammatory agents [e.g., aspirin, nonsteroidal antiinflammatory drugs (NSAIDs): naprosyn or indomethacin]. Consider cardiology consult (there is a high incidence of heart block and aortic insufficiency), rheumatology consult, and physical therapy consult.

   Inflammatory bowel disease Often benefits from systemic steroids or sulfadiazine or both and supplemental vitamin A. Needs a medical or gastrointestinal consult.

   Reiter's syndrome If urethritis is present, then the patient and sexual partners are treated for chlamydia (e.g., tetracycline, 250 to 500 mg, q.i.d., doxycycline, 100 mg, b.i.d., or erythromycin, 250 to 500 mg, q.i.d., for 3 to 6 weeks). Obtain medical, rheumatology, or physical therapy consult or a combination of these.

   Psoriatic arthritis Consider a rheumatology or dermatology consult.

   Glaucomatocyclitic crisis See Section 10.12, Glaucomatocyclitic Crisis.

   Lens-induced uveitis Usually requires removal of lens material, see Phacolytic Glaucoma, Section 10.8; Lens-Particle Glaucoma, Section 10.9; and Phacoanaphylactic Endophthalmitis, Section 13.14.

Herpes uveitis   Requires prophylactic topical antivirals when atypical or taking steroids; may benefit from systemic acyclovir. See Herpes Simplex Virus, Section 4.15; or Herpes Zoster Virus, Section 4.16.

UGH   See Postoperative Glaucoma, Section 10.15.

Behçet's disease   Often needs systemic steroids or immunosuppressive agents (responds well to chlorambucil); consider a medical or rheumatology consult.

Lyme disease   See Section 14.4, Lyme Disease.

JRA   The steroid dosage is adjusted according to the degree of cells, not flare, present in the anterior chamber; prolonged cycloplegic therapy (e.g., tropicamide, 0.5%, qhs) may be required. A rheumatology or pediatric consult for possible aspirin or systemic steroid therapy is usually obtained.

❖ **Note** *There is a high complication rate with cataract surgery.*

Chronic iridocyclitis of children   Same as JRA.

Fuchs' heterochromic iridocyclitis   Usually does not respond to or require steroids (a trial of steroids may be attempted, but they should be tapered quickly if there is no response); cycloplegics are rarely necessary.

❖ **Note** *Patients usually do well with cataract surgery.*

Sarcoidosis   Often needs periocular and systemic steroids; a medicine or pulmonary consult is advisable for systemic evaluation (see Section 13.4, Sarcoidosis).

Syphilis   See Acquired Syphilis, Section 14.2, or Congenital Syphilis, Section 14.3.

Tuberculosis   Avoid systemic steroids. Refer the patient to an internist for consideration of systemic antituberculous treatment.

Follow-up

Every 1 to 7 days in the acute phase, depending on the severity; every 1 to 6 months when stable. At each visit, the anterior-chamber reaction and IOP should be evaluated. A vitreous and fundus examination should be performed for all flare-ups, when vision is affected, or every 3 to 6 months. If the anterior-chamber reaction is improving, then the steroid drops can be slowly tapered [usually 1 drop per day every 3 to 7 days (e.g., q.i.d. for 1 week, then t.i.d. for 1 week, then b.i.d. for 1 week)]. Steroids are usually discontinued once all cells have disappeared from the anterior chamber (flare is often still present). Rarely long-term low-dose steroids every day or every other day are required to keep the inflammation from recurring. The cycloplegic agents also can be tapered as the anterior-chamber reaction improves. Cycloplegics should be used at least qhs until the anterior chamber is free of cells.

❖ **Note** *As with most ocular and systemic diseases requiring steroid therapy, the steroid (be it topical or systemic) should never be discontinued abruptly. Sudden discontinuation of steroids can lead to severe rebound inflammation.*

13.2 POSTERIOR UVEITIS

Symptoms
Blurred vision, floaters; occasionally redness, pain, and photophobia.

Critical Signs
White blood cells and opacities in the vitreous (vitritis), retinal or choroidal infiltrates, edema, vascular sheathing.

Other Signs
Disc swelling, retinal hemorrhages or exudates, or signs of anterior-segment inflammation (e.g., aqueous cells and flare, posterior synechiae) may be present. Glaucoma, cataract, choroidal neovascularization, or retinal detachment may develop.

Etiology
A. More common
- Toxoplasmosis [A yellow–white, fuzzy retinal lesion, in the posterior pole or periphery. It may be difficult to see the lesion because of a severe accompanying vitritis. A chorioretinal scar is frequently seen adjacent to the acute, active lesion. May be associated with retinal vascular occlusive disease. A negative antitoxoplasma antibody titer (undiluted) in an immunocompetent host usually rules out toxoplasmosis. See Section 13.3, Toxoplasmosis.]
- Sarcoidosis [White–yellow exudates or sheathing around retinal veins, retinal or vitreous white nodules, and other retinal or choroidal abnormalities may be present. Vitritis and granulomatous uveitis are common. Patients are frequently African-American and may have pulmonary, skin, central nervous system (CNS), or other systemic involvement. An elevated angiotensin converting enzyme (ACE) level is often present. See Section 13.4, Sarcoidosis.]

- Syphilis (Produces an acute chorioretinitis and vitritis that may mimic almost any other condition. A concomitant skin rash on the palms, soles, or both may be present. Retinal pigment clumping, sometimes similar to retinitis pigmentosa, may later occur. May be associated with retinal vascular occlusive disease. Congenital syphilis typically produces a salt-and-pepper fundus. Positive fluorescent treponemal antibody, absorbed (FTA-ABS). Patients may also have only an iritis. See Sections 14.2, Acquired Syphilis, and 14.3, Congenital Syphilis.)
- Pars planitis [Considered an intermediate uveitis. Usually a bilateral vitritis in patients age 15 to 40 years with white exudative material covering the inferior ora serrata and pars plana. Cellular clumps in the vitreous (appearing as "snowballs") and peripheral vascular sheathing may be present. See Section 13.5, Pars Planitis.]
- Ocular histoplasmosis (Common in temperate river valleys, especially the Ohio–Mississippi River Valley area. Yellow–white choroidal scars, usually <1 mm in diameter, macular degenerative changes, sometimes with choroidal neovascularization, and peripapillary atrophy or scarring is seen. Minimal-to-no vitreous or aqueous cells are seen. See Section 12.11, Ocular Histoplasmosis Syndrome.)

B. After surgery or trauma: See Postoperative Uveitis, Section 13.9; Postoperative Endophthalmitis, Section 13.10; Traumatic Endophthalmitis, Section 13.11; and Sympathetic Ophthalmia, Section 13.15.

C. Immunocompromised host [e.g., acquired immunodeficiency syndrome (AIDS), patients being treated with chemotherapy]
- Cytomegalovirus (CMV) (Whitish patches of necrotic retina are mixed with retinal hemorrhage. Also seen in neonates. See Acquired Immunodeficiency Syndrome, Section 14.1.)
- Candida (Seen also in hospitalized patients being treated with prolonged antibiotic therapy, i.v. drug abusers, and patients with long-standing catheters. Yellow–white, fluffy, retinal or preretinal lesions are found initially. Later, associated "cotton balls" develop in the vitreous. Candida may be cultured from the blood, urine, or an i.v. site.)
- Herpetic retinitis (Clinically similar to acute retinal necrosis, but may not have vitreous cells and may spare retinal vessels. May involve deep retina. Rapidly progressive. Treat like acute retinal necrosis.)
- Endogenous endophthalmitis (Patients are typically septic, and many have an anterior-chamber reaction or hypopyon in addition to the vitritis. See Section 13.12, Endogenous Bacterial Endophthalmitis.)
- Others (Herpes simplex, varicella-zoster, fungi, mycobacteria, others.)

D. Less common

- Acute posterior multifocal placoid pigment epitheliopathy (AMPPE) (Acute visual loss, typically in young adults, sometimes after a viral illness. Multiple gray–white subretinal lesions with indistinct margins, approximately one half of a disc diameter in size, are usually found in the posterior poles of both eyes. Vitreous cells, disc edema, serous retinal detachment, and rarely CNS signs may be present. Vision usually returns to normal in 2 to 6 weeks.)

- Acute retinal necrosis (Frequently seen as acute iridocyclitis. Unilateral or bilateral multiple opaque white patches of thickened retina with vascular sheathing, usually in the retinal periphery. The patches of necrotic retina gradually enlarge and coalesce. Vitreous cells are abundant. Retinal detachment is a common sequela in untreated patients. See Section 13.6, Acute Retinal Necrosis.)

- Acute retinal pigment epithelitis (Krill's disease) (Young adults with sudden visual loss. Gray spots are seen at the level of the retinal pigment epithelium in the macula, each of which is surrounded by a lighter-colored halo. The spots occur in two to four distinct clusters. The condition may be unilateral or bilateral. It resolves in 6 to 12 weeks without treatment.)

- Behçet's disease (Usually a bilateral ocular disease of young adult men. Retinal and optic disc edema, vascular sheathing, and occasionally hemorrhages or exudate may accompany a vitritis and anterior uveitis, sometimes with a hypopyon. The eye is typically not red. Recurrent oral or genital ulcers or both, erythema nodosum, or arthritis may be noted. See Anterior Uveitis, Section 13.1.)

- Birdshot (vitiliginous) retinochoroidopathy [Usually middle-aged women with bilateral multiple creamy yellow spots deep to the retina, approximately 1 mm in diameter, scattered around the equator of the fundus. Occasionally, the spots coalesce and spread to the macula. Vitreous cells are more abundant than aqueous cells. Retinal or optic nerve edema or both may be present. Positive HLA-A29 in most patients. Visual loss may also occur from cystoid macular edema (CME) and choroidal neovascular membranes.]

- Cat-scratch disease (Unilateral, stellate macular exudates, optic nerve swelling, vitreous cells, positive Bartonella serology. See Section 5.3, Parinaud's Oculoglandular Conjunctivitis)

- Diffuse unilateral subacute neuroretinitis (Unilateral visual loss in children and young adults, thought to be caused by a nematode. Optic nerve swelling, vitreous cells, and deep gray–white retinal lesions are present initially. Later, optic atrophy, narrowing of retinal vessels, and atrophic pigment epithelial changes develop. Vision and visual fields deteriorate with time.)

- Septic (embolic) retinitis [Sudden onset of decreased vision in a systemically ill patient. Retinal edema, vascular sheathing, and hemorrhages with white centers (Roth's spots) may be accompanied by vitreous cells. Diseased heart valves are common sources.]
- Lyme disease (Produces varied forms of posterior uveitis. More common in New England and Middle Atlantic states, particularly in patients who camp outdoors. A history of a tick bite, skin rash, Bell's palsy, or arthritis may be elicited. See Section 14.4, Lyme Disease.)
- Multiple evanescent white-dot syndrome (Acute unilateral visual loss, often after a viral illness, usually in young women. May be bilateral or sequential. Multiple creamy white lesions at the level of the retinal pigment epithelium are accompanied by a granularity of the fovea. There are few vitreous cells and occasional sheathing of retinal vessels. There is often an enlarged blind spot on formal visual-field testing. Vision typically returns to normal within weeks without treatment.)
- Recurrent multifocal choroiditis (multifocal choroiditis with panuveitis) [Unilateral visual loss in young women, who often have bilateral fundus involvement. Multiple, small, round, pale inflammatory lesions at the level of the pigment epithelium and choriocapillaris are found (similar to "histo-spots"), sometimes associated with choroidal neovascularization. Vitreous cells, mild disc edema, and less commonly, anterior-chamber cells and flare may be present. The lesions are predominantly in the macular area and frequently respond to oral or periocular steroids, but typically recur. Chronic cases may exhibit nominal or extensive subretinal fibrosis. Myopia is common. Laser photocoagulation may be considered in the presence of a choroidal neovascular membrane.]
- Rubella (Usually seen in infants whose mothers developed rubella during the pregnancy. Salt-and-pepper pigmentation of the retina is typical. Microphthalmos, cataract, or iris transillumination defects may be present. The optic nerve may be pale. An increased anti-rubella antibody titer can usually be demonstrated.)
- Serpiginous choroidopathy [Typically bilateral, recurrent chorioretinitis characterized by acute lesions (yellow–white subretinal patches with indistinct margins) bordering old atrophic scars; however, one third may begin peripherally. The chorioretinal changes usually extend from the optic disc outward. Patients are typically aged 30 to 60 years. A choroidal neovascular membrane may develop, requiring laser photocoagulation to prevent visual loss.]
- Toxocariasis (Usually occurs in children, affecting only one eye. The most common presentations are a macular granuloma with poor vision, unilateral pars planitis with peripheral granuloma, or

endophthalmitis. A granuloma appears as an elevated, white retinal lesion. A peripheral lesion may be associated with a fibrous band extending to the optic disc, sometimes dragging the macular vessels away from their normal course. A severe vitritis and anterior uveitis may be present. A negative undiluted toxocara titer in an immunocompetent host usually rules out this disease. See Section 9.1, Leukocoria.)

- Tuberculosis [Produces varied clinical manifestations. The diagnosis is usually made by ancillary laboratory tests. Miliary tuberculosis may produce multifocal, small, yellow–white choroidal lesions. Most patients have concomitant anterior granulomatous or nongranulomatous uveitis. A 2-week therapeutic trial of isoniazid, 300 mg, p.o., daily, and pyridoxine (vitamin B_6), 10 mg/day, may be given. If the uveitis is the result of tuberculosis, it should improve significantly in patients on this regimen.]

- Vogt–Koyanagi–Harada (VKH) syndrome (Serous retinal detachment with vitreous cells, a swollen optic disc, or atrophic patches at the level of the retinal pigment epithelium may accompany an anterior-chamber reaction. Patients are darkly pigmented, typically of Asian or Native American ancestry, and have or develop systemic signs including meningeal signs, vitiligo, alopecia, and poliosis. Harada's disease implies posterior pole involvement with neurologic involvement. See Section 13.7, Vogt–Koyanagi–Harada Syndrome.)

- Whipple's disease (Rare. Small white vitreous opacities, retinal hemorrhages and exudates, or exudative material over the pars plana in a patient with diarrhea, arthralgia, and weight loss. The diagnosis is made by intestinal biopsy or, less commonly, by pars plana vitrectomy.)

- Others [*Nocardia, Coccidioides* species, *Aspergillus* species, *Cryptococcus* species, meningococcus, ophthalmomyiasis, onchocerciasis and cystericercosis (seen in Africa and Central and South America), measles, Eales' disease, Crohn's disease, multiple sclerosis, subacute sclerosing panencephalitis, and age-related vitritis.]

Differential Diagnosis
(Masquerade syndromes.)

- Reticulum cell sarcoma (large cell lymphoma) (Persistent vitreous cells in patients older than 50 years, which usually do not respond completely to systemic steroids. Yellow–white subretinal infiltrates, retinal edema and hemorrhage, anterior-chamber inflammation, or neurologic signs may be present. See Section 13.8, Reticulum Cell Sarcoma.)
- Malignant melanoma (A retinal detachment and associated vitritis may obscure the underlying tumor. B-scan ultrasound will usually detect the

tumor in cases not detectable by indirect ophthalmoscopy. See Section 8.3, Malignant Melanoma of the Choroid.)
- Retinitis pigmentosa (Vitreous cells and macular edema may accompany "bone-spicule" pigmentary changes and attenuated retinal vessels. Drusen of the optic disc may be mistaken for disc swelling. Electroretinography aids in diagnosis. See Section 12.24, Retinitis Pigmentosa.)
- Rhegmatogenous retinal detachment (RRD) (A small number of pigmented anterior vitreous cells and an anterior uveitis frequently accompany a RRD. See Section 12.19, Retinal Detachment.)
- Retained intraocular foreign body [Persistent inflammation after a penetrating ocular injury. May have iris heterochromia. Diagnosed by indirect ophthalmoscopy, B-scan ultrasound, ultrasound biomicroscopy, or computed tomography (CT) scan of the globe. See Section 3.15, Intraocular Foreign Body.]
- Posterior scleritis [May or may not have an accompanying anterior scleritis. Vitritis is accompanied by a subretinal mass or thickening and sometimes an exudative retinal detachment. Chorioretinal folds may be seen. Fluorescein angiography and B-scan ultrasonography (showing T sign) are helpful in diagnosis.]
- Retinoblastoma (Almost always occurs in young children. May be seen with a pseudohypopyon and vitreous cells. One or more elevated white retinal lesions are usually, but not always, present. A retinal detachment, iris neovascularization, or both may be found. Fluorescein angiography, CT scan, and B-scan ultrasonography may aid in diagnosis. See Section 9.1, Leukocoria.)
- Leukemia (Unilateral retinitis and vitritis may occur in patients already known to have leukemia.)
- Amyloidosis (Rare. Vitreous globules or membranes without any signs of anterior-segment inflammation. A serum protein electrophoresis and diagnostic vitrectomy confirm the diagnosis.)
- Asteroid hyalosis [Small, white refractile particles (calcium soaps) adherent to collagen fibers and floating in the vitreous] (Usually asymptomatic and of no clinical significance.)

Workup
1. History: Systemic disease or infection, skin rash, i.v. drug abuse, indwelling catheter, risk factors for AIDS? Recent eye trauma or surgery? Travel to the Ohio–Mississippi River Valley, Southwestern United States, New England, or Middle Atlantic area? Tick bite?
2. Complete ocular examination, including intraocular pressure (IOP) measurement and careful ophthalmoscopic examination. Indirect ophthalmoscopy with scleral depression of the entire ora serrata is essential.

3. Consider fluorescein angiography to help in diagnosis or plan for therapy.
4. Blood tests (any of the following are obtained, depending on the suspected diagnosis): Toxoplasma titer, ACE level, FTA-ABS, rapid plasma reagin (RPR), erythrocyte sedimentation rate (ESR), anti-nuclear antibody (ANA), HLA-B5 (Behçet's), HLA-A29 (birdshot), Toxocara titer, Lyme immunofluorescent assay or enzyme-linked immunosorbent assay (ELISA), and in neonates or immunocompromised patients, titers for CMV, herpes simplex, varicella-zoster, or rubella virus. Cultures of blood and i.v. sites may be helpful when infectious etiologies are suspected.
5. PPD (purified protein derivative of *tuberculin*) with anergy panel.
6. Chest x-ray.
7. Urine for cytomegalovirus (CMV) in immunocompromised patients.
8. CT scan of the brain and lumbar puncture when reticulum cell sarcoma is suspected and when human immunodeficiency virus (HIV)-associated opportunistic infections indicate a potential for systemic, and in particular, CNS involvement.
9. Diagnostic vitrectomy when appropriate (see individual sections).

See the individual sections for more specific guidelines for workup and treatment.

13.3 TOXOPLASMOSIS

Symptoms
Blurred vision, floaters, may have pain, redness, photophobia.

Critical Signs
Unilateral white–yellow retinal lesion associated with a hazy vitreous as a result of the presence of vitreous cells. An old chorioretinal scar can often be seen adjacent to the new white–yellow lesion but is not always present. Sometimes disc edema may be present.

Other Signs
Vitreous precipitates on the posterior surface of the detached vitreous, vitreous debris, optic-disc swelling, neuroretinitis, mild granulomatous iritis, localized vasculitis, retinal artery or vein occlusion in the area of the inflammation. Chorioretinal scars are occasionally found in the uninvolved eye. Large visual field loss may result from peripapillary toxoplasmosis. Cystoid macular edema (CME) or macular star may be present. A choroidal (subretinal) neovascular membrane develops on rare occasions as a late sequela.

❖ **Note** *Toxoplasmosis can also develop in the deep retina, in which case, few to no vitreous cells may be present. Toxoplasmosis is the most common cause of posterior uveitis.*

Differential Diagnosis

See Posterior Uveitis, Section 13.2, for a complete list. The following may closely simulate toxoplasmosis.

- Syphilis [Positive fluorescent treponemal antibody, absorbed (FTA-ABS). See Section 14.2, Acquired Syphilis.]
- Tuberculosis [Positive PPD (purified protein of *tuberculin*) with possible abnormal chest x-ray. Rare.]
- Toxocariasis [Usually affects children. A fibrous band may be seen radiating from a white retinal mass. Old chorioretinal scars are not typically seen. May have a history of exposure to puppies or eating dirt. Positive Toxocara enzyme-linked immunosorbent assay (ELISA).]

Workup

See Posterior Uveitis, Section 13.2, for a nonspecific workup when the diagnosis is in doubt.

1. History: Does the patient eat raw meat or has he or she been exposed to cats (sources of acquired infection)? Inquire about risk factors for AIDS in atypical cases (e.g., several active lesions without old chorioretinal scars).
2. Complete ocular examination, including a dilated fundus evaluation.
3. Serum antitoxoplasma antibody titer. Should have a positive titer from current or previous infection (the dilution is unimportant), but a negative titer on any dilution does not exclude the diagnosis. Immunoglobulin M (IgM) is found approximately 2 to 6 months after initial infection, after which only IgG remains.

❖ **Note** *Ask the laboratory to do a 1:1 dilution, as only a positive result is necessary in the setting of classic fundus findings.*

4. FTA-ABS, PPD with anergy panel, chest radiograph, and a Toxocara ELISA when the diagnosis is uncertain.
5. Fluorescein angiogram if a choroidal neovascular membrane is suspected.
6. Consider an HIV test in atypical cases or when the patient is a high-risk candidate for AIDS.

Treatment

A. The disease is self-limited in an immunocompetent patient. Mild peripheral retinochoroiditis may not require treatment. If an anterior-chamber reaction is present, a topical cycloplegic (e.g., cyclopentolate, 2%, t.i.d.) with or without a topical steroid (e.g., prednisolone acetate, 1%) q.i.d., is given. No additional treatment is indicated. The drops are tapered as the anterior-chamber reaction resolves.

B. Treatment should be considered in an immunocompetent patient if the lesion is present within the temporal arcade, the lesion is within 2 to 3 mm of the disc, threatening a large retinal vessel, a lesion that is associated with a large hemorrhage, or if the vitritis is severe enough to cause a two-line decrease in vision. Immunocompromised patients should be treated because the disease will not resolve spontaneously. Dosing for the nonpregnant adult is listed below.

1. Usual first-line therapy (for 3 to 6 weeks):
   a. Pyrimethamine, 200 mg, p.o. load (or two 100-mg doses, p.o., 12 hours apart), and then 25 mg, p.o., b.i.d.
   b. Folinic acid, 10 mg, p.o., twice weekly (to minimize bone marrow toxicity of pyrimethamine).
   c. Sulfadiazine, 2 g, p.o. load and then 1 g, p.o., q.i.d.
2. Prednisone may be added, after initiation of antibiotic therapy, at a dose of 20 to 40 mg, p.o., daily beginning 12 to 24 hours after antimicrobial therapy has begun. Periocular steroids should never be given.
3. Clindamycin, 450 to 600 mg, p.o., q.i.d., may be used with pyrimethamine as alternative therapy (if the patient is sulfa allergic) or as an adjunct to previously discussed therapy.
4. Other alternative therapies are used with success. Atovaquone (e.g., Mepron) has been used with good results and is able to kill toxoplasma cysts in vitro. Its ability to prevent recurrences in vivo is not yet known. Another alternative treatment is trimethoprim/sulfamethoxazole (160 mg/800 mg) one tablet orally, b.i.d., with or without clindamycin and prednisone.
5. Anterior-segment inflammation is treated with cycloplegia (e.g., cyclopentolate, 1% to 2%, t.i.d.) and topical steroid (e.g., prednisolone acetate, 1%, q.i.d.).

❖ **Note** *Systemic steroids should never be used without antimicrobial treatment and rarely used in immunocompromised patients. Before systemic steroid use, evaluation of fasting blood sugar and studies to rule out tuberculosis are prudent.*

If a patient is given pyrimethamine, a platelet count and CBC must be obtained once or twice per week to check for a low platelet count and a low red or white blood cell count (pyrimethamine can depress the bone marrow). If the platelet count decreases below 100,000, then reduce the dosage of pyrimethamine and increase the folinic acid.

Patients taking pyrimethamine should not take vitamins that contain folic acid. The medication should be given with meals to reduce anorexia. A small amount of pyrimethamine pills should be given at each visit to ensure compliance.

Patients on clindamycin should be warned about pseudomembranous colitis, and the medication should be stopped if diarrhea develops.

C. Laser photocoagulation, cryotherapy, and vitrectomy have been used as adjunctive treatment modalities.

D. Maintenance therapy (if patient is immunosuppressed)
    1. Pyrimethamine, 25 to 50 mg, p.o., qd.
    2. Sulfadiazine, 500 to 1,000 mg, p.o., q.i.d.
    3. Folinic acid, 10 mg, p.o., qd.
    4. If sulfa allergic, may use clindamycin, 300 mg, p.o., q.i.d.

Follow-up

In 3 to 7 days for blood tests or ocular assessment or both, and then every 1 to 2 weeks on therapy.

❖ Notes

1. *If a patient cannot use or must discontinue clindamycin, tetracycline, 2 g load, p.o., followed by 250 mg, p.o., q.i.d., is used alternatively. Do not give tetracycline to children or pregnant or breast-feeding women.*
2. *Pyrimethamine should not be given to pregnant or breast-feeding women.*
3. *Only women who develop toxoplasmosis during pregnancy can transmit it to their fetuses. A woman cannot transmit congenital toxoplasmosis.*
4. *Indocyanine green angiography has demonstrated that toxoplasma retinochoroiditis is more widespread than can be appreciated clinically and can be used to assess the extent of the disease.*

See AIDS, Section 14.1, for additional information.

REFERENCES

Engstrom RE, Holland GN, Nussenblatt RB, Jabs DA. Current practices in the management of ocular toxoplasmosis. *Am J Ophthalmol* 1991;111:601–610.

Opremcak EM, Scales DK, Sharpe MR. Trimethoprim-sulfamethoxazole therapy for ocular toxoplasmosis. *Ophthalmology* 1992;99:920–925.

de Boer JH, Verhagen C, Bruinenberg M, et al. Serologic and polymerase chain reaction analysis of intraocular fluids in the diagnosis of infectious uveitis. *Am J Ophthalmol* 1996;121:650–658.

Auer C, Bernasconi O, Herbort CP. Toxoplasmic retinochoroiditis: new insights provided by indocyanine green angiography. *Am J Ophthalmol* 1997;123:131–133.

13.4 SARCOIDOSIS

Symptoms

Pain, photophobia, decreased vision. Typically affects African-Americans in the 20- to 50-year age group.

Critical Ocular Signs

Granulomatous iritis with large "mutton-fat" keratic precipitates on the corneal endothelium (or less commonly, a nongranulomatous iritis), vitritis with white, fluffy opacities in the inferior vitreous or yellow–white nodules or exudates ("candle-wax drippings") and sheathing along peripheral retinal veins.

Other Ocular Signs

Iris or choroidal nodules or both, retinal hemorrhage, conjunctival granuloma, band keratopathy, posterior synechiae, glaucoma, cataract, lacrimal-gland enlargement, dry eye, optic disc swelling, optic nerve granuloma, optic neuritis, extraocular muscle palsy, and proptosis. Neovascularization (of the iris, optic nerve, and retina) and cystoid macular edema (CME) may occur.

Systemic Signs

Facial nerve palsy, salivary gland enlargement, hilar adenopathy on chest radiograph, erythema nodosum (erythematous, tender nodules beneath the skin, often in the anterior tibial area), arthritis, lymphadenopathy, hepato-splenomegaly, and other skin, CNS, and bone changes may be found.

❖ **Note** *Uveitis, secondary glaucoma, cataracts, and macular edema are the most common as well as the most significant vision-threatening complications of ocular sarcoid.*

Differential Diagnosis

- Sickle-cell disease (May also produce peripheral retinal neovascularization in young African-American individuals, but it is more commonly "sea-fan" in appearance. There is no uveitis, and a hemoglobin electrophoresis is abnormal in sickle-cell disease. See Section 12.23, Sickle-Cell Disease.)
- Tuberculosis (TB) (Rare. May appear identical to sarcoidosis. Positive PPD, may have abnormal chest x-ray.)
- Idiopathic pars planitis (White, fluffy vitreous opacities and cells and white exudative material accumulating along the ora serrata and pars plana, typically inferiorly. See Section 13.5, Pars Planitis.)

- Others (See Anterior Uveitis, Section 13.1, and Posterior Uveitis, Section 13.2.)

Workup

The following are the tests that are obtained when sarcoidosis is suspected clinically. See Anterior Uveitis, Section 13.1, and Posterior Uveitis, Section 13.2, for nonspecific uveitis workups.

1. Chest x-ray.
2. Serum angiotensin converting enzyme (ACE): Usually, but not always increased in active systemic sarcoidosis. May also be increased in TB, diabetes, leprosy, histoplasmosis, and other conditions that do not produce uveitis. Normal ACE values vary with age, requiring comparison with age-matched controls. Oral steroids and ACE inhibitors usually suppress the ACE level soon after starting treatment.
3. PPD with anergy panel: Used to distinguish TB (induration of 10 mm or more in most cases) from sarcoidosis (anergy in 50% of cases).
4. Biopsy of any conjunctival granuloma or the palpebral lobe of the lacrimal gland when it is enlarged. (An acid-fast stain and a methenamine–silver stain should be performed at the time of biopsy to rule out TB and fungal infection.) A "blind conjunctival" biopsy has an extremely low yield and generally is not recommended.

If this workup is inconclusive, yet sarcoidosis is still suspected, the following tests may be obtained:

5. Gallium scan of the head, neck, and mediastinum (often shows increased uptake in patients with active systemic sarcoidosis).

❖ **Note** *Serum ACE level and whole-body gallium scan used together increase the specificity for diagnosis to greater than 99% in patients with normal or equivocal chest radiographs.*

6. Serum lysozyme (may be increased) and serum protein electrophoresis (may show hypergammaglobulinemia).
7. Directed biopsy. Skin, lymph node, or lung biopsy by the appropriate physician.
8. Kveim's skin test (rarely available).
9. Pulmonary function tests may be indicated.

Serum calcium levels are sometimes obtained in patients diagnosed with sarcoidosis to ascertain that the blood calcium is not dangerously high.

Treatment

All patients are referred to an internist for systemic evaluation and medical management.

   A. Uveitis
1. Cycloplegic (e.g., cyclopentolate, 2%, or scopolamine, 0.25%, t.i.d.).
2. Topical steroid (e.g., prednisolone acetate, 1%, q 1 to 6 hours, depending on the degree of inflammation).
3. Periocular steroids (e.g., triamcinolone, 40 mg in 0.5 ml, subtenons every 3 to 4 weeks) may be required when the uveitis does not respond to q1h topical steroids. See Appendix 7 for the technique.
4. Systemic steroids (e.g., prednisone, 20 to 100 mg, p.o., daily) and a histamine H_2 blocker (e.g., ranitidine, 150 mg, p.o., b.i.d.) are often required in the presence of posterior uveitis (including optic neuritis). See Drug Glossary when considering systemic steroids.
5. Cyclosporin A has been used effectively in patients who are intolerant of or refractory to systemic steroids.
   B. Cystoid macular edema: See Section 12.14, Cystoid Macular Edema.
   C. Glaucoma: See Inflammatory Open-Angle Glaucoma, Section 10.4; Steroid-Response Glaucoma, Section 10.5; Acute Angle-Closure Glaucoma, Section 10.10; or Neovascular Glaucoma, Section 10.13, depending on the origin of the glaucoma.
   D. Retinal neovascularization: May require panretinal photocoagulation.
   E. Orbital disease is managed with systemic steroids as described previously.
   F. Pulmonary disease, seventh-nerve palsy, CNS disease, and renal disease require systemic steroids and management by an internist. Hypercalcemia also may require medical treatment.

Follow-up

Patients are reexamined in 3 to 7 days. The steroid dosages are adjusted in accordance with the patient's response to treatment. As the inflammation subsides, the steroids and cycloplegic agent are tapered slowly. Intraocular presure is monitored, and fundus reevaluation is performed at each visit. Asymptomatic patients with quiet eyes are seen every 6 months. Patients being treated with steroids need to be monitored more closely (e.g., every 1 to 3 months). Children with sarcoidosis are reexamined every 3 months because of the frequent occurrence of asymptomatic but damaging uveitis.

REFERENCES

Power WJ, Neves Ra, Rodriguez A, Pedroza-Seres M, Foster CS. The value of combined serum angiotensin-converting enzyme and gallium scan in diagnosing ocular sarcoidosis. *Ophthalmology* 1995;102(12):2007–2011.

13.5 PARS PLANITIS (INTERMEDIATE UVEITIS)

Symptoms

Floaters and cloudy vision, rarely red eye, pain, or photophobia. Usually age 15 to 40 years and bilateral.

Critical Signs

"Snowbanking" (white exudative material over the inferior ora serrata and pars plana), vitreous cells.

❖ **Note** *Snowbanking can often be seen only with indirect ophthalmoscopy and scleral depression.*

Other Signs

Cellular aggregates in the vitreous, especially inferiorly ("snowball" opacities), peripheral retinal vascular sheathing, anterior-chamber inflammation, cystoid macular edema (CME), posterior subcapsular cataract, secondary glaucoma, posterior vitreous detachment, vitreous hemorrhage, retinal detachment, retinal tears, or peripapillary edema may develop.

Differential Diagnosis

Usually idiopathic. Rarely may be associated with sarcoidosis, multiple sclerosis, Lyme disease, ocular lymphoma, and chronic *Propionibacterium acnes* infection.

See Posterior Uveitis, Section 13.2.

Workup

See Posterior Uveitis, Section 13.2.

Treatment

No treatment is necessary for patients who have a visual acuity of 20/40 or better. For patients with a visual acuity worse than 20/40 as a result of CME or vitreous opacities, any or all of the following may be tried [although (2) and (3) are not generally given simultaneously].

1. Topical prednisolone acetate, 1% (e.g., Pred Forte) q 1 to 2 hours may serve a dual purpose, relieving discomfort from an anterior-chamber reaction, and frequently improving the CME.
2. Periocular repository steroids (e.g., methylprednisolone, 40 mg in 0.5 ml subtenons). Repeat the injections every 1 to 2 months until the vision and CME are no longer improving, and then slowly taper the fre-

quency of injections. Contraindicated in patients with steroid-responsive intraocular pressure (IOP). See Appendix 7 for the technique.
3. If there is no improvement after the first three subtenons injections, then consider systemic steroids (e.g., prednisone, 40 to 60 mg, p.o., daily for 4 to 6 weeks), tapering gradually according to the patient's response. See Drug Glossary before starting systemic steroids.

❖ **Note** *In bilateral cases, systemic steroid therapy is often preferred to bilateral periocular injections.*

4. In patients who fail to respond to either oral or subtenons corticosteroids, transcleral cryotherapy to the area of snowbanking may be tried. If cryotherapy fails, pars plana vitrectomy can be considered.
5. As a last resort, some physicians advocate the use of systemic immunosuppressive agents (e.g., cyclophosphamide, cyclosporin A).

❖ **Notes**
1. *Some physicians delay periocular repository steroid therapy for several weeks to observe whether the patient is a steroid responder (i.e., develops a significant IOP increase caused by the topical steroids). If a steroid response is found, then the periocular steroid may need to be withheld.*
2. *Acetazolamide, 500 mg, p.o., daily may be tried in refractory CME patients.*
3. *Cataracts are a frequent complication. If cataract extraction is performed, systemic steroids are required after surgery because of increased inflammation. Patients may do better without an intraocular lens and with an aphakic contact lens.*

Follow-up
In the acute phase, patients are reevaluated every 1 to 4 weeks, depending on the severity of the condition. In the chronic phase, reexamination is performed every 3 to 6 months.

13.6 ACUTE RETINAL NECROSIS (ARN)

Symptoms
Blurred vision (often with floaters), ocular pain, photophobia. Most patients are in good systemic health, but underlying AIDS should be considered.

Critical Signs
Multiple white opaque patches of thickened retina, usually in the periphery, which gradually enlarge and coalesce. The posterior pole tends to be spared until later. There is a sharp demarcation line between the involved

and normal retina. Vitreous cells are often abundant. Involvement is bilateral (simultaneously or sequentially) in one third of patients.

Other Signs

Anterior-chamber reaction (sometimes granulomatous); increased intraocular pressure (IOP); sheathed retinal arterioles and sometimes venules, especially in the periphery; retinal hemorrhages (minor finding); optic disc edema; rhegmatogenous retinal detachments (RRD) occur in approximately 70% of patients. (The RRD typically has multiple, large, irregular posterior breaks and is usually a late finding.) An optic neuropathy (disc edema or pallor with an afferent pupillary defect, decreased color vision, and a central scotoma) sometimes develops.

Differential Diagnosis

Herpes virus family (varicella-zoster or herpes simplex)
See Posterior Uveitis, Section 13.2.

Workup

See Posterior Uveitis, Section 13.2, for a nonspecific uveitis workup.

1. History: Risk factors for AIDS? Immunocompromised? If yes, the differential diagnosis includes cytomegalovirus (CMV) retinitis and syphilis.
2. Complete ocular examination: Evaluate the anterior chamber and the vitreous for cells, measure the IOP, and perform a dilated retinal examination by using indirect ophthalmoscopy and scleral depression.
3. Consider a complete blood count (CBC) with differential, fluorescent treponemal antibody, absorbed (FTA-ABS), rapid plasma reagin (RPR), erythrocyte sedimentation rate (ESR), toxoplasmosis titers, PPD with anergy panel, and chest radiograph to rule out other etiologies.
4. Consider testing for HIV.
5. Consider acute and convalescent serum titers for herpes simplex, varicella-zoster, and CMV (limited utility).
6. Consider a fluorescein angiogram (limited utility).
7. An orbital CT scan or B-scan ultrasound to look for an enlarged optic nerve in cases of suspected optic nerve dysfunction.
8. CT scan or magnetic resonance imaging (MRI) of the brain and lumbar puncture if large cell lymphoma, tertiary syphilis, or encephalitis is suspected.

Treatment

1. Admit to the hospital. The goal of treatment is to decrease the incidence of the disease in the fellow eye. Treatment does not reduce the rate of retinal detachment in the first eye.
2. Acyclovir,* 1,500 mg/m^2 of body surface area/day, i.v., in three divided doses for 7 to 10 days. Then oral acyclovir (400 to 600 mg 5 times daily)

---

*The dosage of acyclovir needs to be reduced in patients with renal insufficiency. Blood urea nitrogen and creatinine levels are followed closely.

for up to 6 weeks from the onset of infection.* Regression of the retinitis is usually seen within 4 days. The lesions may progress during the first 48 hours of treatment. Famciclovir may be useful in cases that do not respond to acyclovir.

3. Topical cycloplegic (e.g., atropine, 1%, t.i.d.) and topical steroid (e.g., prednisolone acetate, 1%, q 2 to 6 hours) in the presence of anterior-segment inflammation.

4. Consider anticoagulation (e.g., heparin or warfarin for a total of 2 to 3 weeks) or antiplatelet therapy (aspirin, 125 to 650 mg, daily).

5. Systemic steroids (controversial): Some physicians administer steroids aggressively at the time of diagnosis (e.g., methylprednisolone, 250 mg, i.v., q.i.d., for 3 days followed by prednisone, 60 mg, p.o., b.i.d., for 1 to 2 weeks), particularly when the optic nerve is thought to be involved. Others delay steroid therapy for one or more weeks until the retinitis begins to clear. A typical oral corticosteroid regimen (initial or delayed therapy) is prednisone, 60 to 80 mg/day, for 1 to 2 weeks followed by a taper over 2 to 6 weeks. See Drug Glossary before starting systemic steroids.

6. See Inflammatory Open-Angle Glaucoma, Section 10.4, for treatment of increased IOP.

7. Consider prophylactic laser photocoagulation (confluent laser spots posterior to active retinitis) to wall-off or prevent subsequent RRD.

8. Pars plana vitrectomy, with long-acting gas or silicone oil, is the best way to repair the associated complex RRD. Proliferative vitreo-retinopathy is common.

9. Consider optic nerve sheath decompression surgery for ARN optic neuropathy when the optic nerve is enlarged and the patient's condition worsens or does not improve with medical therapy.

Follow-up

Patients are seen daily in the hospital and are then examined every few weeks to months for the following year. A careful fundus evaluation with scleral depression is performed at each visit to rule out retinal holes that may lead to a detachment. If the retinitis crosses the margin of prior laser treatment, consider applying additional laser therapy. A pupillary examination should always be performed, and optic neuropathy should be considered if the retinopathy does not explain the amount of visual loss.

REFERENCES

Duker JS, Blumenkranz MS. Diagnosis and management of the acute retinal necrosis syndrome. *Surv Ophthalmol* 1991;35:327–343.

Figueroa MS, Garabito I, Gutierrez C, Fortun J. Famciclovir for the treatment of acute retinal necrosis (ARN) syndrome. *Am J Ophthalmol* 1997;123:255–257.

*Six weeks of treatment is based on the observation that occurences in the second eye most often begin within 6 weeks of the onset in the first eye.

13.7 VOGT–KOYANAGI–HARADA (VKH) SYNDROME

Symptoms

Bilaterally decreased vision, photophobia, pain, and red eyes, accompanied by or preceded by a headache, stiff neck, nausea, vomiting, fever, and malaise. Hearing loss, dysacusia, and tinnitus frequently occur.

Critical Signs

Bilateral serous retinal detachments with underlying choroidal infiltrates, posterior vitreous cells and opacities, retinal hemorrhages, optic disc edema, anterior-chamber flare and cells, and graunlomatous ("mutton fat") keratic precipitates. Perilimbal vitiligo is common. Alopecia, vitiligo, and poliosis may develop later.

Other Signs

May see mottling and atrophy of the retinal pigment epithelium after the serous retinal detachment resolves (sunset fundus), hyphema, iris nodules, peripheral anterior and posterior synechiae, scleritis, hypotony, venous engorgement, retinal vasculitis, or choroidal neovascularization. Neurologic signs, including loss of consciousness, paralysis, and seizures, may occur. Typically, patients are aged 20 to 50 years and are of a darkly pigmented heritage such as Asian or Native American.

Differential Diagnosis

See Posterior Uveitis, Section 13.2, for a complete list. In particular, consider the following:

- Sympathetic ophthalmia (History of trauma or surgery to the uninvolved eye. Generally no CNS, skin, or hair manifestations. See Section 13.15, Sympathetic Ophthalmia.)
- Acute posterior multifocal placoid pigment epitheliopathy (AMPPE) (Ophthalmoscopic and fluorescein angiographic features may be very similar, but there is less vitreous inflammation and no anterior-segment involvement.)
- Other granulomatous panuveitides (e.g., syphilis, sarcoidosis, tuberculosis)

Workup

See Posterior Uveitis, Section 13.2, for a nonspecific uveitis workup.

1. History: Neurologic symptoms, hearing loss, or hair loss? Previous eye surgery or trauma?
2. Complete ocular examination, including a dilated retinal evaluation.
3. Complete blood count (CBC), rapid plasma reagin (RPR), fluorescent treponemal antibody, absorbed (FTA-ABS), angiotensin converting ezyme

(ACE), and PPD (purified protein derivative of *tuberculin*) with anergy panel and possibly chest radiograph to rule out similar-appearing disorders.

4. Consider a CT scan with and without contrast or MRI of the brain during attacks with neurologic signs to rule out a CNS disorder.
5. Lumbar puncture during attacks with meningeal symptoms for cell count and differential, protein, glucose, VDRL, Gram's and methenamine-silver stains, and culture. (Lymphocytosis is often seen in VKH and AMPPE.)
6. Fluorescein angiogram may help in diagnosis.

Treatment

Inflammation is controlled with steroids; the dose depends on the severity of the inflammation. In moderate-to-severe cases, the following regimen can be used initially. Steroids are tapered slowly as the condition improves.

1. Topical steroids (e.g., prednisolone acetate, 1%, q1h).
2. Systemic steroids (e.g., prednisone, 60 to 80 mg, p.o., daily) and a histamine H_2 blocker (e.g., ranitidine, 150 mg, p.o., b.i.d.). See Drug Glossary for a systemic steroid workup.
3. Topical cycloplegic (e.g., scopolamine, 0.25%, t.i.d.).
4. Treatment of any specific neurologic disorders (e.g., seizures or coma).
5. Immunosuppressive agents (e.g., methotrexate, azathioprine, chlorambucil, cyclosporine) can be used under the supervision of a medical consultant in patients who cannot tolerate or are unresponsive to systemic steroids.

Follow-up

Initial management may require hospitalization. Weekly, then monthly reexamination is performed, watching for recurrent inflammation and increased intraocular pressure. The steroids are tapered slowly. Inflammation may recur up to 9 months after the steroids have been discontinued. If this occurs, the previously described treatment regimen should be reinstituted.

13.8 RETICULUM CELL SARCOMA
(LARGE CELL LYMPHOMA)

Symptoms

Painless decrease in vision, floaters. Usually no history of uveitis.

Critical Signs

Large amount of vitreous cells and debris in a patient older than 40 years (typically older than 50 years) that do not respond well to systemic steroids. Usually bilateral.

Other Signs

May see patches of yellow–white chorioretinal or subretinal pigment epithelial infiltrates, retinal edema and hemorrhages, or a mild anterior-chamber reaction with fine keratic precipitates. Neurologic manifestations may be present.

Differential Diagnosis

See Posterior Uveitis, Section 13.2.

Workup

See Posterior Uveitis, Section 13.2, for a nonspecific uveitis workup. Evaluate for CNS disorders and visceral lymphoma.

1. History: Previous uveitis? Recent intraocular surgery? Immunocompromised or risk group for AIDS? Concomitant systemic symptoms or signs (e.g., skin rash, difficulty breathing, diarrhea)? If yes, see Posterior Uveitis, Section 13.2.
2. Complete ocular examination.
3. CT scan (axial and coronal views) with and without contrast or MRI of the orbit and head (and a body CT scan, if indicated).
4. Lumbar puncture for cell count, cytology, VDRL, protein, glucose, culture, and Gram's and methenamine–silver stains.
5. Consider a diagnostic vitrectomy with cytologic and immunohistologic studies.
6. Perform biopsy of suggestive lymph nodes as needed.
7. Bone marrow biopsy, if indicated.

Treatment

In cooperation with an oncologist and radiation therapist.

1. Ocular and brain radiation therapy.
2. Intravenous chemotherapy.
3. Systemic radiation therapy (if there is visceral involvement).
4. Intrathecal chemotherapy, if indicated.

Follow-up

In conjunction with the oncologist and radiation therapist.

13.9 POSTOPERATIVE UVEITIS

Postoperative inflammation is typically mild-to-moderate, usually resolving within 6 weeks. This section presents several etiologies of postoperative uveitis and a workup that may be considered when postoperative inflammation is atypical.

Etiology

A. Severe intraocular inflammation in the early postoperative course
   - Infectious endophthalmitis [Progressive and often severe ocular pain (but not always), deteriorating vision, corneal edema, eyelid swelling, chemosis, sometimes a hypopyon, and commonly vitreous inflammation and blunting of the red reflex. See Section 13.10, Postoperative Endophthalmitis.)
   - Phacoanaphylactic endophthalmitis (A severe granulomatous inflammation with mutton-fat keratic precipitates, resulting from an autoimmune reaction to lens protein exposed during surgery. See Section 13.14, Phacoanaphylactic Endophthalmitis.)
   - Aseptic endophthalmitis (A severe sterile postoperative uveitis caused by excess tissue manipulation, especially vitreous manipulation, during surgery. A hypopyon and a mild vitreous cellular reaction may develop. Generally not characterized by profound or progressive pain or visual loss. Eyelid swelling and chemosis are atypical. Usually resolves with topical steroid therapy.)

B. Persistent postoperative inflammation (e.g., beyond 6 weeks)
   - Patient noncompliance with steroid drops (e.g., not taking the drops or not shaking them properly)
   - Steroid drops tapered too abruptly
   - Iris or vitreous incarceration in the wound
   - Uveitis–glaucoma–hyphema (UGH) syndrome (Irritation of the iris or ciliary body by an intraocular lens. Increased intraocular pressure (IOP) and red blood cells in the anterior chamber accompany the anterior-segment inflammation.)
   - Retinal detachment (Often produces a low-grade anterior-chamber reaction. See Section 12.19, Retinal Detachment.)
   - Low-grade endophthalmitis (e.g., *Proprionibacterium acnes*, fungal, or partially treated bacterial endophthalmitis)
   - Inflammatory reaction to contaminants on the intraocular lens (e.g., polishing substances or substances used to sterilize the lens) or to the viscoelastic substance
   - Epithelial downgrowth or fibrous ingrowth (Corneal or conjunctival epithelium or fibrous tissue grows into the eye through a corneal wound and may be seen on the posterior corneal surface. The iris may appear flattened because of the spread of the membrane over the anterior-chamber angle onto the iris. Large cells may be seen in the anterior chamber, and glaucoma may be present. The diagnosis of epithelial downgrowth can be confirmed by observing the immediate appearance of white spots after medium-power argon laser treatment to the areas of iris covered by the membrane.)
   - Preexisting uveitis (see Anterior Uveitis, Section 13.1)

C. Sympathetic ophthalmia (Diffuse granulomatous inflammation in both eyes, after trauma or surgery to one eye. See Section 13.15, Sympathetic Ophthalmia.)

Workup

1. History: Is the patient taking and shaking the steroid drops properly? Did the patient stop the steroid drops abruptly? Was there a postoperative wound leak allowing epithelial downgrowth or fibrous ingrowth? Previous history of uveitis?
2. Complete ocular examination of both eyes, including a slit-lamp assessment of the anterior-chamber reaction, a determination of whether vitreous or residual lens material is present in the anterior chamber, and an inspection of the posterior lens capsule looking for posterior capsular opacities (as is seen in some cases of *P. acnes*). Gonioscopy (checking for iris or vitreous to the wound), an IOP measurement, a dilated indirect ophthalmoscopic examination (to rule out a retinal detachment or signs of chorioretinitis), and a posterior vitreous evaluation with a slit-lamp and a 60-diopter, Hruby, or Goldmann's contact lens looking for inflammatory cells should be performed.
3. Obtain a B-scan ultrasound when the fundus view is obscured.
4. A diagnostic surgical vitrectomy is usually performed for smears and cultures when nonpostoperative infectious endophthalmitis is suspected. For postoperative endophthalmitis, see Section 13.10, Postoperative Endophthalmitis. Anaerobic cultures, using both solid media and broth, should be obtained to isolate *P. acnes* (routine cultures also are obtained, see Postoperative Endophthalmitis, Section 13.10). The anaerobic cultures should be incubated in an anaerobic environment as rapidly as possible and allowed to grow for at least 2 weeks.
5. Consider an anterior-chamber paracentesis for diagnostic smears and cultures.
6. Consider diagnostic medium-power argon laser treatment to the areas of iris thought to be covered by epithelial downgrowth.

If this workup is negative, no underlying etiology can be elicited, and a trial of steroids only transiently reduces the inflammation, surgical removal of the capsular bag and intraocular lens should be considered in an effort to isolate *P. acnes*.

See Anterior Uveitis, Section 13.1; Posterior Uveitis, Section 13.2; Postoperative Endophthalmitis, Section 13.10; Phacoanaphylactic Endophthalmitis, Section 13.14; and Sympathetic Ophthalmia, Section 13.15 for more specific information on diagnosis and treatment.

13.10 POSTOPERATIVE ENDOPHTHALMITIS

Acute (One to Several Days after Surgery)

Symptoms

Sudden onset of progressively decreasing vision, redness, and increasing eye pain.

Critical Signs

More ocular inflammation than would be expected after the ocular procedure performed. Intense flare and cell in the anterior chamber and vitreous, with or without hypopyon, eyelid edema, chemosis, and a reduced red reflex.

❖ **Note** *Pain and a hypopyon may not be present.*

Other Signs

Corneal edema, iris hyperemia, purulent discharge.

Organisms

Most common   Staphylococcus epidermidis.
Common   Staphylococcus aureus, streptococcal species (except *Pneumococcus,* which is not a common cause).
Less common   Gram-negative bacteria (Pseudomonas species, *Aerobacter* species, *Proteus* species, *Haemophilus influenzae, Klebsiella* species, *Escherichia coli, Bacillus* species, *Enterobacter* species) and anaerobes.

Differential Diagnosis

See Postoperative Uveitis, Section 13.9.

Workup

1. Complete ocular history and examination.
2. Consider a B-scan ultrasound, which may confirm the clinical suspicion by revealing marked vitreous cells, and establishes a baseline against which the success of therapy can be measured. Also used to evaluate for retinal breaks if media is too cloudy adequately to visualize the retina.
3. If vision is light perception or worse, a diagnostic (and therapeutic) vitrectomy is often performed. Cultures (blood, chocolate, Sabouraud's, thioglycolate) and smears (Gram's and Giemsa stains) are obtained, and intravitreal antibiotics are given as described in the following section. Otherwise, an anterior-chamber paracentesis combined with vitreous aspiration of 0.3 ml is performed.
4. Consider CBC with differential and serum electrolytes.

Treatment
1. Hospitalization.
2. Intravitreal antibiotics are the treatment of choice, (e.g., amikacin, 0.4 mg in 0.1 ml, or ceftriaxone, 2 mg in 0.1 ml, and vancomycin, 1.0 mg in 0.1 ml; clindamycin, 1 mg in 0.1 to 0.2 ml may be used in place of vancomycin) combined with topical antibiotics; the benefit of subconjunctival antibiotics is controversial and is not frequently used.
3. Immediate pars plana vitrectomy is beneficial if visual acuity on presentation is light perception or worse. Otherwise, vitreous aspiration ("tap") combined with placement of intravitreal antibiotics (and possibly steroid) is usually performed.
4. Topical fortified antibiotics (e.g., fortified cefazolin or fortified vancomycin q1h and fortified gentamicin or tobramycin q1h alternating every half hour). See Appendix 9, which describes fortified drop preparation.
5. Often combined with topical, subconjunctival, or intravitreal steroids or a combination of these because fungi are unlikely in the early postoperative setting. Use topical prednisolone acetate, 1% q1h, and subconjunctival triamcinolone, 40 mg, at the time of vitrectomy. Intravitreal dexamethasone, 0.4 mg, at time of vitreous tap or vitrectomy is at surgeon's discretion.
6. Topical cycloplegic (e.g., atropine, 1%) 3 to 4 times per day.

❖ **Note** *Vitrectomy offers the theoretic advantages of reducing bacterial load as well as providing material for diagnostic studies.*

Follow-up
1. Monitor the clinical course every 4 to 8 hours.
2. The antibiotic regimen is refined according to the patient's response to treatment and to the culture and sensitivity results. If a patient is getting worse or an identified organism is found to be resistant to the intravitreal antibiotics injected, an additional intravitreal injection of one antibiotic can be given 48 hours after the initial injection.
3. If the patient is responding well to treatment, topical fortified antibiotics may be slowly tapered after 48 hours and then switched to regular strength or a fluoroquinolone. Close outpatient follow-up is warranted.

❖ **Note** *Some physicians administer a systemic steroid (e.g., prednisone, 60 to 100 mg, p.o., daily) once the responsible organism has been treated appropriately for 24 hours. This regimen is maintained for 7 to 10 days and then tapered. We do not generally do this.*

Delayed-Onset (A Week to a Month or More After Surgery)

Symptoms
Insidious decreased vision, increasing redness and pain.

Critical Signs
Reduced visual acuity, anterior-chamber and vitreous inflammation, vitreous abscesses, hypopyon; clumps of exudate in the anterior chamber, on the iris surface, or along the pupillary border.

Other Signs
Corneal infiltrate and edema; may have a surgical bleb.

Etiology/Organisms
- Fungi (*Aspergillus* > *Candida, Cephalosporium* > *Penicillium* species; others)
- *Propionibacterium acnes* (Recurrent, granulomatous anterior uveitis, often with a hypopyon, but with minimal conjunctival injection and pain. A white plaque or opacities on the posterior lens capsule may be evident. There is only a transient response to steroids.)
- Other bacteria [Related to a filtering bleb (often streptococci), vitreous wick, or partial suppression with antibiotics during or after surgery.)

Differential Diagnosis
See Postoperative Uveitis, Section 13.9.

Workup
1. Complete ocular history and examination.
2. Vitreous material for smears (Gram's, Giemsa, and methenamine–silver) and cultures [blood, chocolate, Sabouraud's, thioglycolate, and a solid medium for anaerobic culture (e.g., *Brucella* or blood agar); *P. acnes* will be missed unless proper anaerobic cultures are obtained]. Intravitreal antibiotics are given as described in the following section.
3. Consider CBC with differential, serum electrolytes, liver-function studies.

Treatment
1. Initially treat as acute postoperative endophthalmitis, as described previously, but do not start steroids.
2. Immediate pars plana vitrectomy is beneficial if visual acuity on presentation is light perception or worse up to 6 weeks after surgery. Benefit beyond 6 weeks is not known.
3. If a fungal infection is suspected or an intraoperative smear is consistent with fungus, administer intravitreal amphotericin B, 5 to 10 µg at the time of vitrectomy. If fungus is identified on Gram stain, Giemsa, or Calcofluor white, then use combination of topical and systemic antifungal medications. Use topical natamycin, 5%, q1h, and flucytosine, 37.5 mg/kg, p.o., q6h, until specific organism is known. Role of systemic amphotericin B and fluconazole is unclear. Dosing information is provided later.

a. Amphotericin B, 0.25 to 0.3 mg/kg/day, i.v., initially (in test doses of 1 mg), and then increase the dose slowly to 0.75 to 1.0 mg/kg/day i.v. in divided doses.

b. Consider miconazole, 10 mg in 1 ml, subconjunctivally.

c. A therapeutic vitrectomy should be performed if it was not done with the initial cultures. Antifungal therapy is modified in accordance with sensitivity testing, clinical course, and tolerance to antifungal agents.

4. Removal of the lens and capsular remnants may be required for diagnosis and treatment of *P. acnes,* which may be sensitive to intravitreal penicillin, cefoxitin, clindamycin, or vancomycin.

5. If mild *S. epidermidis* is isolated, intraocular vancomycin alone may be sufficient.

Follow-up

Dependent on the organism. In general, follow-up is as described previously for acute postoperative endophthalmitis. Repeat CBC, serum electrolytes, and liver-function tests 2 times per week during treatment for fungal endophthalmitis.

REFERENCES

Endophthalmitis Vitrectomy Study Group. Results of the endophthalmitis vitrectomy study. *Arch Ophthalmol* 1995;113:1479–1496.

13.11 TRAUMATIC ENDOPHTHALMITIS

This condition constitutes an emergency. If suspected, prompt action is required.

Symptoms and Signs

Same as Acute Postoperative Endophthalmitis, Section 13.10.

❖ **Note** *Patients with* Bacillus *endophthalmitis may develop a high fever, leukocytosis, proptosis, a corneal abscess in the form of a ring, and rapid visual deterioration.*

Organisms

Bacillus species, *S. epidermidis,* gram-negative species, fungi, *Streptococcus* species, others. A mixed flora may be present.

Differential Diagnosis

- Sterile inflammatory response from a retained intraocular foreign body or blood in the vitreous
- Sterile inflammation as a result of surgical complications
- Phacoanaphylactic endophthalmitis (A sterile autoimmune inflammatory reaction as a result of exposed lens protein. See Section 13.14, Phacoanaphylactic Endophthalmitis.)

Workup

Same as for Acute Postoperative Endophthalmitis, Section 13.10. An orbital CT scan (axial and coronal views) and ultrasound also are performed to rule out an intraocular foreign body.

Treatment

1. Hospitalization.
2. Management for a ruptured globe or penetrating ocular injury if present (see Section 3.14, Ruptured Globe and Penetrating Ocular Injury).
3. Topical fortified gentamicin or tobramycin, q1h, and fortified cefazolin or fortified vancomycin, q1h, alternating every half hour. See Appendix 9, which describes fortified drop preparation.
4. Benefit of subconjunctival antibiotics is limited, and they are not often used; if used, may consider gentamicin and clindamycin, 34 mg, which can be repeated qd.
5. Systemic antibiotics (e.g., gentamicin, 2.0 mg/kg, i.v. load, followed by 1.0 mg/kg i.v., q8h, and clindamycin, 600 mg, i.v., q8h with or without cefazolin, 500 to 1,000 mg, i.v., q8h.)*
6. Intravitreal antibiotics (amikacin, 0.4 mg in 0.1 ml, or ceftriaxone, 2 mg in 0.1 ml, and vancomycin, 1 mg in 0.1 ml, or clindamycin, 1 mg in 0.1 ml). These may be repeated every 48 to 72 hours, as needed.
7. The benefit of pars plana vitrectomy (PPV) is unknown for this type of endophthalmitis. However, PPV offers the benefit of reducing infectious load and providing sufficient material for diagnostic culture and pathology.
8. If tetanus immunization not up to date, give tetanus toxoid, 0.5 ml, i.m.
9. Steroids should **NOT** be used until fungal organisms are ruled out. If no fungi are isolated, may use prednisolone acetate, 1%, q4h, and subconjunctival dexamethasone, 4 mg. Prednisone, 40 to 80 mg, p.o., qd, is at the discretion of the surgeon. If fungus is isolated, specific antifungal regimens may be used.

---

*Drug doses may need to be reduced in children and patients with renal disease. Check gentamicin peak and trough levels one-half hour before and after the fifth dose, and follow the blood urea nitrogen and creatinine levels.

❖ **Notes** *Antibiotics are usually withheld until after the vitrectomy is performed unless a prolonged delay until surgery is expected.*

Follow-up

Same as for Postoperative Endophthalmitis, Section 13.10. The specific antibiotics and the frequency of their administration should be modified in accordance with the patient's response to treatment, as well as the culture and sensitivity results.

13.12 ENDOGENOUS BACTERIAL ENDOPHTHALMITIS

Symptoms

Decreased vision in an acutely ill (e.g., septic) patient, an immunocompromised host, or an i.v. drug abuser. No history of recent intraocular surgery.

Critical Signs

Vitreous cells and debris, anterior-chamber cell and flare, or a hypopyon in a high-risk patient.

Other Signs

Iris microabscess, absent red fundus reflex, retinal inflammatory infiltrates, flame-shaped retinal hemorrhages with or without white centers, corneal edema, eyelid edema, chemosis, conjunctival injection. Panophthalmitis [orbital involvement (proptosis, restricted ocular motility) and endophthalmitis] may develop.

Etiology

Bacillus cereus (especially in i.v. drug abusers), streptococci, *Neisseria meningitidis, S. aureus, H. influenzae,* others).

Differential Diagnosis

- Endogenous fungal endophthalmitis (May see fluffy, white vitreous opacities. Fungi grow on cultures. See Candida Retinitis/Uveitis/Endophthalmitis, Section 13.13.)
- Retinochoroidal infection (e.g., toxoplasmosis and toxocariasis) (Yellow or white retinochoroidal lesion present.)

- Noninfectious posterior uveitis (e.g., sarcoidosis, pars planitis) (May have a known history of uveitis. Unlikely to get coincidentally the first episode during sepsis.)
- Neoplastic conditions [e.g., reticulum cell sarcoma (usually older than 50 to 55 years), retinoblastoma (usually in the first few years of life)]

Workup

1. History: Duration of symptoms? Underlying disease or infections? i.v. drug abuse? Immunocompromised?
2. Complete ocular examination, including a dilated fundus examination.
3. B-scan ultrasound to determine the extent of posterior segment ocular involvement if it cannot be determined on clinical examination.
4. Complete medical workup by an infectious disease expert.
5. Cultures of blood, urine, and all indwelling catheters and i.v. lines, as well as Gram's stain of any discharge. A lumbar puncture is indicated when meningeal signs are present.
6. Vitrectomy with intraocular antibiotics (e.g., amikacin, 0.4 mg in 0.1 ml, or ceftriaxone, 2 mg in 0.1 ml, and vancomycin, 1 mg in 0.1 ml; clindamycin, 1 mg in 0.1 ml, may be used in place of vancomycin): The timing of this procedure is controversial. We perform it as soon as possible. Other physicians initially perform aqueous and vitreous aspirations when the systemic cultures are negative and the organism remains unknown.

Treatment

In conjunction with a medical internist.

1. Hospitalize the patient.
2. Broad-spectrum antibiotics are started after appropriate smears and cultures are obtained. Antibiotic choices vary according to the suspected source of septic infection (e.g., gastrointestinal tract, genitourinary tract) and are determined by an infectious disease expert. Dosages recommended for meningitis and severe infections are used.

❖ **Note** *Intravenous drug abusers are given an aminoglycoside and clindamycin to eradicate* Bacillus cereus.

3. Topical cycloplegic (e.g., atropine, 1%, t.i.d.).
4. Topical steroid (e.g., prednisolone acetate, 1%, q1 to 6 hours, depending on the degree of anterior-segment inflammation).
5. Periocular antibiotics (e.g., subconjunctival or subtenons injections) are sometimes used. See Appendix 7 for injection techniques.
6. Intravitreal antibiotics offer higher intraocular concentrations.
7. Vitrectomy offers the benefit of reducing infective load and providing sufficient material for diagnostic culture and pathology.

Follow-up

Daily in the hospital. Peak and trough levels for many antibiotic agents are examined every few days. Blood urea nitrogen and creatinine levels are monitored during aminoglycoside therapy. The antibiotic regimen is guided by the culture and sensitivity results, as well as the patient's clinical response to treatment. Intravenous antibiotics are maintained for at least 2 weeks and until the condition has resolved.

13.13 CANDIDA RETINITIS/UVEITIS/ ENDOPHTHALMITIS

Symptoms

Decreased vision, floaters, pain, often bilateral. Patients typically are i.v. drug abusers, immunocompromised hosts (e.g., as a result of cancer, immunosuppressive agents, AIDS, long-term antibiotics, or systemic steroids) or possess a long-term indwelling catheter (e.g., for hyperalimentation or hemodialysis).

Critical Signs

Multifocal, yellow–white, fluffy retinal lesions from one to several disc diameters in size. With time, the lesions increase in size, spread into the vitreous, and appear as "cotton balls."

Other Signs

Vitreous cells and haze, vitreous abscesses, retinal hemorrhages with or without pale centers (pale centers indicate Roth's spots), aqueous cells and flare, hypopyon. Retinal detachment may develop.

Differential Diagnosis

The following should be considered in immunocompromised hosts.

- Cytomegalovirus (CMV) retinitis (Minimal-to-mild vitreous reaction, more retinal hemorrhage, tends to concentrate along vessels; consider strongly in AIDS patients. See Section 14.1, Acquired Immunodeficiency Syndrome.)
- Toxoplasmosis (Yellow–white lesion confined to the retina. An adjacent chorioretinal scar may or may not be present. Vitreous cells and debris are common, but vitreous abscesses or "cotton balls" are not. See Section 13.3, Toxoplasmosis.)
- Others (e.g., herpes simplex; *Mycobacterium avium-intracellulare; Nocardia, Aspergillus,* and *Cryptococcus* species; coccidioidomycosis)

Workup

1. History: Medications? Medical problems? i.v. drug abuse? Other risk factors for AIDS?
2. Search the skin for scars from i.v. drug injection.
3. Complete ocular examination, including a dilated retinal evaluation.
4. Blood, urine, and catheter site (if present) cultures for *Candida* species; these often need to be repeated several times and may be negative despite ocular candidiasis.
5. Diagnostic (and therapeutic) vitrectomy is indicated when a significant amount of vitreous involvement is present. Cultures and smears are taken at the time of vitrectomy to confirm the diagnosis and to evaluate the organisms' sensitivity to antifungal agents. Amphotericin B, 5 µg in 0.1 ml, is injected into the central vitreous cavity at the conclusion of the procedure.
6. Baseline CBC, blood urea nitrogen, creatinine, and liver-function tests.

Treatment

1 Hospitalize all unreliable patients, systemically ill patients, or those with moderate-to-severe vitreous involvement.
2. An infectious-disease specialist or internist familiar with antifungal therapy should be consulted.
3. Fluconazole, 200 to 400 mg, p.o., qd.
4. In resistant cases, amphotericin B may be administered. For the first few days, amphotericin B, 1 mg i.v., is given 5 times per day, then larger doses totaling 20 mg/day are administered. Therapy is discontinued when a total dose of 1,000 mg has been given. Patients with endophthalmitis can be given up to 1 mg/kg/day for several weeks, not to exceed a total dose of 2 g.
5. Topical cycloplegic agent (e.g., atropine, 1%, t.i.d.).
6. See Inflammatory Open-Angle Glaucoma, Section 10.4, for intraocular pressure (IOP) control. Note, however, that steroids are generally contraindicated in candidiasis.

Follow-up

Patients are seen daily. Visual acuity, IOP, and the degree of anterior-chamber and vitreous inflammation are assessed. Serum blood urea nitrogen levels, creatinine levels, and CBC are repeated a few times per week. Liver-function tests are repeated periodically. Serum levels of antifungal agents are followed, and dosages are adjusted accordingly.

❖ **Note:** *Systemic antifungal agents may not be necessary if no systemic disease is uncovered.*

13.14 PHACOANAPHYLACTIC ENDOPHTHALMITIS

Definition
A sterile autoimmune inflammatory reaction to exposed lens protein. It usually occurs 1 day to a few weeks after surgical, traumatic, or spontaneous disruption of the lens capsule.

Symptoms
Pain, photophobia, red eye, decreased vision.

Critical Signs
A greater anterior-chamber inflammatory reaction than is typically seen after a surgical procedure (more cells and flare; sometimes, a hypopyon and mutton-fat keratic precipitates). Lens material may be seen in the anterior chamber.

Other Signs
Eyelid edema, chemosis, increased intraocular pressure (IOP), posterior synechiae.

Differential Diagnosis
See Postoperative Uveitis, Section 13.9.

Workup
See Postoperative Uveitis, Section 13.9, for a generalized uveitis workup in a postoperative patient.

1. History: Recent ocular surgery or trauma?
2. Complete ocular examination: Look for lens particles in the anterior chamber, measure the IOP, and search for any inflammatory reaction in the vitreous. The red fundus reflex should be assessed during a dilated retinal examination.
3. If infectious endophthalmitis cannot be ruled out, cultures are obtained and antibiotics started (see Postoperative Endophthalmitis, Section 13.10).
4. B-scan ultrasound to help in diagnosis and follow-up.

Treatment
1. Topical steroids (e.g., prednisolone acetate, 1%) q 1 to 2 hours.
2. Subconjunctival steroids (e.g., methylprednisolone, 40 mg in 0.5 ml). See Appendix 7 for the technique.

3. If the IOP is increased, see Inflammatory Open-Angle Glaucoma, Section 10.4, and Steroid-Response Glaucoma, Section 10.5, for management.

If severe:

4. Systemic steroids (e.g., prednisone, 80 to 100 mg, p.o., daily) and an antacid or histamine H_2 blocker (e.g., ranitidine, 150 mg, p.o., b.i.d.). See Drug Glossary before starting systemic steroids.
5. After the inflammation has subsided, surgery may be indicated to remove residual lens material and capsule.

Follow-up
Every 1 to 7 days, depending on the severity of the condition (some patients may need to be hospitalized).

- Check the IOP: Watch for glaucoma.
- Assess the degree of inflammation. Taper the steroids slowly as the inflammation subsides.

13.15 SYMPATHETIC OPHTHALMIA

Symptoms
Bilateral eye pain, photophobia, decreased vision (near vision is often affected before distance vision), red eye. A history of penetrating trauma or intraocular surgery to one eye (usually 4 to 8 weeks before, but the range is from 5 days to 66 years, with 90% occurring within 1 year) may be elicited.

Critical Signs
Any inflammation in the uninvolved eye after unilateral ocular trauma is suspicious. Bilateral severe anterior-chamber reaction with large mutton-fat keratic precipitates, small depigmented nodules at the level of the retinal pigment epithelium (Dalen–Fuchs' nodules), and thickening of the uveal tract. Signs of previous injury or surgery in one eye are usually present, including indications of previous laser therapy or cryotherapy.

Other Signs
Nodular infiltration of the iris, peripheral anterior synechiae, neovascularization of the iris, occlusion and seclusion of the pupil, cataract, exudative retinal detachment, papillitis. The earliest sign may be loss of accommodation or a mild anterior or posterior uveitis in the uninjured eye.

Differential Diagnosis
- Vogt–Koyanagi–Harada syndrome (VKH) (Similar signs, but often no history of ocular trauma or surgery. Other symptoms and signs may include headache, nausea, vomiting, fever, malaise, vertigo, bizarre behavior, focal neurologic symptoms, alopecia, vitiligo, or poliosis. Darkly pigmented persons, especially Asians, are more commonly affected. See Section 13.7, Vogt–Koyanagi–Harada Syndrome.)
- Phacoanaphylactic endophthalmitis (Severe anterior-chamber reaction from injury to the lens capsule, usually from trauma or surgery. No posterior uveitis is present. Contralateral eye is uninvolved. See Section 13.14, Phacoanaphylactic Endophthalmitis.)
- Sarcoidosis (May cause a granulomatous panuveitis with exudates over retinal veins or white clumps in the anterior vitreous inferiorly. Concomitant pulmonary disease is common. No history of trauma. See Section 13.4, Sarcoidosis.)
- Syphilis (Granulomatous panuveitis may be accompanied by interstitial keratitis, dilated capillary nests on the iris, or a diffuse pigmentary retinopathy. Positive fluorescent treponemal antibody, absorbed (FTA-ABS). No history of trauma. See Section 14.2, Acquired Syphilis.)

Workup
1. History: Any prior eye surgery or injury? Venereal disease? Difficulty breathing?
2. Complete ophthalmic examination, including a dilated retinal examination.
3. Complete blood count (CBC), rapid plasma reagin (RPR), FTA-ABS, with or without angiotensin converting enzyme (ACE) level if sarcoidosis is a serious consideration.
4. Consider a chest radiograph to evaluate for tuberculosis or sarcoidosis.
5. Fluorescein angiography or B-scan ultrasonography or both to help confirm the diagnosis.

Treatment
1. Prevention: Enucleation of a blind, traumatized eye before a sympathetic reaction can develop (usually considered within 7 to 14 days of the trauma). If sympathetic ophthalmia develops, enucleation may still be beneficial, regardless of the time since the trauma.

Inflammation is controlled with steroids; the dose depends on the severity of the inflammation. In moderate-to-severe cases, the following regimen can be used initially. Steroids are tapered slowly as the condition improves.

2. Topical steroids (e.g., prednisolone acetate, 1%, q 1 to 2 hours).
3. Periocular steroids (e.g., subconjunctival dexamethasone, 4 to 5 mg in 0.5 ml, 2 to 3 times per week). See Appendix 7 for the administration technique.

4. Systemic steroids [e.g., prednisone, 60 to 80 mg, p.o., daily, and an antacid or histamine H_2 blocker (e.g., ranitidine, 150 mg, p.o., b.i.d.)]. Before using systemic steroids, should consider evaluation of fasting blood sugar, PPD (purified protein derivative of *tuberculin*), and chest x-ray (CXR).

5. Cycloplegic (e.g., scopolamine, 0.25%, t.i.d.).

6. If steroids are ineffective or contraindicated, an immunosuppressive agent (e.g., methotrexate or cyclosporin) may be tried, usually in conjunction with a medical consultant.

Follow-up

Every 1 to 7 days initially, to monitor the effectiveness of therapy. As the condition improves, the follow-up interval may be extended to every 3 to 4 weeks. Intraocular pressure must be monitored closely. Steroids should be maintained for 3 to 6 months after all signs of inflammation have resolved. Because of the possibility of recurrence, periodic checkups are important.

SYSTEMIC DISORDERS

14.1 ACQUIRED IMMUNODEFICIENCY SYNDROME (AIDS)

Description

AIDS results from end-stage infection with the human immunodeficiency virus (HIV), which ultimately depletes the immune system of CD4+ T lymphocytes. At risk for HIV infection are homosexual or bisexual men, i.v. drug abusers, hemophiliacs and transfusion recipients, sexual partners of HIV-infected (HIV+) individuals, prostitutes and their sexual partners, and infants born to HIV+ mothers.

Laboratory Testing

For initial diagnosis (establishes HIV+ status):

1. Serum enzyme-linked immunosorbent assay (ELISA) for HIV antibody (highly sensitive, less specific).
2. If ELISA is positive, Western blot to confirm (highly specific). If Western blot is positive, patient is considered HIV+.

For monitoring the patient's clinical status:

3. CD4+ cell counts.
4. HIV viral titers.

❖ **Note** *A diagnosis of AIDS is made on the basis of CD4+ counts less than 200 cells/mm³ or the presence of an AIDS-defining illness, in an HIV+ patient.*

Ocular Complications of AIDS

Cornea and External Diseases

HERPES ZOSTER OPHTHALMICUS (HZO)

May be the initial clinical manifestation of HIV infection. HZO in patients older than 40 years without known immunocompromise should raise the clinical suspicion for AIDS.

Signs

Vesicular lesions of the face in the distribution of the ophthalmic division of the trigeminal nerve. May be associated with almost any ocular abnormality, including keratitis, uveitis, scleritis, and cranial nerve palsies. (See Herpes Zoster Virus, Section 4.16).

Workup

1. Complete ophthalmic examination, including dilated fundus examination. AIDS patients with HZO should be screened for progressive outer retinal necrosis (PORN), a rapidly progressive retinitis characterized by clear vitreous and sheet-like opacification deep to normal-looking retinal vessels. PORN also may be seen with spontaneous vitreous hemorrhage. This condition frequently leads to blindness due either to the infection itself or to secondary retinal detachment, making prompt diagnosis and treatment essential. (See Section 13.6, Acute Retinal Necrosis).
3. Herpes zoster virus (HZV) retrobulbar optic neuritis may precede clinical retinitis. Profound visual loss may develop despite i.v. antiviral treatment.

Treatment

1. Nucleoside analog antiviral medications, tailored to the individual patient. The location and extent of the lesions as well as the stage of the HIV infection are all factors that play a role in selecting an appropriate therapy. Intraocular plus intravenous antivirals may be used for PORN or HZV retrobulbar optic neuritis.
   See Table 14-1 for treatment details.
2. When intraocular inflammation is present, a topical cycloplegic (e.g., scopolamine, 0.25%, t.i.d.) and a topical steroid (e.g., prednisolone acetate, 1%, q 1 to 2 hours) are given.
3. Bacitracin ointment to the skin lesions, b.i.d.
4. Steroid treatment for retrobulbar optic neuritis is absolutely contraindicated in HIV+ patients until infectious etiology is excluded.

❖ **Note** *Patients should not receive oral steroids because of the risk of further immunosuppression and extension of the infection.*

TABLE 14-1. *Herpes Zoster Ophthalmicus*

Drug	Dosing Information	Toxicities	Contraindications
Acyclovir (e.g., Zovirax)	10 mg/kg i.v. q8 h (q12 h if creatinine >2.0) × 7–10 days. Consider maintenance with 800 mg p.o. 5×/day to prevent reactivation	i.v.: reversible renal and neurologic toxicity	Use with caution in patients with a history of renal impairment
Famciclovir (e.g., Famvir)	500 mg p.o. q8 h. Adjust dosage for creatinine clearance <60 ml/min	Headache, nausea, diarrhea, dizziness, fatigue	Use with caution in patients with a history of renal impairment
Valacyclovir HCl (e.g., Valtrex)	1 g p.o. q8 h. Adjust dosage for creatinine clearance <60 ml/min	Headache, nausea, vomiting, diarrhea	See comment.[a]

[a]Comment: In patients with advanced HIV disease and/or AIDS, thrombotic thrombocytopenic purpura/hemolytic uremic syndrome (TTP/HUS) has been reported in association with valacyclovir doses of 8 g/day.

KAPOSI'S SARCOMA (KS)

KS of the ocular adnexal tissues occurs in approximately 5% of patients with AIDS. See Section 8.1, Conjunctival Tumors.

Signs

Skin lesions are more common than conjunctival lesions. Eyelid lesions are purple–red, nontender nodules and can have associated edema, trichiasis, or entropion formation. Bright-red subconjunctival lesions are most commonly located in the inferior cul-de-sac. (These may be mistaken for benign subconjunctival hemorrhage.) Orbital lesions with associated periorbital edema occur rarely.

Treatment

1. Vinblastine and vincristine have had some success in causing remission of KS.
2. Local treatment by excision, cryotherapy, or irradiation may be performed for single lesions if systemic chemotherapy is not used or has failed.

❖ **Note** *KS lesions may resolve when patients are given HIV protease inhibitors.*

OTHER CORNEA AND EXTERNAL DISEASE

- Molluscum contagiosum:
  Chronic follicular conjunctivitis, umbilicated eyelid nodules. (See Section 5.2, Chronic Conjunctivitis.)
- Microsporidial keratoconjunctivitis:
  Chronic superficial punctate keratitis and conjunctival injection not responsive to conservative treatment. Diagnosed with Giemsa stain of corneal scraping. Treated with topical fumagillin or oral itraconazole or both. Epithelial debridement followed by topical antibiotic ointment (e.g., bacitracin, t.i.d.) may be useful for mild cases.
- Fungal keratitis:
  May occur without prior corneal injury.
  (See Section 4.13, Fungal Keratitis.)
- Herpes simplex virus (HSV) keratitis:
  May be associated with more frequent recurrence and prolonged, peripheral ulceration.
  (See Section 4.15, Herpes Simplex Virus.)
- Herpes zoster disciform keratitis:
  May occur without preceding skin eruption.
  (See Section 4.16, Herpes Zoster Virus.)
- Cytomegalovirus (CMV) keratitis:
  Stellate keratic precipitates are suggestive of concomitant CMV retinitis and CMV keratitis. Treatment for CMV keratitis is not well established.

Uveitis

- Acute retinal necrosis (ARN). (See Section 13.6, Acute Retinal Necrosis.)
- CMV infection. (See Posterior Segment Disease.)
- Syphilis. (See Section 14.2, Acquired Syphilis.)
- Toxoplasmosis. (See Posterior Segment Disease.)
- Drug-induced uveitis. Several agents used in HIV patients may cause uveitis/hypopyon, including rifabutin, cidofovir, sulfonamides, streptokinase, and various interleukins. If rifabutin is the inciting agent, reduce the dose, and add topical steroids to control the uveitis. For all others, stop the inciting agent.
- Pseudohypopyon secondary to lymphoma.
- HIV infection–associated uveitis. Consider this if inflammation is poorly responsive to steroids and no other etiology is present (e.g., drug reaction).

Posterior Segment Disease

NONINFECTIOUS RETINAL MICROVASCULOPATHY ("HIV RETINOPATHY")

Noninfectious retinopathy is the most common ocular manifestation of HIV infection and AIDS. Additionally, it may be the presenting sign of AIDS.

Symptoms

Usually asymptomatic.

Signs

Cotton-wool spots, intraretinal hemorrhages, microaneurysms (resembles diabetic retinopathy, not specific for AIDS). An ischemic maculopathy may occur, causing significant visual loss in 3% of patients.

Workup

HIV retinopathy is a marker of low CD4+ counts; thus the presence of retinal microvasculopathy should prompt a complete slit-lamp and dilated fundus examination looking for concomitant opportunistic infections (e.g., CMV retinitis).

CYTOMEGALOVIRUS (CMV) RETINITIS

The most common ocular opportunistic infection in patients with AIDS (34% prevalence) and the leading cause of AIDS-related blindness. CMV is generally seen in patients with CD4+ counts ≤50 cells/mm^3. Because active retinitis may be asymptomatic, dilated fundus examination should be performed at least every 3 months in patients with CD4+ counts ≤50 cells/mm^3 to rule out opportunistic disease.

Symptoms

The presence of floaters is the most common symptom. Patients may also notice a scotoma or decreased vision in one or both eyes. Pain or photophobia is generally not found.

Critical Signs

Two clinical forms are observed:

Indolent form   Peripheral granular opacities with occasional hemorrhage.
Fulminant form   Confluent areas of necrosis with associated hemorrhage, starting along the major retinal vascular arcades. Progressive retinal atrophy may also indicate active CMV.

Other Signs

The eye is typically quiet and white with little to no aqueous or vitreous cells. Retinal pigment epithelial (RPE) atrophy and pigment clumping result once the active process resolves. Rhegmatogenous retinal detachment (RRD) occurs in about one third of patients with CMV retinitis. (There is an increased risk of RRD when more than 25% of the retina is affected by retinitis.)

Workup

1. History and complete ocular examination, including dilated fundus examination.

2. Serial fundus photographs are useful to document progression and should be taken at each visit.
3. Refer the patient to an internist for a systemic CMV evaluation and treatment.

Treatment

1. Intravenous ganciclovir, cidofovir, and foscarnet are used individually or in combination. The goal of treatment is quiescent retinitis: nonprogressive areas of RPE atrophy with a stable opacified border.
   See Table 14-2 for treatment details.
2. Under the direction of an internist, protease inhibitors are often helpful. Regression of CMV has been documented without anti-CMV therapy in patients taking protease inhibitors.
3. CMV-associated retinal detachments are managed as follows:
   A RRD that spares the macula may be treated with laser demarcation. Pars plana vitrectomy with silicone oil is indicated for detachments involving the macula.
4. When ganciclovir implants are used, an RRD also may occur as a complication of implantation.
5. The role of oral ganciclovir prophylaxis against CMV is controversial.

Follow-up

- Ganciclovir resistance (reflected by positive blood or urine CMV cultures) may occur at any point during treatment.
- Almost all patients will relapse eventually. Because relapse may be difficult to recognize clinically, serial fundus photographs are highly recommended. Relapse is defined as recurrent or new retinitis, movement of opacified border, or expansion of the atrophic zone.
- Relapse does not necessarily indicate drug resistance. Reinduction with the same medication is the first line of treatment. Subtherapeutic intraocular drug levels may occur in patients on maintenance and allow for relapse.
- Clinical resistance is defined as persistent or progressive retinitis in spite of induction-level medication for 6 weeks (usually, induction lasts 2 weeks).
- Laboratory confirmation is possible for ganciclovir resistance (screen for UL97 mutation).
- If resistance is recognized, a change in therapy is indicated.
- Cross-resistance may be a problem. Because ganciclovir, foscarnet, and cidofovir are all DNA polymerase inhibitors, viral polymerase mutations may lead to resistance to several drugs within this class. Cross-resistance between ganciclovir and cidofovir is especially common. Ganciclovir–foscarnet cross-resistance is uncommon.

TABLE 14-2. *CMV Retinitis*

Drug	Dosing Information	Toxicities	Contraindications
Ganciclovir (e.g., Cytovene)	i.v. induction: 5 mg/kg i.v. b.i.d. × 2–3 weeks i.v. maintenance: 5 mg/kg i.v. qd, OR 6 mg/kg i.v. 5 days/week	Neutropenia,[a] thrombocytopenia, anemia, renal toxicity	ANC <500/mm^3 platelets <25,000/mm^3; potentially embryotoxic. Discontinue nursing
Ganciclovir implant	4.5 mg sustained-release device implanted in the anterior vitreous. Lasts 6–10 months	Well tolerated[b]	Surgical complications occur (e.g., retinal detachment, vitreous hemorrhage)
Foscarnet (e.g., Foscavir)	i.v. induction: 90 mg/kg i.v. bid × 2 weeks i.v. maintenance: 120 mg/kg i.v. qd[c] Monitor creatinine/ electrolytes and adjust dosing as needed	Renal impairment; neutropenia; anemia; electrolyte imbalances	Use caution with renal impairment or electrolyte imbalances
Cidofovir, HPMPC (e.g., Vistide)	i.v. induction: 5 mg/kg i.v. weekly × 3 weeks i.v. maintenance: 3–5 mg/kg biweekly Intravitreal: 20 µg q 5–6 weeks	Dose- and schedule-dependent nephrotoxicity, hypotony (necessitates discontinuation), iritis (steroid responsive)	Intravitreal injection in the fellow eye is contraindicated if permanent hypotony develops in the first (treated) eye

CMV, cytomegalovirus; ANC, absolute neutrophil count.
[a]Concomitant use of granulocyte colony-stimulating factor (g-CSF, also known as Neupogen) can reduce the incidence of neutropenia.
[b]Compared with i.v. ganciclovir, with implant therapy, there is an increased risk of systemic disease (30%) and fellow eye involvement (50%) after 6 months. However, the relapse-free interval is greatly increased.
[c]During induction phase, each dose is delivered in 500 ml of normal saline. During maintenance: 1,000 ml of saline should be used.

- Discontinuation of anti-CMV maintenance therapy may be considered in selected patients taking protease inhibitors with other antiretroviral agents who have CD4+ counts >100 cells/mm^3 and completely quiescent CMV retinitis. In these patients whose immune system can control CMV, stopping maintenance therapy may prevent drug toxicity and forestall development of drug-resistant organisms.

Toxoplasmosis (*Toxoplasma gondii*)

Symptoms

Decreased vision, floaters, photophobia, pain, red eye.

Signs

Retinochoroidal lesions clinically indistinguishable from CMV. Unlike CMV, significant vitreous response is typically present, and patients typically have higher CD4+ counts. Adjacent retinochoroidal scars are usually not observed. The lesions may be single or multifocal, discrete or diffuse, and unilateral or bilateral.

Workup

1. Complete ocular examination with special emphasis on the neuro-ophthalmic aspects.
2. Referral to an internist for a complete medical evaluation, which must include central nervous system (CNS) imaging because of a high association with CNS disease.
3. Toxoplasmosis antibody titers may be unreliable in HIV patients.
4. Because many infectious organisms (e.g., CMV, *Toxoplasma*, HSV, HZV, syphilis, cryptococcus) and lymphoma can cause a similar-appearing necrotizing retinitis, diagnostic vitrectomy may be necessary.

Treatment

1. Sulfadiazine and pyrimethamine together are the preferred treatment. Long-term maintenance therapy may be necessary to prevent recurrence.
2. Folinic acid, 5 to 10 mg, p.o., qd minimizes pyrimethamine toxicity.
3. For patients who cannot take sulfonamides, clindamycin is substituted (not recommended for maintenance therapy).
4. Topical steroid (e.g., prednisolone acetate, 1%, q 1 to 6 hours). The dosage depends on the degree of anterior-segment inflammation.
5. Topical cycloplegic (e.g., scopolamine, 0.25%, t.i.d.) in the presence of anterior-segment inflammation.
6. Systemic steroids are contraindicated for ocular toxoplasmosis in AIDS. See Table 14-3 for treatment details.

Pneumocystis carinii Choroidopathy

A rare ocular manifestation of AIDS in patients with widely disseminated *P. carinii* infection.

Symptoms

Mild decrease in visual acuity; may be asymptomatic.

TABLE 14-3. *Toxoplasmosis (Toxoplasma Gondii)*

Drug	Dosing Information	Toxicities	Contraindications
Sulfadiazine	Loading dose: 2 g p.o. × 1 Maintenance dose: 1 g p.o. q.i.d. for 3–6 weeks[a]	Hypersensitivity, crystalluria, hematuria, renal stones, anemia	Pregnancy, nursing mothers
Pyrimethamine	Loading dose: 100–200 mg p.o. × 1 Maintenance dose: 25 mg p.o. b.i.d. for 3–6 weeks.[a] Check CBC weekly. Reduce dose if platelet count <100,000/mm^3	Hypersensitivity, megaloblastic anemia, leukopenia, thrombocytopenia	Use with caution in pregnant and nursing women. Megaloblastic anemia due to folate deficiency
Clindamycin	300–600 mg p.o. q.i.d. for 3–6 weeks[a]	Pseudomembranous colitis, renal and hepatic toxicity	Use with caution in patients with GI, renal, or hepatic disease

CBC, complete blood count; GI, gastrointestinal.
[a]May need chronic maintenance therapy.

Signs

Multifocal, yellow, round, deep choroidal lesions about one-half to two disc diameters in size, located in the posterior pole. Typically, no retinal vascular changes or vitritis. Patients are often very ill.

Workup

1. Elicit history of *P. carinii* pneumonia and associated treatment (e.g., aerosolized pentamidine).
2. Complete dilated ocular examination.
3. Refer the patient to an internist for medical evaluation and management consultation.

Treatment

In conjunction with an internist or infectious disease specialist, the following treatments may be used.

1. Intravenous trimethoprim/sulfamethoxazole (TMP/SMX), or
2. Intravenous pentamidine.
   See Table 14-4 for treatment details.

TABLE 14-4. *Pneumocystis Carinii Choroiditis*

Drug	Dosing Information	Toxicities	Contraindications
Trimethoprim (TMP)/ sulfamethoxazole (SMX)	i.v.: 5 mg/kg TMP and 25 mg/kg SMX i.v. q8 h for 3 weeks	Megaloblastic anemia, leukopenia, thrombocytopenia, Stevens–Johnson syndrome. Discontinue if any skin rashes or toxicities occur— fatalities have been reported	History of hypersensitivity to related drugs. Megaloblastic anemia due to folate deficiency. Use with caution in pregnant and nursing women
Pentamidine	4 mg/kg i.v. qd infused over 2 h	Leukopenia, hypoglycemia, thrombocytopenia, hypotension, renal failure, hypocalcemia, Stevens–Johnson syndrome	No absolute contraindications

SYPHILIS

Strictly speaking, syphilis is not an opportunistic infection (because it may be found in patients with CD4+ counts >200 cells/mm^3). Nonetheless, there is an increased incidence of neurosyphilis in the AIDS population. Therefore, lumbar puncture (LP) is mandatory in all HIV+ patients with syphilis. In patients with AIDS, the rapid plasma reagin (RPR) may be negative despite active syphilis, but the specific treponemal antibody test (e.g., FTA-ABS, MHA-TP) is usually positive. (See Acquired Syphilis, Section 14.2.)

❖ **Note** *Ocular syphilis can mimic CMV retinitis in clinical appearance.*

Neuro-Ophthalmologic Disease

Two percent to 12% of AIDS patients may develop neuro-ophthalmologic abnormalities (e.g., cranial nerve palsies, pupillary abnormalities, brainstem ocular motility defects, ischemic or infectious optic neuropathy, visual-field defects, visual hallucinations) resulting from CNS infection (e.g., toxoplasmosis), lymphoma, or primary HIV disease. Steroids are absolutely contraindicated in AIDS patients with retrobulbar optic neuritis or other optic neuropathies until infection is ruled out. Syphilis, cryptococcus, and HZV are the primary causes of infectious retrobulbar optic neuritis. (See the appropriate sections of Chapter 11.)

14.2 ACQUIRED SYPHILIS

Systemic Signs

STAGES

Primary Chancre (ulcerated, painless lesion), regional lymphadenopathy.
Secondary Skin or mucous membrane lesions, generalized lymphadenopathy, constitutional symptoms (e.g., sore throat, fever), other less common but more severe abnormalities including symptomatic or asymptomatic meningitis.
Latent No clinical manifestations.
Tertiary Cardiovascular disease (e.g., aortitis), central nervous system disease (e.g., meningovascular disease, general paresis, tabes dorsalis).

Ocular Signs
Primary A chancre may occur on the eyelid or conjunctiva.
Secondary Uveitis, optic neuritis, active chorioretinitis, retinitis, retinal vasculitis, conjunctivitis, dacryoadenitis, dacryocystitis, episcleritis, scleritis, monocular interstitial keratitis, others.
Tertiary Optic atrophy, old chorioretinitis, interstitial keratitis, chronic iritis, Argyll Robertson pupil (will not react to light, but will accommodate; see Section 11.3, Argyll Robertson Pupil), and other signs seen in secondary disease.

❖ **Note** *Patchy hyperemia of the iris with the development of fleshy, pink nodules near the iris sphincter is pathognomonic of syphilis.*

Differential Diagnosis
See Anterior Uveitis, Section 13.1, and Posterior Uveitis, Section 13.2.

Workup
See Sections 13.1 Anterior Uveitis, and 13.2, Posterior Uveitis, for a nonspecific uveitis workup.

1. Complete ophthalmic examination, including pupillary evaluation, slit-lamp examination, and dilated fundus examination.
2. Venereal Disease Research Laboratories test (VDRL) or rapid plasma reagin (RPR) reflects the activity of the disease and is important in

monitoring the patient's response to treatment. Used for screening, but many false-negatives can occur in early primary, latent, or late syphilis. Not as specific as fluorescent treponemal antibody, absorbed (FTA-ABS) or MHA-TP.

3. FTA-ABS or MHA-TP are very sensitive and specific in all stages of syphilis. Once reactive, these tests do not revert to normal and therefore cannot be used to assess the patient's response to treatment.

4. HIV serology: Should be offered to patients with sexually transmitted diseases.

5. Lumbar puncture (LP). The indications are controversial. We consider LP in the following situations:

a. Positive FTA-ABS and neurologic or neuro-ophthalmologic signs, papillitis, active chorioretinitis, or anterior or posterior uveitis.

b. Patients who are HIV-positive as well as FTA-ABS positive.

c. Those for whom treatment has failed.

d. Patients to be treated with a nonpenicillin regimen (as a baseline).

e. Patients with untreated syphilis of unknown duration or longer than 1 year duration.

Treatment Indications

1. FTA-ABS negative: No treatment indicated. Patient probably does not have syphilis. Consider retesting if clinical circumstances are compelling.

2. FTA-ABS positive and VDRL-negative
   - If appropriate past treatment cannot be documented, treatment is indicated.
   - If appropriate past treatment can be documented, treatment is not indicated.

3. FTA-ABS positive and VDRL-positive: A VDRL titer of 1:8 or greater (e.g., 1:64) is expected to decline at least fourfold within 1 year of appropriate treatment, and should revert to negative (or at least to 1:4 or less) within 1 year in primary syphilis, 2 years in secondary syphilis, and 5 years in tertiary syphilis. A VDRL of <1:8 (e.g., 1:4) often does not decrease fourfold. Therefore, the following recommendations are made:
   - If appropriate past treatment cannot be documented, treatment is indicated.
   - If appropriate past treatment can be documented, and
     a. if a previous VDRL titer greater than or equal to 4 times the current titer can be documented, no treatment is indicated (unless 5 years have passed and the titer is still >1:4).
     b. if a previous VDRL titer was ≥1:8 and did not decrease fourfold, treatment is indicated.
     c. if the previous VDRL titer was <1:8, treatment is not indicated, unless the current titer has increased fourfold.

d. if a previous VDRL is unavailable, treatment is not required unless treatment was more than five years earlier and the VDRL is still >1:4.

❖ **Notes**
- *If active syphilitic signs (e.g., active chorioretinitis, papillitis) are present despite appropriate past treatment (regardless of the VDRL titer), LP and treatment may be needed.*
- *Patients with concurrent HIV and active syphilis may have negative serologies (FTA-ABS, RPR) because of their immunocompromised state. These patients manifest aggressive, recalcitrant syphilis. They should be treated with neurosyphilis dosages, usually over longer treatment periods. Consultation with an infectious-disease specialist is recommended.*

Treatment
1. Neurosyphilis [positive FTA-ABS in the serum and either cell count >5 WBC/mm^3, protein >45 mg/dl, or positive cerebrospinal fluid (CSF)-VDRL on LP]: i.v. aqueous crystalline penicillin (PCN) G, 2 to 4 million U, q4h, for 10 to 14 days, followed by benzathine PCN, 2.4 million U i.m., weekly, for 3 weeks (1.2 million U in each buttock).
2. Syphilis with abnormal ocular but normal CSF findings: Benzathine PCN, 2.4 million U, i.m. weekly for 3 weeks.
3. If anterior-segment inflammation is present, treatment with a cycloplegic (e.g., cyclopentolate, 2%, t.i.d.) and topical steroid (e.g., prednisolone acetate, 1%, q.i.d.) may be beneficial.

❖ **Notes**
- *Treatment for possible chlamydia infection with tetracycline, 250 mg, p.o., q.i.d., doxycycline, 100 mg, p.o., b.i.d., or erythromycin, 250 mg, p.o., q.i.d. for 3-6 weeks, is typically indicated.*
- *Therapy for PCN-allergic patients is not well established. Tetracycline, 500 mg, p.o., q.i.d., for 30 days, is used by some for both late syphilis and neurosyphilis, but better CSF penetration may be obtained with doxycycline (200 mg, p.o., b.i.d., for 30 days) or a third-generation cephalosporin.*

Follow-up
1. Neurosyphilis: Repeat LP every 6 months for 2 years, less if the cell count returns to normal sooner. The cell count should decrease to a normal level within this period, and the CSF VDRL titer should decrease fourfold (these changes typically occur within 6 to 12 months). An increased cerebrospinal fluid (CSF) protein decreases more slowly. If these indices do not decrease as expected, retreatment may be indicated.

2. Other forms of syphilis: Repeat the VDRL titer at 3 and 6 months after treatment. If a VDRL titer of 1:8 or more does not decline fourfold within 6 months, or if the VDRL titer increases fourfold at any point, or if clinical symptoms or signs of syphilis persist or recur, LP and retreatment are indicated. If a pretreatment VDRL titer is less than 1:8, retreatment is indicated only when the titer increases during follow-up or when symptoms or signs of syphilis recur.

See Congenital Syphilis, Section 14.3, for additional information.

14.3 CONGENITAL SYPHILIS

Presenting Ocular Signs

Any of the following may be present.

Interstitial keratitis (IK)   Usually presents acutely in the first or second decade of life with cellular infiltration and superficial and deep vascularization of the cornea (corneal "salmon patch"). Both eyes eventually become affected. As the inflammation resolves, the cornea may thin, opacify, or exhibit blood vessels containing no blood within their lumens (ghost vessels).

Anterior uveitis   Cells and flare in the anterior chamber.

Chorioretinitis   Typically appears as a salt-and-pepper fundus (pigmented areas interspersed among atrophic white areas).

Optic atrophy   A pale optic nerve.

Systemic Signs

Widely spaced, peg-shaped teeth (Hutchinson's teeth), frontal bossing, depressed nasal bridge (saddle nose), nerve deafness, recurrent arthropathy, linear scars at the angles of the mouth, mental retardation, others.

Differential Diagnosis

• Other congenital infections [toxoplasmosis, rubella, cytomegalovirus, herpes simplex or zoster virus, rubeola (measles)] [Specific serologic titers will usually be positive; rapid plasma reagin (RPR) and fluorescent treponemal antibody, absorbed (FTA-ABS) will usually be negative.]

Workup

1. History: Maternal syphilis? Medical problems since birth (persistent runny nose, rash, deafness, scars on the skin, others)? Previous treatment for syphilis?

2. Complete ocular examination, including a pupillary assessment, a slit-lamp examination if possible, and a dilated fundus examination (in interstitial keratitis, the fundus may not be well visualized).
3. B-scan ultrasound should be considered when no fundus view is obtained to rule out a retinal detachment and mass lesion.
4. Blood tests: RPR (or VDRL) and FTA-ABS (or MHA-TP)*; consider viral and toxoplasma titers when the diagnosis is uncertain.
5. Consider darkfield examination of scrapings from skin lesions, if available.
6. Lumbar puncture (LP) for routine studies including a VDRL is indicated in all cases of active disease or in cases of inactive disease not previously treated.

Treatment
See Acquired Syphilis, Section 14.2, for treatment indications.

1. Systemic antibiotic (one of the following):
   a. Aqueous crystalline PCN G, 50,000 U/kg/day, i.m. or i.v., in two divided doses for 10 to 14 days.
   b. Aqueous procaine PCN G, 50,000 U/kg, i.m. daily for 10 to 14 days.
   c. For PCN-allergic patients: Erythromycin, 50 mg/kg/day, p.o., in four divided doses for 2 weeks.
2. In the presence of acute IK or anterior-chamber inflammation, a topical steroid (prednisolone acetate, 1%, 4 to 8 times per day) and a cycloplegic (e.g., scopolamine, 0.25%, t.i.d.) should be used.
3. Intraocular pressure (IOP) control (e.g., if >30 mm Hg, consider levobunolol or timolol, 0.25% to 0.5%, b.i.d., or acetazolamide, 5 mg/kg, p.o., q6h, or both).

Follow-up
Patients are seen daily until their systemic therapy is completed, and then in 1 to 2 weeks. When the LP is abnormal (e.g., positive cerebrospinal fluid, VDRL, white blood cell count >5 WBC/mm^3 or protein >45 mg/dl), follow-up is as described for neurosyphilis (see Acquired Syphilis, Section 14.2). Otherwise, follow-up is as described for other forms of acquired syphilis (see Section 14.2). The FTA-ABS typically remains reactive despite treatment.

---

*Both the RPR (or VDRL) and FTA-ABS (or MHA-TP) can be positive in a syphilis-free infant born to a mother with the disease. The RPR usually converts to negative by age 3 months in a disease-free child; the FTA-ABS is usually found to be negative by age 6 months. A positive immunoglobulin M (IgM)–FTA-ABS in an infant suggests active disease.

14.4 LYME DISEASE (*BORRELIA BURGDORFERI*)

Symptoms

Decreased vision, double vision, pain, photophobia, facial weakness. Patients may also complain of headache, malaise, fatigue, fever, chills, palpitations, or muscle or joint pains. A history of a tick bite within the previous few months may be elicited.

Ocular Signs

Optic neuritis; vitritis; iritis; stromal keratitis; choroiditis; exudative retinal detachment; third, fourth, or sixth cranial nerve palsy, bilateral optic nerve swelling; conjunctivitis; episcleritis; exposure keratopathy; other rare abnormalities, including orbital inflammatory pseudotumor.

Critical Systemic Signs

One or more flat erythematous or "bull's-eye" skin lesions, which enlarge in all directions (erythema migrans); unilateral or bilateral facial nerve palsies; arthritis. The skin lesions and arthritis may be transient and migratory. These findings may not be present at the time the ocular signs develop. A high serum antibody titer against the causative agent, Borrelia burgdorferi, is often, but not always present.

Other Systemic Signs

Meningitis, peripheral radiculoneuropathy, synovitis, joint effusions, cardiac abnormalities, or a low false-positive fluorescent treponemal antibody, absorbed (FTA-ABS) titer, or a combination of these.

Differential Diagnosis

- Syphilis (High positive FTA-ABS titer may produce a low false-positive antibody titer against *B. burgdorferi*. No history of a tick bite. History of chancre, maculopapular rash on palms and soles, exposure to or risk factors for sexually transmitted disease. May have interstitial keratitis, uveitis, optic neuritis, patchy iris hyperemia, a salt-and-pepper chorioretinitis, or pigmented "bone spicules" on fundus examination. See Section 14.2, Acquired Syphilis.)
- Others (Rickettsial infections, acute rheumatic fever, juvenile rheumatoid arthritis.)

Workup

1. History: Does patient live in endemic area? Prior tick bite, skin rash, Bell's palsy, joint or muscle pains, flu-like illness? Meningeal symptoms? Prior positive Lyme titer?

2. Complete systemic (especially neurologic) and ocular examinations.
3. Two-step diagnosis with a screening assay and confirmatory Western blot for *B. burgdorferi*.
4. Serum rapid plasma reagin (RPR) and FTA-ABS.
5. Consider lumbar puncture when meningitis is suspected or neurologic signs or symptoms are present.

Treatment

EARLY LYME DISEASE

(including Lyme-related uveitis, keratitis, or seventh nerve palsy)

1. Doxycycline, 100 mg, p.o., b.i.d., for 10 to 21 days.
2. In children, pregnant women, and those who cannot take doxycycline, substitute amoxicillin, 500 mg, p.o., t.i.d.
3. Other alternatives include cefuroxime axetil (e.g., Ceftin) 500 mg, p.o., b.i.d., clarithromycin, 500 mg, p.o., b.i.d., or azithromycin, 500 mg, p.o., qd.

PATIENTS WITH NEURO-OPHTHALMIC SIGNS OR RECURRENT OR RESISTANT INFECTION

1. Ceftriaxone, 2 g, i.v., daily for 2 to 3 weeks.
2. Alternatively, penicillin G, 20 million units, i.v., daily for 2 to 3 weeks.

Follow-up
Every 1 to 3 days until improvement is demonstrated, and then weekly until resolved.

14.5 CHICKEN POX [VARICELLA ZOSTER VIRUS (VZV)]

Symptoms
Facial rash, red eye, foreign-body sensation.

Ocular Signs
Early Acute conjunctivitis with vesicles or papules at the limbus, on the eyelid, or on the conjunctiva. Pseudodendritic corneal epithelial lesions, stromal keratitis, anterior uveitis, optic neuritis, retinitis, and ophthalmoplegia occur rarely.

Late (weeks to months after the outbreak) Immune stromal or neurotrophic keratitis may occur.

Treatment

A. Conjunctival involvement: Cool compresses and erythromycin ointment to the eye and periorbital lesions, t.i.d.

B. Corneal epithelial lesions: Same as for conjunctival involvement.

C. Stromal keratitis with uveitis: Topical steroid (e.g., prednisolone acetate, 1%, q.i.d.), cycloplegic (e.g., scopolamine, 0.25%, b.i.d.), and erythromycin ointment qhs.

D. Neurotrophic keratitis: (uncommon) See Neurotrophic Keratopathy, Section 4.5.

E. Canalicular obstruction: (uncommon) Managed by intubation of puncta.

❖ **Notes**

• *Do not give aspirin to these children because of the possible risk of Reye's syndrome.*

• *Immunocompromised children with chicken pox may require i.v. acyclovir.*

• *VZV vaccination is now available for children and is likely preventive of ophthalmic complications of chicken pox in immune competent patients if given at least 8 to 12 weeks before exposure.*

Follow-up

Follow up in 1 to 7 days, depending on the severity of ocular disease. Taper the topical steroids slowly. Watch for stromal or neurotrophic keratitis about 4 to 6 weeks after the chicken pox resolves. VZV stromal keratitis can have a chronic course requiring long-term topical steroids with a very gradual taper.

14.6 DIABETES MELLITUS

Diabetic Retinopathy

Signs

Mild nonproliferative diabetic retinopathy (NPDR)   Dot-and-blot hemorrhages, microaneurysms, and hard exudates, generally most prominent in the posterior pole. Nearly always bilateral.

Moderate NPDR   Same findings as mild NPDR, plus cotton-wool spots, venous beading and loops, and moderate capillary nonperfusion (seen on fluorescein angiography).

Severe NPDR   Same findings as moderate NPDR, plus four quadrants of intraretinal hemorrhages, or two quadrants of venous beading, or one quadrant of intraretinal microvascular abnormalities (IRMA).

Proliferative diabetic retinopathy (PDR) The findings in mild, moderate, or severe NPDR, or a combination of these, are often present *plus* neovascularization on or within one disc diameter of the optic disc (NVD), neovascularization elsewhere (retina) (NVE), or neovascularization of the iris (NVI). Fibrovascular tissue along the posterior surface of or extending into the vitreous and adherent to the retina, traction retinal detachment (TRD), or vitreous hemorrhage (VH) also may be present. Usually bilateral, but can be asymmetric. Almost always in the posterior pole.

❖ **Note** *Macular edema may be present in any of the stages listed.*

Differential Diagnosis

NONPROLIFERATIVE

- Central retinal vein occlusion (CRVO) (Optic disc swelling is present, veins are more tortuous, hard exudates are usually not found, hemorrhages are more prominent, and CRVO is generally unilateral and of more sudden onset. See Section 12.3, Central Retinal Vein Occlusion.)
- Branch retinal vein occlusion (BRVO) [The hemorrhages are distributed along the course of a vein, and do not extend across the horizontal raphé (midline). See Section 12.4, Branch Retinal Vein Occlusion.]
- Ocular ischemic syndrome (The hemorrhages are larger and mostly in the midperiphery; exudate is absent. See Section 12.7, Ocular Ischemic Syndrome.)
- Hypertensive retinopathy (The hemorrhages are more commonly flame-shaped and rarely abundant, microaneurysms occur less frequently, and the retinal arterioles are narrowed. See Section 12.5, Hypertensive Retinopathy.)
- Radiation retinopathy (Microaneurysms are rarely present. Follows radiation therapy to the eye or adnexal structures such as the brain, sinus, or nasopharynx, when the eye is irradiated inadvertently. May develop anytime after the radiation therapy, but occurs most commonly within a few years. Generally, 3,000 cGy is necessary, but it has been noted to occur with 1,500 cGy.)

PROLIFERATIVE

- Neovascular complications of BRVO, CRVO, or central retinal artery occlusion (History of one of these events. See previous discussion.)
- Sickle-cell retinopathy (Retinal neovascularization occurs peripherally, generally not in the macula. "Sea-fans" of peripheral retinal neovascularization are present. See Section 12.23, Sickle-Cell Disease.)
- Embolization from i.v. drug abuse (e.g., talc retinopathy) (History of i.v. drug abuse, peripheral retinal neovascularization, may see particles of talc in macular vessels.)

- Sarcoidosis [May have uveitis, exudates around veins ("candle-wax drippings") or systemic findings. See Section 13.4, Sarcoidosis.]
- Ocular ischemic syndrome (Generally accompanied by pain; mild anterior-chamber reaction; corneal edema; episcleral vascular congestion; a middilated, poorly reactive pupil; iris neovascularization; and pulsations of the central retinal artery induced by light digital pressure. See Section 12.7, Ocular Ischemic Syndrome.)
- Radiation retinopathy (See prior discussion.)

Workup

1. Examine the iris carefully for neovascularization, preferably before pharmacologic dilation. [Check the angle with gonioscopy, especially if intraocular pressure (IOP) is increased.]
2. Dilated fundus examination by using a 90- or 60-diopter or fundus contact lens with a slit lamp to obtain a stereoscopic view of the posterior pole. Rule out neovascularization and macular edema. Use indirect ophthalmoscopy to examine the retinal periphery.
3. Fasting blood sugar, glycosylated hemoglobin and, if necessary, a glucose tolerance test if the diagnosis is not established.
4. Check the blood pressure.
5. Consider fluorescein angiography to determine areas of perfusion abnormalities, foveal ischemia, microaneurysms, and clinically inapparent neovascularization.
6. Consider blood tests for hyperlipidemia if extensive exudate is present.

Treatment

CLINICALLY SIGNIFICANT MACULAR EDEMA (CSME)

Focal or grid laser treatment should be considered when any of the following forms of macular edema are present (Fig. 14-1):

- Retinal thickening within 500 μm (one third of disc diameter) of the center of the macula.
- Hard exudates within 500 μm of the center of the macula, if associated with thickening of the adjacent retina.
- Retinal thickening greater than one disc area in size, part of which is within one disc diameter of the center of the macula.

❖ **Note** *Patients with enlarged foveal avascular zones on fluorescein angiography are treated lightly, away from the regions of foveal ischemia, if they are treated at all. Patients with extensive, frank foveal ischemia are poor candidates for treatment. Younger patients and diet-controlled diabetics tend to have a better treatment response.*

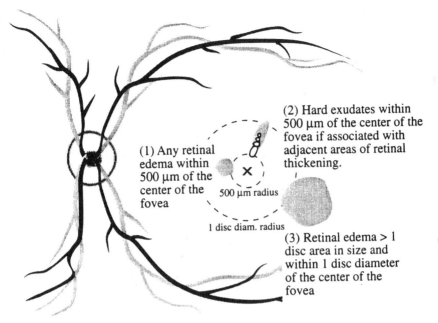

Figure 14-1
Clinically significant macular edema in diabetic retinopathy that warrants grid-pattern photocoagulation.

PROLIFERATIVE DIABETIC RETINOPATHY

Panretinal laser photocoagulation is indicated for any one of the following high-risk characteristics (Fig. 14-2):

- NVD greater than one fourth to one third of the disc area in size.
- Any degree of NVD when associated with preretinal or vitreous hemorrhage.
- NVE greater than one half of the disc area in size when associated with a preretinal or vitreous hemorrhage.
- Any NVI.

❖ **Note** *Some physicians treat NVE or any degree of NVD without preretinal or vitreous hemorrhage, especially in unreliable patients.*

❖ **Note** *If the ocular media are too hazy for an adequate fundus view, yet one of these conditions is met, peripheral retinal cryotherapy may be indicated, if there is no vitreous traction. Pars plana vitrectomy and endolaser therapy with or without lensectomy and posterior-chamber intraocular lens is another alternative.*

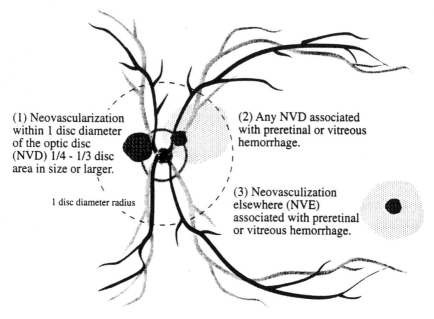

(1) Neovascularization within 1 disc diameter of the optic disc (NVD) 1/4 - 1/3 disc area in size or larger.

1 disc diameter radius

(2) Any NVD associated with preretinal or vitreous hemorrhage.

(3) Neovasculization elsewhere (NVE) associated with preretinal or vitreous hemorrhage.

Figure 14-2

High-risk characteristics for visual loss in proliferative diabetic retinopathy that warrants panretinal photocoagulation.

INDICATIONS FOR VITRECTOMY

Vitrectomy may be indicated for any one of the following conditions:

- Dense vitreous hemorrhage causing decreased vision, especially when present for several months.
- Traction retinal detachment involving and progressing within the macula.
- Macular epiretinal membranes or recent-onset displacement of the macula.
- Severe retinal neovascularization and fibrous proliferation that are unresponsive to laser photocoagulation.
- Dense premacular hemorrhage.

❖ **Note** *Juvenile type 1 diabetics are known to have more aggressive proliferative diabetic retinopathy and therefore may benefit from earlier vitrectomy and laser photocoagulation. B-scan ultrasonography may be required to rule out tractional detachment of the macula in eyes with dense vitreous hemorrhage obscuring a fundus view.*

Follow-up

Diabetes without retinopathy. Annual dilated examination.

Mild NPDR. Dilated examination every 6 months.

Moderate to Severe NPDR. Dilated examination every 2 to 4 months.
PDR (not meeting high-risk criteria). Dilated examination every 1 to 3
months.

See Section 14.8 for the follow-up of diabetic retinopathy in pregnant
women.

❖ **Note** *The Diabetes Control and Complications Trial showed that intensive
control of blood sugar with insulin (in type I diabetes) decreases the progression of diabetic retinopathy (as well as nephropathy and neuropathy).**

Neuro-Ophthalmic Problems
Cranial Nerve Abnormalities

An isolated third, fourth, or sixth cranial nerve palsy, often associated with
pain in or around the eye, may result from diabetic microvascular disease.
Only very rarely are two nerves involved simultaneously. Typically, third-
nerve involvement spares the pupil (i.e., it does not become dilated). A diabetic cranial nerve paralysis usually resolves within 3 months. No treatment
is indicated.

Acute Disc Edema (Diabetic Papillopathy)

Benign disc edema may occur in one or both eyes of a diabetic, most commonly with mild visual loss. There is no correlation with the severity of diabetic retinopathy. In addition to disc edema, disc hyperemia due to telangiectasias of the disc vessels may also occur, simulating neovascularization. This
entity is more common in juvenile-onset diabetics. No treatment is indicated.
Spontaneous resolution generally occurs after 3 to 4 months.

   Idiopathic anterior ischemic optic neuropathy also may occur in diabetics.
Usually it is associated with more dramatic visual loss than in nondiabetics
(manifested as a decrease in acuity and visual-field loss).

Glaucoma
Primary Open-Angle Glaucoma

Diabetics are probably at an increased risk for this form of glaucoma. When
treating with a topical β-blocker, additional care must be exercised in monitoring for side effects. β-Blockers may mask the warning symptoms of hypoglycemia (e.g., sweating, shaking, nightmares, restlessness).

---

*N Engl J Med 1993; 329(14):977-986.

Neovascular Glaucoma

As discussed previously, neovascularization of the iris and glaucoma are complications of diabetes, and panretinal photocoagulation is indicated as soon as possible.

Miscellaneous

Refractive Changes

Acute hyperglycemia may produce a sudden hyperopic or myopic shift, causing bilateral blurred vision. Glasses should not be prescribed until the patient's blood sugar has been stable for several months.

Cataract

Diabetics are at an increased risk of cataract, especially posterior subcapsular cataracts.

Mucormycosis

A rare, life-threatening orbital infection caused by this ubiquitous fungus can occur in diabetics, particularly those with ketoacidosis. Any diabetic or compromised host with the appearance of orbital cellulitis (eyelid edema, proptosis, external ophthalmoplegia, and fever) should be further examined for necrosis of the skin, nasal mucosa, or palate. An emergency computed tomography (CT) scan of the sinuses, orbit, and brain should be performed to aid in diagnosis. A biopsy should be obtained from any necrotic tissue as well as the nasopharynx and paranasal sinuses if this condition is suspected. Treat with liposomal amphotericin B. (See Cavernous Sinus/Superior Orbital Fissure Syndrome, Section 11.9.)

REFERENCES

The Early Treatment Diabetic Retinopathy Research Study Group. Early photocoagulation for diabetic retinopathy: ETDRS Report 9. *Ophthalmology* 1991;98(suppl):766–785.

The Diabetes Control and Complications Trial Research Group. The effect of intensive treatment of diabetes on the development and progression of long-term complications in insulin-dependent diabetes mellitus. *N Engl J Med* 1993;329:977–986.

14.7 ALBINISM

Symptoms

Decreased vision and photophobia.

Signs

Nystagmus (starting at age 2 to 3 months), iris transillumination defects, visible choroidal vasculature, absent foveal pit, absence of macula lutea pigment, absence of macular hyperpigmentation, failure of the retinal vessels to wreathe the fovea, pink reflex through an undilated pupil.

Types

I. Oculocutaneous albinism: Hair, skin, and eye affected.
   A. Tyrosinase positive: Some pigment as adults.
   B. Tyrosinase negative: No pigment, ever.
II. Ocular: Decreased ocular pigment only. Skin may be lighter than that of siblings, but appears essentially normal. Usually inherited as X-linked recessive (Nettleship–Falls). Carrier females will have partial iris transillumination and mottled areas of hypopigmentation in peripheral retina.

❖ **Note** *The only reliable ocular finding (always present) is foveal hypoplasia.*

Associated Disorders

- Hermansky–Pudlak syndrome (An autosomal recessive bleeding disorder caused by platelet dysfunction. There is a high incidence in patients of Puerto-Rican descent.)
- Chediak–Higashi syndrome (An autosomal recessive disorder affecting white blood cell function, causing a high susceptibility to infection and a predisposition for a lymphoma-like condition.)

Workup

1. History: Early bruisability? Is patient of Puerto Rican heritage? Frequent nosebleeds? Prolonged bleeding after dental work? Frequent infections?
2. Family history.
3. External examination (check hair and skin color).
4. Complete ocular examination including a slit-lamp evaluation (nystagmus, iris color, and iris transillumination) and a dilated fundus examination.
5. Obtain a bleeding time if the patient is planning to undergo surgery. Some physicians believe that a bleeding time should be obtained in all albinos. If the Hermansky–Pudlak syndrome is suspected, bleeding time, platelet-aggregation studies, and platelet electron microscopy are indicated.
6. If the Chediak–Higashi syndrome is suspected, polymorphonuclear leukocyte function should be evaluated by a hematologist.
7. If the patient's presentation is atypical, molecular analysis can establish the diagnosis for several subtypes of albinism.

Treatment

There is currently no effective treatment for albinism, but the following may be helpful:

1. Tinted eyeglasses may reduce photophobia.
2. Low-vision aids may be helpful in adults.
3. Eye muscle surgery may be considered for patients with significant strabismus or an abnormal head position due to nystagmus (Kestenbaum-type procedure).
4. Genetic counseling.
5. Dermatologic consultation.

❖ **Notes**

• *Albinos with strabismus rarely achieve binocularity after strabismus surgery, possibly because of a lack of the necessary neuronal connections.*

• *Albinos do poorly after retinal-detachment repair because of nystagmus and inherently weak retinal pigment epithelium–neurosensory retina adherence.*

• *Patients with the Hermansky–Pudlak syndrome may require platelet transfusion before surgery.*

14.8 PREGNANCY

Many ocular problems can arise as a result of pregnancy. We list some of the complaints that induce pregnant women to seek eye care and some of the disorders that should be considered in pregnancy.

Blurred or Decreased Vision

CHANGE IN REFRACTIVE ERROR

(Visual acuity decreased with current glasses, but can be improved to normal status with a new refraction or a pin hole. No other findings on examination.)

The patient's change in refraction is probably the result of a shift in fluid, hormonal status, or both, and will most likely revert to normal after delivery. Some of this change is attributable to the increased corneal thickness and secondary change in corneal refractive index during pregnancy. A transient loss of accommodation also may occur. Unless the patient has a strong desire (e.g., occupational need) to change her glasses prescription, it is best to wait until several weeks after birth before giving a new prescription.

PREECLAMPTIC/ECLAMPTIC HYPERTENSIVE RETINOPATHY

(Occurs after 20 weeks of gestation. Same clinical findings as hypertensive retinopathy of other etiologies: Focal or generalized narrowing of the arterioles, flame-shaped hemorrhages, cotton-wool spots; disc swelling may or may not be present. An exudative retinal detachment can occur. Bilateral occipital lobe infarction and cortical blindness rarely can occur.)

The severity of retinal changes correlates with the risk of fetal mortality and possibly with the risk of damage to the mother's kidneys. If severe retinopathy is present and progressing, strong consideration should be given to early delivery or terminating the pregnancy. Sometimes the clinical findings (e.g., exudative retinal detachment) resolve with blood pressure control. (See Section 12.5, Hypertensive Retinopathy.)

CENTRAL SEROUS CHORIORETINOPATHY

(Localized detachment of the sensory retina from the underlying pigment epithelium by clear serous fluid in the macular area. The margins of the detachment are sloping and merge gradually into attached retina. No blood is present.)

With rare exception, observation is the treatment of choice, with most cases resolving postpartum. A more hyperopic correction may be provided as a temporary visual aid. Focal laser therapy is rarely needed. (See Section 12.8, Central Serous Chorioretinopathy.)

RETINAL DETACHMENT

Usually exudative, resolving a few weeks after delivery. The visual prognosis is generally good, and no treatment is indicated. The pregnancy does not have to be terminated if preeclampsia/eclampsia can be ruled out. (See Section 12.19, Retinal Detachment.)

DIABETIC RETINOPATHY

Visual loss from diabetes may occur in patients who had diabetes before gestation. The following are our recommendations for management based on prepregnancy diagnosis.

A. Gestational diabetes only: Not at risk for retinopathy. No retinal treatment or follow-up is required.
B. No retinopathy or only minimal background retinopathy before pregnancy: The vast majority of patients do not experience progression, and few of those patients who do progress have any visual impairment. Baseline examination in the first trimester and a repeated examination in the third trimester. No treatment is needed.
C. Mild to moderate nonproliferative retinopathy (microaneurysms, dot-and-blot hemorrhages, hard exudates): Up to 50% of patients may

experience progression, with many regressing after birth. Examination every trimester. No treatment is needed unless high-risk proliferative changes occur.

D. High-risk nonproliferative retinopathy (cotton-wool spots, venous beading and loops, intraretinal microvascular abnormalities): Up to 50% may experience progression, with some showing regression postpartum. Examine every month. No treatment is indicated unless high-risk proliferative changes occur.

E. Proliferative retinopathy (during any stage of pregnancy; neovascularization of the disc, retina, or iris): Laser panretinal photocoagulation as per current treatment recommendations. In earlier stages, more aggressive institution of therapy is important in pregnant women because proliferative diabetes tends to progress rapidly. This is not an indication to terminate pregnancy. (See Section 14.6, Diabetes Mellitus.) Examine monthly.

❖ **Note** *Active proliferative retinopathy at the time of labor may be an indication for cesarean section, because Valsalva's maneuver at the time of delivery can cause vitreous hemorrhage.*

PURTSCHER'S RETINOPATHY

Decreased vision, usually 20/200 or worse, with extensive cotton-wool spots and nerve-fiber layer hemorrhages in the posterior pole. Preretinal hemorrhage may occur. Unknown etiology (may be related to sudden increases in venous pressure, fat or amniotic fluid embolization, or release of inflammatory mediators at the time of labor and delivery). Classically occurs in the setting of major trauma. Visible fundus changes resolve in several weeks, but some visual impairment persists in about 50% of cases. No treatment has been established.

Headache

PITUITARY ADENOMA

Pituitary adenomas may enlarge during pregnancy, producing a visual-field disturbance (classically a bitemporal hemianopsia) or headache. Because subclinical pituitary adenomas may produce amenorrhea, women who underwent treatment to induce ovulation should be examined with a high index of suspicion.

A possible cause of pituitary adenoma enlargement during pregnancy is pituitary apoplexy, a potentially life-threatening event. Therefore, any woman with a diagnosis of pituitary adenoma with a headache or a new visual-field defect should receive magnetic resonance imaging (MRI) with or without lumbar puncture to rule out subarachnoid hemorrhage from the tumor. Women with growing pituitary adenomas (especially those with evidence of subarachnoid blood on imaging) should be delivered by cesarean section to avoid the risk of apoplexy during the delivery. Postpartum hemorrhage or shock can cause an infarction of the pituitary gland leading to hypopituitarism (Sheehan's syndrome).

PSEUDOTUMOR CEREBRI

Recent reports suggest the incidence of this entity is not increased in pregnant women relative to age-matched controls. Headache, papilledema, a normal MRI scan of the head, and a high opening pressure on LP with a normal spinal fluid composition confirm the diagnosis. Treatment may be difficult, because many of the medications generally used to treat this entity are contraindicated in pregnant women. The visual outcome of pregnant women with this entity is no different than that of nonpregnant women with this disorder. (See Section 11.14, Pseudotumor Cerebri.)

PREECLAMPTIC/ECLAMPTIC HYPERTENSIVE DISEASE

As discussed previously. Refer to the obstetrician for blood pressure control.

MIGRAINE HEADACHE

Usually worse during pregnancy and immediately postpartum. (See Section 15.4, Migraine.)

MENINGIOMA OF PREGNANCY

Very aggressive growth pattern. Difficult to treat.

OTHERS

For example, cortical venous thrombosis.

❖ **Note** *All pregnant women complaining of a headache should have their blood pressure, visual fields, and fundus checked (particularly looking for papilledema). As mentioned, MRI with or without LP is often required if a hemorrhage or cortical venous thrombosis is suspected.*

Difficulty Wearing Contact Lenses

CORNEAL CHANGES

Physiological changes in the cornea may hinder contact lens wear. As corneal sensitivity is also known to decrease during pregnancy (possibly increasing the risk of infection), discontinuation of contact lenses is often advisable.

REFERENCES

Sunness JS. The pregnant woman's eye. *Surv Ophthalmol* 1988;32:219–238.

14.9 STEVENS–JOHNSON SYNDROME
(ERYTHEMA MULTIFORME MAJOR)

Symptoms

Acute onset of fever, rash, red eyes, often with generalized malaise and arthralgias.

Critical Signs

"Target" lesions on the skin (red-centered vesicles surrounded by a pale ring surrounded by a red ring), hemorrhagic crusting of the lips, bilateral conjunctivitis.

Other Signs

Skin vesicles, bullae, and maculopapular lesions concentrated on the hands and feet; ruptured bullae of the mouth; ulcerative stomatitis. Patients may appear toxic. The mortality rate is 10% to 33%. Later-onset: corneal neovascularization; scarring of the conjunctiva, cornea, or both; dry eyes; symblepharon; trichiasis; eyelid deformities; corneal ulcers; corneal perforation may develop.

Etiology

May be precipitated by many agents, including any of the following:

- Drugs (e.g., sulfonamides, barbiturates, chlorpropamide, thiazide diuretics, phenytoin, salicylates, tetracycline, codeine, penicillins, cancer chemotherapeutic agents.)
- Infectious agents (e.g., various bacteria, viruses, and fungi, especially herpes and mycoplasma)

Differential Diagnosis

- Ocular cicatricial pemphigoid (Slowly progressive scarring of the conjunctiva with symblepharon formation, forniceal shortening, and dry eye. Mucous membrane vesicles or ruptured or formed bullae are evident. Occurs in older patients. See Section 5.9, Ocular Cicatricial Pemphigoid.)

Workup

1. History: Attempt to determine the precipitating factor.
2. Slit-lamp examination: Be certain to evert the eyelids and examine the fornices.
3. Conjunctival and corneal scrapings for stains and cultures if infection is suspected (see Infectious Corneal Infiltrate/Ulcer, Section 4.12).
4. Electrolyte profile, complete blood count (CBC).

Treatment

1. Hospitalize the patient.
2. Treat the precipitating factor (e.g., remove the antibiotic, treat the infection).
3. Topical steroid drops (e.g., prednisolone acetate, 1%, 4 to 8 times per day) or ointment (e.g., dexamethasone) depending on the severity of the anterior-segment inflammation.
4. Systemic steroids (e.g., prednisone, 80 to 100 mg, p.o., daily; controversial) and a histamine H_2 blocker (e.g., ranitidine, 150 mg, p.o., b.i.d.). See Medical Glossary for a systemic steroid work-up.
5. Topical antibiotic (e.g., erythromycin or bacitracin ointment, 2 to 3 times per day).
6. Artificial tears (e.g., Refresh Plus drops, q 1 to 2 hours) prn and punctal occlusion as needed. Moisture chambers or tarsorrhaphy may be necessary.
7. Cycloplegic (e.g., atropine, 1%, t.i.d.).
8. Break symblepharon with a glass rod b.i.d. after instilling a topical anesthetic (e.g., proparacaine).
9. Supportive systemic care (e.g., hydration, local mouth and skin care, systemic antibiotics) as needed. Dermatologic or internal medicine consultation as required (treated like burn patient).

Follow-up

- Examine the patient daily in the hospital, watching for the development of an infectious ulcer or increased intraocular pressure (IOP). When the acute phase has resolved, weekly outpatient follow-ups are initiated, watching for long-term ocular complications.
- Steroid and antibiotic treatment are maintained for 48 hours after the eye is healed, and then tapered.
- Artificial tears and lubricating ointment may need to be maintained indefinitely if the conjunctiva has been severely scarred.
- If trichiasis develops, repeated epilation, cryotherapy, or surgical repair may be indicated.
- Consider a permanent keratoprosthesis in a scarred, end-stage eye with visual potential.

14.10 VITAMIN A DEFICIENCY

Symptoms

Dry eye, foreign-body sensation, ocular pain, night blindness, severe loss of vision. Gradual onset in most cases.

Critical Signs

Patients often appear malnourished or are victims of a process causing defective vitamin A absorption or utilization. Bilateral conjunctival and corneal dryness with lack of normal luster, keratinized areas (Bitot's spots: paralimbal silvery white dots in a triangular patch), and a decreased tear-film break-up time are typical.

Other Signs

Sterile corneal ulceration with a sharp delineation between normal and abnormal stroma; corneal perforation or secondary bacterial infection may occur. There may be loss of pigment in the retinal periphery.

Etiology

Primary   Dietary lack of vitamin A (usually from malnutrition or an extreme dietary habit: relatively uncommon in developed countries).

Secondary   Vitamin A deficiency in the presence of an adequate dietary intake, often from cystic fibrosis in children and young adults, chronic pancreatitis, postgastrectomy surgery, inflammatory bowel disease, intestinal bypass surgery for obesity, chronic liver disease, abetalipopro-teinemia (Bassen–Kornzweig syndrome), others.

Differential Diagnosis

*   Keratoconjunctivitis sicca (See Dry-Eye Syndrome, Section 4.2.)

Workup

1. History: Malnutrition? Poor or extreme diet? Gastrointestinal or liver disease? Previous surgery?
2. Complete ophthalmic examination: Be certain to test eyelid closure, inspect the eyelid margins, and pull down the lower eyelids to examine the inferior fornices.
3. Serum vitamin A level before treatment is initiated (typically <20 to 80 μg/dl).
4. Consider impression cytology of the conjunctiva if available, looking for decreased conjunctival goblet cell density.
5. Dark-adaptation electroretinogram (may be more sensitive than the serum vitamin A level, which may not decrease until the body's reserves are depleted).

6. If a corneal ulcer exists and appears infected, scrapings for stains and cultures are obtained (see Infectious Corneal Infiltrate/Ulcer, Section 4.12).

Treatment
1. Vitamin A replacement therapy: Vitamin A palmitate in oil 200,000 IU (60,000 μg) p.o., daily for 2 days (an additional dose is usually given 1 to 4 weeks later to "top up" liver reserves).
   - One-half dose for children younger than 1 year and for pregnant women.
   - If unable to use the oral route (e.g., due to gastric disease) the equivalent dose is given intramuscularly in the water-dispersible form.
2. Intensive ocular lubrication with artificial tears (e.g., Refresh Plus drops) q 15 to 60 minutes and artificial tear ointment (e.g., Refresh PM) qhs.
3. Topical vitamin A ointment 2 to 4 times per day may be of some benefit.
4. Treatment of malnutrition if present.
5. Consider supplementing the patient's diet with zinc.
6. Consider a penetrating keratoplasty or keratoprosthesis for corneal scars in eyes with potentially good vision.

Follow-up
Determined by the clinical presentation and response to treatment. Some patients need to be admitted to the hospital, but others can be followed up every few days to weeks.

14.11 NEUROFIBROMATOSIS
(VON RECKLINGHAUSEN'S SYNDROME)

Criteria for Diagnosis
Type I   Two or more of the following:
   - Six or more café-au-lait macules whose greatest diameter is >5 mm in prepubertal patients and >15 mm in postpubertal patients.
   - Two or more neurofibromas of any type or one plexiform neurofibroma.
   - Intertriginous freckling.
   - Optic nerve glioma.
   - Two or more Lisch's nodules (iris hamartomas).
   - Distinctive osseous lesion (e.g., sphenoid dysplasia or thinning of long-bone cortex).
   - Parent, sibling, or child of the patient has the diagnosis.

Type II   One of the following:
- Bilateral acoustic nerve masses (diagnosed by CT or MRI).
- Parent, sibling, or child of the patient has type II neurofibromatosis and either unilateral acoustic nerve mass or any two of the following: neurofibroma, meningioma, glioma, schwannoma, or juvenile posterior subcapsular cataract.

Other Ocular Signs

Neurofibroma or plexiform neuroma of the eyelid and conjunctiva, glaucoma, pulsating proptosis (absence of the greater wing of the sphenoid bone with a herniated encephalocele), prominent corneal nerves, astrocytoma of the retina, myelinated nerve fibers, diffuse uveal thickening, choroidal nevus or melanoma or both, optic nerve meningioma, orbital neurofibroma, orbital schwannoma.

Other Systemic Signs

Intracranial astrocytoma (glioma), pituitary adenoma or other tumor, cranial or spinal nerve schwannoma (with potential for malignant degeneration), mental deficiency, pheochromocytoma, gastrointestinal malignancy, genitourinary malignancy (including Wilms' tumor).

❖ **Note** *The presence of Lisch's nodules is a highly sensitive and specific sign for type I neurofibromatosis. Moreover, Lisch's nodules often precede the development of cutaneous neurofibromas. (These iris nodules are highly unusual in type II neurofibromatosis.)*

Inheritance

Autosomal dominant with incomplete penetrance (type I, chromosome 17; type II, chromosome 22).

Workup

1. Family history: Examination of family members is important.
2. Complete general and ophthalmic examinations.
3. CBC, electrolytes.
4. CT scan (axial and coronal views) or MRI of the orbit and brain.
5. IQ and psychological testing.
6. Electroencephalogram.
7. Audiography.
8. Urine tests for levels of epinephrine and norepinephrine.

Treatment

1. Depends on findings.
2. Genetic counseling.
3. Psychological support and counseling.

Follow-up

Every 6 to 12 months in the absence of a disorder requiring therapy. Neonates with an eyelid plexiform neurofibroma should be seen more frequently, because about 50% develop early glaucoma.

14.12 TUBEROUS SCLEROSIS
(BOURNEVILLE'S SYNDROME)

Ocular Signs

Astrocytic harmartoma of the retina or optic disc (a white, semitransparent or mulberry-appearing tumor in the superficial retina that may undergo calcification with age; no prominent feeder vessels, no associated retinal detachment.)

Critical Systemic Signs

Adenoma sebaceum (yellow–red papules in a butterfly distribution on the upper cheeks, apparent in the prepubertal years), astrocytic hamartomas of the brain with seizures or subnormal intelligence or mental retardation or a combination of these.

Other Systemic Signs

Subungual angiofibromas (yellow–red papules around and beneath the nails of the fingers or toes); shagreen patches; ash-leaf sign (depigmented macules on the skin); café-au-lait spots; renal angiomyolipoma; cardiac rhabdomyoma; pleural cysts causing spontaneous pneumothorax; cystic bone lesions; hamartomas of the liver, thyroid, pancreas, or testes.

Inheritance

Autosomal dominant with incomplete penetrance.

Differential Diagnosis

- Retinoblastoma (Flat or elevated white retinal tumor that has prominent feeder vessels; may be bilateral or multifocal or both. Vitreous seeding, retinal detachment, pseudohypopyon, iris neovascularization, or vitreous hemorrhage may be present. No systemic signs, initially.)

Workup

1. Family history: Examination of the family members is important.
2. Complete general physical and ophthalmic examinations.
3. CBC, electrolytes.

4. CT scan (axial and coronal views) or MRI of the brain.
5. Electroencephalogram.
6. Echocardiogram.
7. Chest x-ray.
8. Abdominal CT scan.

Treatment

1. Retinal astrocytomas generally require no treatment.
2. Genetic counseling.

Follow-up

Yearly in the absence of a disorder requiring therapy.

14.13 STURGE–WEBER SYNDROME
(ENCEPHALOFACIAL CAVERNOUS HEMANGIOMATOSIS)

Ocular Signs

Diffuse choroidal hemangioma ("tomato catsup" fundus: the lesion obscures all detail of the choroidal vasculature and produces a uniform red fundus background; best appreciated when compared with the other eye), unilateral glaucoma (facial hemangioma of the upper eyelid increases the risk of glaucoma), iris heterochromia, blood in Schlemm's canal (seen on gonioscopy), secondary serous retinal detachment, secondary retinal pigment epithelial alterations (retinitis pigmentosa-like picture).

Critical Systemic Sign

Port-wine stain or nevus flammeus (congenital facial hemangioma along the first and second divisions of the trigeminal nerve).

Other Signs

Subnormal intelligence or mental retardation, Jacksonian-type seizures, peripheral arteriovenous communications, facial hemihypertrophy ipsilateral to nevus flammeus, leptomeningeal angiomatosis, cerebral calcifications.

Inheritance

Sporadic.

Workup

1. Complete general and ophthalmic examinations.
2. CT scan (axial and coronal views) or MRI of the brain.
3. Electroencephalogram.

Treatment

1. Treat glaucoma if present: First-line drugs are aqueous suppressants (e.g., timolol or levobunolol and/or brimonidine and/or dorzolamide); latanoprost, pilocarpine, and epinephrine compounds are less effective because of high episcleral venous pressure. Surgery (goniotomy or trabeculectomy or both) is often required at an early stage to control the intraocular pressure (IOP), with moderate to high success. (See Primary Open-Angle Glaucoma, Section 10.1.)
2. Consider treating serous retinal detachments that threaten or involve the macula. Laser photocoagulation has been used, but the success rate is low. Low-dose external beam radiotherapy or plaque radiotherapy will often resolve the subretinal fluid.
3. Anticonvulsants for epilepsy, in concert with neurologist or pediatrician.
4. Tunable dye laser for cutaneous nevus flammeus, in concert with dermatologist.

Follow-up

Every 6 months; watch carefully for glaucoma or a serous retinal detachment.

- If glaucoma is present, closer follow-up may be required.
- If skin involvement is only in the mandibular area, the risk of glaucoma is much lower, and the interval for follow-up may be extended to 1 year.

14.14 VON HIPPEL–LINDAU SYNDROME
(RETINOCEREBELLAR CAPILLARY HEMANGIOMATOSIS)

Critical Ocular Signs

Retinal capillary hemangioma (small, yellow–red tumor with a tortuous dilated feeder artery and a draining vein), sometimes associated with subretinal exudates, a retinal detachment, or both.

Other Signs

Cerebellar hemangioblastoma, hypernephroma (renal cell carcinoma), pheochromocytoma, renal cysts, pancreatic cysts, epididymal cysts, syringomyelia.

Inheritance

Autosomal dominant with incomplete penetrance (chromosome 3p).

Differential Diagnosis

- Racemose hemangiomatosis (No definable tumor present; large, dilated, tortuous vessels form arteriovenous communications.)

- Coats' disease (Characteristic aneurysmal dilatation of blood vessels is found with prominent subretinal exudate. No identifiable tumor is present.)
- Retinoblastoma (Multiple white rather than pink retinal tumors. Subretinal exudate is rare.)

Workup

Indicated when multiple or bilateral retinal capillary hemangiomas are discovered, or when a unilateral retinal capillary hemangioma is found along with characteristic systemic findings or a positive family history.

❖ **Note** *Some physicians work up all patients with retinal capillary hemangiomas.*

1. Family history and examination of family members.
2. Complete general physical and ophthalmic examinations.
3. CBC, electrolytes.
4. MRI of the brain (visualizes the posterior fossa better than CT scan).
5. Urine tests for levels of epinephrine and norepinephrine.
6. Abdominal CT scan.
7. Fluorescein angiogram if treatment of the retinal capillary hemangioma is planned.

Treatment

1. Photocoagulation or cryotherapy of a retinal hemangioma is often indicated if it is affecting or threatening vision.
2. Genetic counseling.
3. Systemic therapy, depending on findings.

Follow-up

Every 3 to 6 months, depending on the retinal condition.

14.15 WYBURN–MASON SYNDROME
(RACEMOSE HEMANGIOMATOSIS)

Ocular Signs

Enormously dilated, tortuous retinal vessels with arteriovenous communications. No distinct mass or subretinal exudate is present. Rarely proptosis from a racemose hemangioma of the orbit is present.

Systemic Signs

Midbrain racemose hemangiomas, seizures, hemiparesis, mental changes, and ipsilateral pterygoid fossa, mandible, and maxillary hemangiomas. Intracranial hemorrhage from a midbrain hemangioma can occur.

Inheritance

Sporadic.

Differential Diagnosis

- Retinal capillary hemangioma (A distinct mass is present, sometimes with subretinal exudate.)
- Coats' disease (The vessels are irregularly dilated, and exudative retinal detachment is found.)

Workup

1. Complete general and ophthalmic examinations.
2. MRI of the brain.
3. Electroencephalogram.

Treatment

1. No treatment is required for the retinal lesions. The condition is congenital and does not progress.
2. Warn the patient of the risk of massive hemorrhage with ipsilateral dental and facial surgery.

Follow-up

Yearly

14.16 ATAXIA TELANGIECTASIA
(LOUIS–BAR SYNDROME)

Ocular Signs

Dilated conjunctival vessels, strabismus, impaired convergence, nystagmus, oculomotor apraxia.

Critical Systemic Signs

Cerebellar ataxia that becomes apparent after the child learns to walk; cutaneous telangiectasias in a butterfly distribution on the face, on the antecubital and popliteal fossa, behind the ears, or at the base of the neck during the first decade of life. Recurrent sinopulmonary infections as a result of IgA deficiency and impaired T-cell function can occur.

Other Systemic Signs

Leukemia or lymphoma (often leading to death in childhood or early adulthood), mental retardation, seborrheic dermatitis, pigmentary changes of the skin, testicular or ovarian atrophy, hypoplastic or atrophic thymus.

Inheritance

Autosomal recessive.

Workup

1. Family history (examination of the family members often aids in the diagnosis).
2. Complete general and ophthalmic examinations.
3. CBC.
4. Chest radiograph.
5. MRI of the brain.

Treatment

1. Systemic treatment, depending on findings.
2. Genetic counseling.

Follow-up

Patients need close medical follow-up. Routine eye examinations should be performed every 1 to 2 years.

GENERAL OPHTHALMIC PROBLEMS

15.1 ACQUIRED CATARACT

Symptoms

Slowly progressive visual loss or blurring, usually over months to years, affecting one or both eyes. Glare, particularly from oncoming headlights while driving at night, and reduced color perception may occur, but not to the same degree of dyschromotopsia as can occur with optic neuropathies. The particular symptoms are based on the location and density of the lens opacity.

Critical Sign

Opacification of the normally clear crystalline lens (see the respective types).

Other Signs

The retina often appears indistinct on funduscopic examination, and the dilated red reflex may be dim on retinoscopy. A direct ophthalmoscope at distances of 3 to 5 feet also may show a decreased red reflex or the hardened nucleus or cortical spokes on retroillumination. The patient may be found to be more myopic than previously noted (so-called "second sight"). A cataract alone does not cause a relative afferent pupillary defect.

Types of Cataracts

A. Nuclear: Yellow or brown discoloration of the central part of the lens on slit-lamp examination. Typically blurs distance vision more than near vision.

B. Posterior subcapsular: Opacities appear near the posterior aspect of the lens, often forming a plaque. They are best seen in retroillumination against a red fundus reflex. Glare and difficulty reading are common complaints. May be associated with ocular inflammation, prolonged steroid use, diabetes, trauma, or radiation. Classically occurs in patients younger than 50 years.

C. Cortical: Radial or spoke-like opacities in the lens periphery that expand to involve the anterior and posterior lens. Often asymptomatic until the changes develop centrally.

❖ **Note** *A mature cataract is defined as anterior cortical changes sufficiently dense to obscure totally the view of the posterior lens and posterior segment of the eye.*

Etiology

- Age-related
- Trauma (Ocular or head contusion, electrocution, others.)
- Toxic [Steroids, anticholinesterases, antipsychotics (e.g., phenothiazines), others.]
- Intraocular inflammation (e.g., uveitis)
- Radiation
- Intraocular tumor (A ciliary body malignant melanoma may produce a sector cortical cataract.)
- Degenerative ocular disease (e.g., retinitis pigmentosa)
- Systemic disease:
  A. Diabetes (The juvenile form is characterized by white "snowflake" opacities in the anterior and posterior subcapsular locations. It often progresses rapidly. Adults develop age-related cataracts as described previously, but at an earlier age.)
  B. Hypocalcemia (Small, white, iridescent cortical changes, usually seen in the presence of tetany.)
  C. Wilson's disease [Red–brown pigment deposition in the cortex beneath the anterior capsule (a "sunflower" cataract). Seen with a corneal Kayser–Fleischer ring.]
  D. Myotonic dystrophy (Multicolored opacities cause a "Christmas-tree cataract" behind the anterior capsule.)
  E. Others (e.g., Down's syndrome, atopic dermatitis)

Workup

Determine the etiology, whether the cataract is responsible for the decreased vision, and whether surgical removal would improve vision.

1. History: Medications? Systemic diseases? Trauma? Ocular disease or poor vision in youth or young adulthood (before the cataract)?

2. Complete ocular examination, including distance and near vision, pupillary examination, and refraction. A dilated slit-lamp examination by using both direct and retroillumination techniques is usually required to view the cataract properly. Fundus examination, concentrating on the macula, is essential in ruling out other causes of decreased vision. It is helpful for preoperative planning to note the degree of pupil dilation, density of the cataract, and presence or absence of pseudoexfoliation syndrome or phacodonesis.

3. B-scan ultrasound when the fundus is obscured by a dense cataract to rule out posterior-segment pathology.

4. The potential acuity meter or laser interferometry can be used to estimate the visual potential when cataract extraction is being considered in an eye with posterior segment pathology.

❖ **Note** *Laser interferometry and the potential acuity meter (PAM) often overestimate the eye's visual potential in the presence of macular holes or macular pigment epithelial detachments. Interferometry also makes an overprediction of results in cases of amblyopia. Near vision is often the most accurate manner of evaluating macular function if the cataract is not too dense. Nonetheless, both laser inferometry and PAM are useful clinical tools.*

5. When surgery is planned, keratometry readings and an A-scan ultrasound measurement of axial length are required for determining the power of the desired intraocular lens. An evaluation of the corneal endothelium, usually done at the slit lamp but occasionally requiring an endothelial cell count, is also needed.

Treatment
1. Cataract surgery may be performed for the following reasons:
   a. To improve visual function in patients with symptomatic visual disability.
   b. As surgical therapy for ocular disease (e.g., lens-related glaucoma or uveitis).
   c. To facilitate management of ocular disease (e.g., to monitor or treat diabetic retinopathy or glaucoma).
2. Correct any refractive error if the patient declines cataract surgery.
3. A trial of mydriasis (e.g., scopolamine, 0.25%, daily) may be used successfully in some patients if the patient desires nonsurgical treatment. The benefits of this therapy are only temporary.

Follow-up
Unless there is a secondary complication from the cataract (e.g., glaucoma; quite rare), a cataract itself does not require urgent action. Patients who

decline surgical removal are reexamined yearly, and sooner if there is a symptomatic decrease in visual acuity.

If congenital, see Congenital Cataract, Section 9.7.

15.2 SUBLUXED OR DISLOCATED LENS

Subluxation   Partial disruption of the zonular fibers; the lens is decentered but remains partially in the pupillary aperture.
Dislocation   Complete disruption of the zonular fibers; the lens is displaced out of the pupillary aperture.

Symptoms
Decreased vision, double vision that persists when covering one eye (monocular diplopia).

Critical Signs
Decentered or displaced lens, iridodonesis (quivering of the iris), phacodonesis (quivering of the lens).

Other Signs
Marked astigmatism, cataract, angle-closure glaucoma as a result of pupillary block, acquired high myopia, vitreous in the anterior chamber, asymmetry of the anterior-chamber depth.

Etiology
- Trauma [Most common cause. Results in subluxation if more than 25% of the zonular fibers are ruptured. Need to rule out a predisposing condition (see other etiologies). Can be associated with syphilis.]
- Marfan's syndrome (Cardiomyopathy, aortic aneurysm, tall stature with long extremities and kyphoscoliosis. Typically, bilateral lens subluxation superiorly and temporally. Patients are at increased risk for a retinal detachment. Often autosomal dominant.)
- Homocystinuria [Frequent mental retardation, skeletal deformities, resembles Marfan's syndrome in stature, high incidence of thromboembolic events (particularly with general anesthesia). Patients with a mild clinical course may be undiagnosed before occurrence of lens subluxation. Typically, bilateral lens subluxation inferiorly and nasally. Increased risk of retinal detachment. Autosomal recessive.)
- Weill–Marchesani syndrome [Short fingers and short stature, seizures, microspherophakia (small, round lens), myopia, no mental retardation.

Often autosomal recessive. The small lens can dislocate into the anterior chamber, causing reverse pupillary block.]

- Others (Acquired syphilis, congenital ectopia lentis, aniridia, Ehlers–Danlos syndrome, Crouzon's disease, hyperlysinemia, sulfite-oxidase deficiency, high myopia, chronic inflammations, hypermature cataract, others.)

Workup

1. History: Family history of the disorders listed? Trauma? Systemic illness (e.g., syphilis, seizures)?
2. Complete ocular examination: At the slit lamp, note whether the condition is unilateral or bilateral and determine the direction of the displaced lens. Evaluation for subtle phacodonesis by having the patient look back and forth while observing the lens at the slit lamp.
3. Systemic examination: Evaluate stature, extremities, hands, and fingers; often in conjunction with an internist.
4. Rapid plasma reagin (RPR) and fluorescent treponemal antibody, absorbed (FTA-ABS), even if there is a history of trauma.
5. Sodium nitroprusside test or urine chromatography to rule out homocystinuria as needed.
6. Echocardiogram to rule out aortic aneurysms associated with Marfan's syndrome as needed.

❖ **Note** *Systemic evaluations of Marfan's and homocystinuria should be performed in conjunction with an internist.*

Treatment

I. Lens dislocated into the anterior chamber

A. Dilate the pupil, place the patient on his or her back, and replace the lens into the posterior chamber by head manipulation. It may be necessary to indent the cornea after topical anesthesia (e.g., proparacaine) with a Zeiss's gonioprism or a cotton swab to reposition the lens. After the lens is repositioned in the posterior chamber, constrict the pupil with chronic pilocarpine, 0.5% to 1%, q.i.d., and perform a peripheral laser iridotomy.

OR

B. Surgically remove the lens (usually performed if the lens is a cataract, if treatment described in A fails, if the patient develops recurrent dislocations, or if there are compliance issues with pilocarpine).

II. Lens dislocated into the vitreous

A. Lens capsule intact, patient asymptomatic, no signs of inflammation: Observe.

B. Lens capsule broken, eye inflamed: Lensectomy either through the pars plana or by using a limbal approach.

III. Subluxation
   A. Asymptomatic: Observe.
   B. High uncorrectable astigmatism or monocular diplopia: Surgical removal of the lens.
   C. Symptomatic cataract: Options include surgical removal of the lens, mydriasis (e.g., scopolamine, 0.25%, daily) and aphakic correction, pupillary constriction (e.g., pilocarpine, 4% gel, qhs) and phakic correction, or a large optical iridectomy (away from the lens).
IV. Pupillary block: Treatment is identical to that for aphakic pupillary block (see Postoperative Glaucoma, Section 10.15).

- If Marfan's syndrome is present: Refer the patient to a cardiologist for an annual echocardiogram and management of any cardiac-related abnormalities. Prophylactic systemic antibiotics are required if the patient undergoes surgery (or a dental procedure), to prevent endocarditis.
- If homocystinuria is present, refer to an internist. The usual therapy consists of:
  1. Pyridoxine, 50 to 1,000 mg, p.o., daily.
  2. Reduce dietary methionine.
  3. Avoid surgery if possible because of the risk of thromboembolic complications. If surgical intervention is necessary, anticoagulant therapy is indicated.

Follow-up
Depends on the etiology, degree of subluxation or dislocation, and symptoms.

15.3 HEADACHE

Most headaches are not dangerous or ominous symptoms; however, they can be symptoms of a life- or vision-threatening problem. We list accompanying signs and symptoms that may indicate a life- or vision-threatening headache and some of the specific signs and symptoms of various headaches.

Warning Symptoms and Signs of a Serious Disorder
- Scalp tenderness, weight loss, pain with chewing, muscle pains, or malaise in patients at least 55 years of age [giant cell arteritis (GCA)].
- Optic nerve swelling
- Fever

- Altered mentation or behavior
- Stiff neck
- Decreased vision
- Neurologic signs
- Subhyaloid (preretinal) hemorrhages on fundus examination

Less Alarming But Suggestive Symptoms and Signs
- Onset in a previously headache-free individual
- A different, more severe headache than the usual headache
- A headache that is always in the same location
- A headache that awakens the person from sleep
- A headache that does not respond to pain medications that previously relieved it
- Nausea and vomiting, particularly projectile vomiting
- A headache followed by migraine visual symptoms (abnormal time course of events)

Etiology

LIFE- OR VISION-THREATENING

- Giant cell arteritis (GCA) [Age older than 55 years, weight loss, fever, malaise, anorexia, muscle aches, scalp tenderness, pain on chewing, palpable tender nodule or cord-like pulseless area along the temporal artery, or decreased vision. May have high erythrocyte sedimentation rate (ESR). See Section 11.16, Giant Cell Arteritis.]
- Acute angle-closure glaucoma [Decreased vision, red and painful eye, cloudy cornea, fixed mid-dilated pupil, high intraocular pressure (IOP). See Section 10.10, Acute Angle-Closure Glaucoma.]
- Ocular ischemic syndrome (Periorbital eye pain, midperipheral retinal hemorrhages, dilated retinal veins, neovascularization of the iris, disc, or retina, spontaneous or easily inducible retinal arterial pulsations, light-induced amaurosis fugax. See Section 12.7, Ocular Ischemic Syndrome.)
- Malignant hypertension (Marked increase of blood pressure, often accompanied by retinal cotton-wool spots, hemorrhages, and when severe, optic nerve swelling. Headaches typically are occipital in location. See Section 12.5, Hypertensive Retinopathy.)
- Increased intracranial pressure (May have papilledema, loss of venous pulsations* in the disc vessels, or a sixth cranial nerve palsy. Headaches

---

*The presence of spontaneous venous pulsations indicates normal intracranial pressure at that moment; however, the absence of pulsations has little significance. A significant number of normal individuals do not have spontaneous venous pulsations. If spontaneous venous pulsation, at that moment, intracranial pressure <180 mm Hg.

usually worse in the morning and worsened with valsalva. See Section 11.13, Papilledema.)
- Infectious central nervous system disorder (meningitis or brain abscess) (Fever, stiff neck, mental status changes, photophobia, neurologic signs.)
- Structural abnormality of the brain [e.g., tumor, aneurysm, arteriovenous malformation (AVM)] (Mental status change, signs of increased intracranial pressure, or neurologic signs during, and often after, the headache episode.)
- Subarachnoid hemorrhage (Extremely severe headache, stiff neck, mental status change; rarely, subhyaloid hemorrhages seen on fundus examination, usually from a ruptured aneurysm.)
- Epidural or subdural hematoma (Follows head trauma; altered level of consciousness; may produce anisocoria.)

OTHERS

- Migraine (See Section 15.4, Migraine.)
- Cluster (See Section 15.5, Cluster Headaches.)
- Tension
- Herpes zoster virus [Headache or pain may precede the herpetic vesicles (see Section 4.16, Herpes Zoster Virus).]
- Sinus disease

❖ **Note** *A "sinus" headache can be a serious headache in diabetics and immunocompromised hosts because mucormycosis may be responsible (see Section 11.9, Cavernous Sinus/Superior Orbital Fissure Syndrome).*

- Tolosa–Hunt syndrome (See Cavernous Sinus/Superior Orbital Fissure Syndrome, Section 11.9.)
- Cervical spine disease
- Temporomandibular joint syndrome
- Dental disease
- Trigeminal neuralgia (tic douloureux)
- Anterior uveitis (See Section 13.1, Anterior Uveitis.)
- After spinal tap
- Paget's disease
- Depression/psychogenic
- Convergence insufficiency (See Section 15.6, Convergence Insufficiency.)
- Accommodative spasm (See Section 15.7, Accommodative Spasm.)

Workup
1. History: Ask about the location, intensity, frequency, possible precipitating factors, and time of day of the headaches. Determine the

patient's age of onset, what relieves the headaches, and whether there are any associated signs or symptoms. Specifically, ask about the serious or suggestive symptoms and signs listed: trauma, medications and birth-control pills, family history of migraine, and whether the patient experienced motion sickness or cyclic vomiting as a child.

2. Complete ocular examination, including pupillary, motility, and visual-field evaluation; IOP measurement, optic disc and venous pulsation assessment, and a dilated retinal examination. Manifest and cycloplegic refractions may be helpful.

3. Neurologic examination (check neck flexibility and other meningeal signs).

4. Palpate the temporal arteries in potential GCA cases (to see if they are swollen, hard, and tender). Ask specifically about jaw claudication, scalp tenderness, temporal headaches, and unexpected weight loss.

5. Temperature and blood pressure.

6. Immediate erythrocyte sedimentation rate (ESR) with or without temporal artery biopsy when GCA is suspected (see Section 11.16, Giant Cell Arteritis).

7. Computed tomography (CT) scan (axial and coronal views) or magnetic resonance imaging (MRI) of the brain when an intracranial abnormality is suspected.

8. Carotid noninvasive flow studies when ocular ischemic syndrome is suspected.

9. Lumbar puncture (in the hospital) is obtained in suspected cases of meningitis or subarachnoid hemorrhage, after CT scan or MRI of the brain.

10. Refer the patient to a neurologist; ear, nose, and throat specialist; internist; or family doctor, as indicated.

Treatment/Follow-up
See individual sections.

15.4 MIGRAINE

Symptoms
Typically unilateral (although it may occur behind both eyes or across the entire front of the head), throbbing or boring head pain accompanied by nausea, vomiting, mood changes, fatigue, or photophobia. Visual disturbances, including flashing (zigzagging) lights, blurred vision, or a visual-field defect lasting 15 to 50 minutes, may precede the migraine. The

migraine is often preceded by an aura (a sensation of an impending migraine). Neurologic deficits may occur. A family history is common, as is a history of car sickness or cyclic vomiting as a child. Migraine in children may be seen as recurrent abdominal pain and malaise. Of these patients, 60% to 70% are girls.

❖ **Note** *The majority of unilateral migraine headaches at some point change sides of the head. Patients who always have a headache on the same side of the head may have a more serious headache disorder.*

❖ **Note** *Pay close attention to temporal order of symptoms: be aware to see if headache precedes visual symptoms. This order of events is more common with arteriovenous malformations, mass lesions with cerebral edema, or seizure focus.*

Signs
Usually none. Complicated migraines may have a permanent neurologic or ocular deficit (see the following discussion).

Classification
Definitions and classifications vary.

I. Common migraine (headache without aura; 80%). Nausea, vomiting, fatigue, and mood changes are associated with this variant.

II. Classic migraine (headache with aura; 10%). The headache is preceded by a 15- to 50-minute visual disturbance or transient focal neurologic change. See Complicated Migraine (listed below) for specific types of visual and neurologic defects.

III. Visual migraine without headache (acephalalgic migraine). The patient experiences the visual aura of a classic migraine without the subsequent headache. Some of these patients have and some have not had migraine headaches in the past.

IV. Complicated migraine. A subset of migraine in which neurologic deficits outlast the headache. Rarely, a deficit may be permanent.

   A. Cerebral: A neurologic deficit involving the motor, sensory, or visual systems. Onset can be at the height of a migraine headache, but more commonly, it follows the headache. Examples include focal motor deficits, speech disorders, and paresthesias of the extremities, face, tongue, or lips. "Hemiplegic migraine" consists of total paralysis or weakness on one side of the body.

   B. Ophthalmoplegic: Ipsilateral paralysis of one or more extraocular muscles, usually occurring during a migraine attack in childhood. The ophthalmoplegia usually occurs as the headache is resolving.

   C. Retinal: Sudden monocular visual loss in a migraine patient. Light flashes and headache do not usually occur.

D. Basilar artery migraine: Mimics vertebrobasilar artery insufficiency with bilateral blurring or blindness, vertigo, gait disturbances, formed hallucinations, and dysarthria in a patient with migraine.

Associations or Precipitating Factors

Birth-control or other hormonal pills, puberty, pregnancy, menopause, foods containing tyramine or phenylalanine (e.g., aged cheeses, wines, chocolate, cashew nuts), nitrates or nitrites, monosodium glutamate, alcohol, fatigue, emotional stress, refractive errors, or bright lights.

Differential Diagnosis

See Headache, Section 15.3.

Workup

See Section 15.3 for a general headache workup.

1. History: May establish the diagnosis.
2. Ocular and neurologic examinations, including refraction.
3. Computed tomography (CT) scan or magnetic resonance imaging (MRI) of the head is indicated for:
   a. Atypical migraines (e.g., migraines that are always on the same side of the head, those with an unusual sequence, such as visual disturbances persisting into or occurring after the headache phase).
   b. Complicated migraines.
4. Consider checking for uncontrolled blood pressure or low blood sugar (hypoglycemic headaches are almost always precipitated by stress or fatigue).

Treatment

1. Avoid agents that precipitate the headaches (e.g., stop using birth-control pills; avoid alcohol and any foods that may precipitate attacks; reduce stress).
2. Correct any significant refractive error.
3. Medications to be used at the onset of the headache (the earlier the better) in patients with infrequent headaches:
   a. Initial therapy: Aspirin or nonsteroidal antiinflammatory agents (e.g., tolfenamic acid, 200 mg, q 3 h, naproxen sodium, 750 mg, in one dose).
   b. More potent therapy (when initial therapy fails):
      Ergotamine,* 2.0 mg in one dose, and then q 30 min for two extra doses if no relief (maximum dose is three tablets or 6 mg total per attack, no more than 10 mg per week)

---

*Contraindicated in elderly patients or those with cardiovascular, cerebrovascular, renal, or hepatic disease, and pregnant patients. Muscle weakness and pain or even cardiac ischemic pain can occur.

Ergotamine* 1.0 mg with caffeine, 100 mg, in one tablet. Two tablets at the onset of symptoms followed by 1 tablet q 30 min ×4 prn (maximum dose, 6 mg of ergotamine per attack, and no more than 10 mg per week).

Dihydroergotamine, 4.0 mg, p.o., in one dose.

Butorphanol nasal spray, one spray in one nostril

Sumatriptan, 6 mg, s.c. ×1 dose. Maximum dose is two injections in 24 hours. Do not give second dose if first is ineffective. Do not use if any ergotamine-containing drug (e.g., ergotamine, dihydroergotamine) has been given in the past 24 hours (because vasoconstriction could be additive).

Sumatriptan, 25 mg, p.o., single dose; if no relief after 2 hours, a second dose of up to 100 mg may be taken. If headache returns, may repeat after 2 hours have passed from previous dose. Maximum oral dose is 300 mg in a 24-hour period.

Sumatriptan, 20 mg, nasal spray, single dose

For prolonged attacks lasting longer than 24 hours, some physicians recommend systemic steroids.

❖ **Note** *Opioid drugs should be avoided.*

4. Prophylactic medication to be used in patients with frequent or severe headache attacks (e.g., two or more headaches per month) or those with neurologic changes:

Propranolol (e.g., Inderal)†, 10 to 80 mg, p.o., daily, in divided doses initially; slowly increase the dose by 10 to 20 mg every 2 to 3 days until the desired effect is obtained (can go up to 160 to 240 mg/day). May also use timolol, p.o., 10 to 15 mg, b.i.d. Metoprolol may have fewer side effects for asthmatics and diabetics (100 mg in one slow-release tablet per day).

Amitriptyline (e.g., Elavil)‡, 25 to 200 mg, p.o., qhs (start at a low dose and increase the dose by 25 mg every 1 to 2 weeks if needed).

Calcium channel blockers (e.g., flunarizine, 5 to 10 mg daily); we rarely use these.

Methylsergide, 2 to 4 mg, p.o., b.i.d. (ergot-containing medication)

5. Antinausea medication as needed for an acute episode (e.g., prochlorperazine, 25 mg rectally, b.i.d.).

---

*Contraindicated in elderly patients or those with cardiovascular, cerebrovascular, renal, or hepatic disease, and pregnant patients. Muscle weakness and pain or even cardiac ischemic pain can occur.

†Do not give to patients with asthma, congestive heart failure, bradycardia, or hypotension. Do not discontinue this drug suddenly; it must be tapered slowly.

‡Do not give to patients taking a monoamine oxidase inhibitor or patients with narrow anterior-chamber angles or benign prostatic hypertrophy.

Follow-up
Patients are generally reevaluated in 4 to 6 weeks to assess the efficacy of the therapy.

15.5 CLUSTER HEADACHE

Symptoms
Typically unilateral, very painful, periorbital, frontal, or temporal headache associated with ipsilateral tearing, rhinorrhea, sweating, nasal stuffiness, or a droopy eyelid or a combination of these. Usually lasts for minutes to hours. Typically recurs once or twice daily for several weeks, followed by a headache-free interval of months to years. The cycle can then repeat itself. Predominantly affects men.

Signs
Ipsilateral conjunctival injection, facial flush, or Horner's syndrome (third-order neuron etiology) may be present. Ptosis may become permanent.

Precipitating Factors
Alcohol, nitroglycerin.

Differential Diagnosis
- Migraine headache (Family history of migraines or a history of car sickness or cyclic vomiting in many cases. The associated symptoms listed previously are typically absent. See Section 15.4, Migraine.)
- Chronic paroxysmal hemicrania (several attacks per day with a dramatic response to oral indomethacin).
- Others (See Headache, Section 15.3.)

Workup
1. History and complete ocular examination.
2. Neurologic examination, particularly a cranial nerve evaluation.
3. Consider an hydroxyamphetamine (e.g., Paredrine) test if Horner's syndrome accompanies a suspected cluster headache to confirm a third-order neuron etiology (see Section 11.2, Horner's Syndrome).
4. Obtain a computed tomography (CT) scan (axial and coronal views) or magnetic resonance imaging (MRI) of the brain when the history is atypical or a neurologic abnormality other than a third-order neuron Horner's syndrome is found.

Treatment
1. No treatment is necessary if the headache is mild.
2. No alcoholic beverages or cigarette smoking during a cluster cycle.
3. Abortive therapy for acute attack:
   - Oxygen, 5 to 8 l/min via face mask for 10 minutes at onset of attack. Relieves pain in 70% of adults.
   - Ergotamine inhalation is the fastest way to reach therapeutic blood levels (e.g, Medihaler, three puffs, 5 minutes apart).
   - Dihydroergotamine, i.m. or i.v. (1.0 mg i.m. in one dose).
   - Corticosteroids (e.g., dexamethasone, 8.0 mg, i.v. in one dose).
4. When headaches are moderate to severe and are unrelieved by nonprescription medication, one of the following drugs may be an effective prophylactic agent during cluster periods:
   - Calcium channel blockers (e.g., verapamil, 360 to 480 mg, p.o., per day in divided doses).
   - Ergotamine, 1.0 to 2.0 mg, p.o., daily.
   - Methysergide, 2 mg, p.o., b.i.d., with meals. Do not use for longer than 3 to 4 months because of the significant risk of retroperitoneal fibrosis. Methysergide is not recommended in patients with coronary artery or peripheral vascular disease, thrombophlebitis, hypertension, pregnancy, or hepatic or renal disease.
   - Oral steroids (e.g., prednisone, 40 to 80 mg, p.o., for 1 week, tapering rapidly over an additional week if possible) and an antiulcer agent (e.g., ranitidine, 150 mg, p.o., b.i.d.). See Medical Glossary (prednisone) for steroid workup.
   - Lithium, 600 to 900 mg, p.o., daily, is administered in conjunction with the patient's medical doctor. Baseline renal (blood urea nitrogen, creatinine, urine electrolytes) and thyroid-function tests [T_3, T_4, thyroid-stimulating hormone (TSH)] are obtained. Lithium intoxication may occur in patients using indomethacin, tetracycline, or methyldopa.

   Some physicians administer an ergotamine inhaler (9 mg/mL, containing 0.36 mg per inhalation), one inhalation q 5 minutes for three inhalations (maximum every 12 to 24 hours) or ergotamine, 2 mg sublingual, q 30 minutes for three times (maximum in 24 hours) to be started at the onset of an attack. Ergotamine pills may be used in prophylaxis. Ergotamine has the same contraindications as methysergide. We do not use ergotamine as a first-line agent.

   If necessary, an acute, severe attack can be treated with i.v. diazepam.

Follow-up
Patients started on systemic steroids are seen within a few days and then every several weeks to evaluate the effects of treatment and monitor intraocular pressure (IOP). Patients taking methysergide or lithium are

reevaluated in 7 to 10 days. Plasma lithium levels are monitored in patients taking this agent.

15.6 CONVERGENCE INSUFFICIENCY (CI)

Symptoms
Eye discomfort, headache, sleepiness, or blurred vision from reading or doing near work. It is most common in teenagers and young adults, but may be seen in presbyopes.

Critical Sign
An inability to maintain fusion at near as a result of a reduced amplitude of fusional convergence power (see Workup).

Other Signs
A distant near point of convergence, an exophoria greater at near than at distance, and a reduced amplitude of accommodation.

Etiology
Fatigue or illness, drugs (parasympatholytics), uveitis, Adie's tonic pupil, glasses inducing a base-out prism effect, postexanthematous encephalitis, or traumatic injury. Often idiopathic.

Differential Diagnosis
Other causes of eyestrain with reading.
- Uncorrected refractive error (especially hyperopia and astigmatism)
- Accommodative insufficiency (AI) [Symptoms develop after 20 to 40 minutes of reading, same age group as convergence insufficiency (CI), but these patients have normal fusional capacities. When a 4-diopter base-in prism is placed in front of the eye while reading, the print is noted to blur in patients with AI, but become clearer in those with CI. Patients with AI usually benefit from reading glasses; those with CI do not.]

Workup
1. Manifest (without cycloplegia) refraction.
2. Determine the near point of convergence: Ask the patient to focus on an accommodative target (e.g., the eraser of a pencil) and to inform you when double vision develops as you bring the target toward him or her; a normal near point of convergence is <6 to 8 cm.

3. Check for exodeviations or esodeviations at distance and near by using the cover tests (see Appendix 2) or the Maddox rod test. See Section 11.6, Isolated Fourth-Nerve Palsy.
4. Measure the patient's fusional ability at near: Have the patient focus on an accommodative target at his or her reading distance. With a prism bar, slowly increase the amount of base-out prism in front of one eye until the patient notes double vision (the break point), and then slowly reduce the amount of base-out prism until a single image is again noted (the recovery point). A low break point (i.e., 10 to 15 prism diopters) or a low recovery point or both are consistent with CI.
5. Place a 4-diopter base-in prism in front of one eye while the patient is reading and determine whether the print becomes clearer or more blurred to rule out AI.
6. Cycloplegic refraction (performed after the previous tests and measurements).

❖ **Note** *These tests are performed with the patient's spectacle correction in place (if glasses are worn for near work).*

Treatment
1. Correct any refractive error (hyperopia should be slightly undercorrected, whereas myopia should be fully corrected).
2. Near-point exercises (e.g., pencil push-ups): The patient is taught to focus on the eraser of a pencil while slowly moving it from arm's length toward the face. The patient must concentrate on maintaining one image of the eraser. When double vision results, the maneuver is repeated. An attempt is made to draw the pencil in closer each time while maintaining single vision. The exercise is repeated 15 times, 5 times per day.
3. Near-point exercises with base-out prisms (for patients whose near point of convergence is satisfactory or for those who have mastered pencil push-ups without a prism): Pencil push-ups as described previously are performed while the patient additionally holds a 6-diopter base-out prism in front of one eye.
4. Encourage use of good lighting and time for relaxation between periods of concentrated close work.
5. For older patients, or those whose condition shows no improvement despite near-point exercises, reading glasses with base-in prism can be useful.

Follow-up
This is not an urgent condition. Patients are reexamined in 1 month.

15.7 ACCOMMODATIVE SPASM

Symptoms

Bilateral blurred distance vision or fluctuating vision, headache, and eyestrain while reading. Typically, patients are teenagers who are under stress. Symptoms may occur after prolonged and intense periods of near work.

Critical Signs

Cycloplegic refraction reveals substantially less myopia (or more hyperopia) than was originally found when the refraction was performed without cycloplegia (the manifest refraction). Manifest myopia may be as high as 10 diopters. Spasm of the near reflex is associated with excess accommodation, excess convergence, and miosis.

Other Signs

Abnormally close near point of focus, miosis, a normal amplitude of accommodation that may appear low.

Etiology

Inability to relax the ciliary muscles. Accommodative spasm is involuntary and is associated with stressful situations or functional neuroses. Fatigue and prolonged reading may also precipitate episodes.

Differential Diagnosis

- Uncorrected hyperopia (Patients accept plus lenses during the manifest refraction.)
- Other causes of pseudomyopia [Hyperglycemia, medication induced (e.g., sulfa drugs and anticholinesterase medications), forward displacement of the lens.]
- Manifestation of iridocyclitis

Workup

1. Complete ophthalmic examination, including an initial manifest refraction. The manifest refraction may be highly variable, but it is important to determine the least amount of minus power or the most amount of plus power that provides clear distance vision.
2. Cycloplegic refraction.

Treatment

1. True refractive errors should be corrected. If a significant amount of esophoria at near is present, additional plus power (e.g., +2.50 diopters) in reading glasses or bifocal form may be helpful for close work.

2. Gentle counseling of the patient and parents to provide a more relaxed atmosphere and avoid stressful situations is important.
3. Cycloplegics, including atropine, have been used to break the spasm, but are rarely needed except in the most resistant cases.

Follow-up
Reevaluate in several weeks. The physician should also be available for additional consultative support.

15.8 HYPOTONY SYNDROME

Definition
Decreased visual function and other ocular symptoms related to low intraocular pressure (IOP).

Symptoms
May have mild-to-severe pain. Vision may be reduced.

Critical Signs
Low IOP, usually <6 mm Hg, but may occur with an IOP as high as 10 mm Hg. Low IOP, even as low as 2 mm Hg, may not cause problems or symptoms.

Other Signs
Corneal edema and folds, aqueous cell and flare, shallow anterior chamber, retinal edema, chorioretinal folds, choroidal detachment, the appearance of optic disc swelling.

Etiology
- Postsurgical [Wound leak, cyclodialysis cleft (disinsertion of the ciliary body from the sclera at the scleral spur), perforation of the sclera from a superior rectus bridle suture or retrobulbar injection, iridocyclitis, retinal or choroidal detachment, others.]
- Posttraumatic (Same causes as postsurgical.)
- Pharmacologic (Usually from a carbonic anhydrase inhibitor in combination with a topical β-blocker.)
- Systemic (bilateral hypotony) [Conditions that cause blood hypertonicity (e.g., dehydration, uremia, exacerbation of diabetes), myotonic dystrophy, others.]
- Vascular occlusive disease (e.g., ocular ischemic syndrome, giant cell arteritis, central retinal vein or artery occlusion. Usually a mild hypotony.)
- Uveitis (causing ciliary body shut-down)

Workup

1. History: Recent ocular surgery or trauma? Other systemic symptoms (nausea, vomiting, twitching, drowsiness, polyuria)? History of renal disease, diabetes, or myotonic dystrophy? Medications?
2. Complete ocular examination, including a slit-lamp evaluation of surgical or traumatic ocular wounds (check for poor wound apposition), IOP check, gonioscopy of the anterior-chamber angle to rule out a cyclodialysis cleft, and indirect ophthalmoscopy to rule out a retinal or choroidal detachment or both and look for signs of a scleral perforation.
3. Seidel's test (with and without gentle pressure) to rule out a wound leak (see Appendix 4).

❖ **Note** *A wound leak may drain under the conjunctiva, producing a filtering bleb. Seidel's test will then be negative.*

4. B-scan ultrasound when the fundus cannot be seen clinically. Consider ultrasound biomicroscopy for evaluation of the anterior-chamber angle.
5. Blood tests in bilateral cases: Glucose, blood urea nitrogen, and creatinine.

Treatment

Repair of the underlying disorder may be needed if symptoms are significant or progressive.

WOUND LEAK

- Large wound leaks: Suture the wound closed.
- Small wound leaks: Can be sutured closed or can be patched with a pressure dressing and an antibiotic ointment (e.g., erythromycin) for 1 night to allow the wound to close spontaneously. A carbonic anhydrase inhibitor and a nonselective topical β-blocker (e.g., acetazolamide, 500 mg sequel p.o., and a drop of levobunolol or timolol, 0.5%) are usually given if patching is to be used.

❖ **Note** *Occasionally, cyanoacrylate glue is applied to small wound leaks and covered with a bandage contact lens.*

- Wound leaks under a conjunctival flap (repaired only if the hypotony is affecting vision or producing a secondary ocular complication such as a flat anterior chamber): Consider cryotherapy or argon laser therapy after painting the conjunctiva with methylene blue or rose bengal, or autologous blood injection.

CYCLODIALYSIS CLEFT

Reattach the ciliary body to the sclera by suturing, cryotherapy, laser photocoagulation, or diathermy.

SCLERAL PERFORATION

The site may be closed by suturing or cryotherapy.

IRIDOCYLITIS

Topical steroid (e.g., prednisolone acetate, 1%, q 1 to 6 hours) and a topical cycloplegic (e.g., scopolamine, 0.25%, t.i.d.).

RETINAL DETACHMENT

Surgical repair.

CHOROIDAL DEETACHMENT

(See also Section 12.21, Choroidal Detachment.)

Treated as iridocyclitis. Surgical drainage of the choroidal effusion along with reformation of the eye and anterior chamber is indicated for any of the following:

1. Retinal apposition ("kissing" choroidal detachments).
2. Lens–corneal touch (needs emergency attention).
3. A flat or persistently shallow anterior chamber accompanied by a failing filtering bleb or an inflamed eye.

PHARMACOLOGIC

Reduce or discontinue the IOP-reducing medications.

SYSTEMIC DISORDER

Refer to an internist.

❖ **Note** *In myotonic dystrophy, the hypotony is rarely severe enough to produce deleterious effects, and treatment of hypotony, from an ocular standpoint, is unnecessary.*

Follow-up
If vision is good, the anterior chamber is well formed, and there is no wound leak, retinal detachment, or kissing choroidal detachments, then the low IOP poses no immediate problem, and treatment and follow-up are not urgent. Fixed retinal folds in the macula may develop from long-standing hypotony.

15.9 BLIND, PAINFUL EYE

A patient with a nonseeing eye and unsalvageable vision may develop mild-to-severe pain in it for a variety of reasons. The etiology, workup, and treatment are discussed.

Causes of Pain
- Corneal decompensation (Fluorescein-staining defect on slit-lamp examination.)
- Uveitis (Anterior-chamber or vitreal white blood cells. If the cornea is opaque, the cells may not be seen.)
- Extremely high intraocular pressure (IOP) (May result from neovascular glaucoma and angle closure, uveitis, or intraocular tumor–related glaucoma. IOP may be difficult to measure if the corneal surface is irregular.)

Workup
1. History: Determine the etiology and duration of the blindness.
2. Ocular examination: Stain the cornea with fluorescein to detect an epithelial defect and measure the IOP. If the cornea is not opaque, look for neovascularization of the iris and angle by gonioscopy, and inspect the anterior chamber for cells and flare. Attempt a dilated retinal examination to rule out an intraocular tumor.
3. B-scan ultrasound of the posterior segment is required to rule out an intraocular tumor when the fundus cannot be adequately visualized.

Treatment
A. Sterile corneal decompensation (if it appears infected, see Infectious Corneal Infiltrate/Ulcer, Section 4.12)
   1. Antibiotic ointment (e.g., erythromycin), cycloplegic (e.g., atropine, 1%), and a pressure patch for 24 to 48 hours.
   2. Antibiotic or lubricating ointment (e.g., Refresh PM) 1 to 4 times per day (after the patch is removed) for weeks to months (or even permanently).
   3. Consider teaching the patient to patch his or her own eye nightly.
   4. Consider a tarsorrhaphy or Gunderson conjunctival flap in refractory cases.
B. Uveitis
   1. Cycloplegic (e.g., atropine, 1%, t.i.d.).
   2. Topical steroid (e.g., prednisolone acetate, 1%, q 1 to 6 hours).
   3. Treat uveitis if it is present or if the cornea is opaque and its presence cannot be ruled out.
C. Markedly increased IOP.
   1. Topical β-blocker (e.g., levobunolol or timolol, 0.5%, b.i.d.) with or without an adrenergic agonist compounds (e.g., brimonidine, 0.2%, or apraclonidine, 0.5%, b.i.d. to t.i.d.). Topical carbonic anhydrase inhibitors (e.g., dorzolamide, 2%, or brinzolamide, 1%, t.i.d.) are effective, but their potential systemic side effects may not warrant their use for pain relief; miotics may increase ocular irritation.

2. If the IOP remains markedly increased and is thought to be responsible for the pain, a cyclodestructive procedure (e.g., YAG or diode laser cyclophotocoagulation or cyclocryotherapy) may be attempted. The potential for sympathetic ophthalmia must be considered.

3. If pain persists despite the previously described treatment, a retrobulbar alcohol block may be given. This is typically effective for approximately 3 to 6 months. Technique: 2 to 3 ml of lidocaine is administered in the retrobulbar region. The needle is then held in place while the syringe of lidocaine is replaced with a 1-ml syringe containing 95% to 100% alcohol (some physicians use 50% alcohol). The contents of the alcohol syringe are then injected into the retrobulbar space through the needle. The syringes are again switched, so a small amount of lidocaine can rinse out the remaining alcohol. The retrobulbar needle is then withdrawn. Patients are warned that transient eyelid droop or swelling, limitation of eye movement, or anesthesia may result.

D. Cause of pain unknown
1. Cycloplegic (e.g., atropine, 1%, t.i.d.).
2. Topical steroid (e.g., prednisolone acetate, 1%, q 1 to 6 hours).
  • When this treatment fails to relieve the pain, enucleation is offered to the patient.
  • The patient should wear protective glasses (e.g., polycarbonate lens) at all times to prevent injury to the contralateral eye.

Follow-up

Depends on the degree of pain and the clinical abnormalities present. Once the pain resolves, patients are reexamined every 6 to 12 months.

USES OF IMAGING IN OPHTHALMOLOGY

General Radiology Studies in Ophthalmology

16.1 PLAIN FILMS

Description

Images of radiopaque tissues obtained by exposure of special photographic plates to ionizing radiation. Not used routinely in ophthalmology at present; previously used to diagnose orbital wall fractures, but computed tomography (CT) is now the gold standard for diagnosis of this condition.

Uses in Ophthalmology

Suspected orbital fractures, intraorbital air, radiopaque foreign body when CT is unavailable or patient unable to tolerate CT scan.

16.2 DACRYOCYSTOGRAPHY

Description

Special application of plain film radiographs to image the nasolacrimal drainage system after injection of radiopaque contrast into the system.

USES IN OPHTHALMOLOGY

1. Suspected nasolacrimal drainage obstruction.
2. May be used for defining lacrimal drainage system anatomy when cause of obstruction is maldevelopment or tumor, but has no ability to comment on physiology.

16.3 COMPUTED TOMOGRAPHY (CT SCAN)

Description

CT uses ionizing radiation and computer-assisted formatting to produce multiple cross-sectional planar images. Possible image planes include axial, coronal, reformatted coronal, and reformatted sagittal images. Views that focus primarily on soft tissues or bony structures are available. Slice width is usually 3 mm unless otherwise specified when ordering the study. Radiodense contrast allows more extensive evaluation of vascular structures and will leak where there is a breakdown of the normal capillary endothelial barrier [as with inflammation (e.g., abscess)].

❖ **Note** *Coronal images are obtained by having the patient hyperextend the neck; this should not be done if there is a strong suspicion of neck injury.*

Uses in Ophthalmology

1. Locating suspected intraorbital or intraocular metallic foreign bodies. Glass, wood, and plastic are less radiopaque and tend to be more difficult to isolate on CT.
2. Excellent for defining bone pathology such as fractures (orbital wall or optic canal) or bony involvement of a soft-tissue mass.
3. Soft-tissue windows are good for determining some soft-tissue pathologic features such as orbital cellulitis/abscess (loss of radiodense margins). May be useful in determining posterior scleral rupture when clinical examination is inconclusive.
4. Excellent for diagnosing sinusitis.
5. Excellent for locating intracranial blood or blood in the subarachnoid, subdural, or epidural space in either acute or subacute setting.
6. Excellent for looking for optic canal fractures in cases of suspected traumatic optic neuropathy.
7. Good for evaluation of leukocoria and proptosis.

Hints for Ordering the Study

1. Request an orbital study (as opposed to looking at the orbits from a head series) when suspecting ocular or orbital pathologic features.
2. Order both axial and coronal views (digitally reconstructed coronal views often have little value).
3. When attempting to diagnose traumatic optic neuropathy, request thin (1-mm) cuts of the optic canal.
4. When attempting to localize either ocular or orbital foreign bodies, order 1-mm cuts.

16.4 NUCLEAR MEDICINE

Description

Nuclear medicine imaging uses radioactive contrast (radionuclide) that emits gamma radiation, which is gathered by a gamma ray detector. The classic types of radionuclide scanning known to ophthalmologists include bone scanning, liver–spleen scanning, and gallium scanning. Radionuclide scintigraphy is rarely if ever performed for intraocular or orbital disease but is requested occasionally by ophthalmologists to screen for systemic disease that might be associated with ophthalmic findings.

Uses in Ophthalmology

1. Scintigraphy (such as with technetium-99): useful for assessing lacrimal drainage physiology. Useful for patients with contradictory or inconsistent irrigation testing.
2. Systemic gallium scan is useful for detecting extraocular sarcoid granulomatous inflammation.
3. P32 test: not currently used in most countries; provides little if any useful differential diagnostic information in most patients with suspected choroidal melanoma.

16.5 MAGNETIC RESONANCE IMAGING (MRI)

Description

1. MRI uses a large magnetic field to excite protons of water molecules. The energy given off as the protons reequilibrate to their normal state

is detected by specialized receivers, and that information is reconstructed into a computer image.

2. May have multiplanar images: axial, coronal, sagittal, etc.
3. Weighting of the image

   T_1-weighted images have good anatomic detail, good for intraorbital structures such as optic nerve, extraocular muscles, and orbital veins, but strong fat signal gives poor resolution of lacrimal gland. T_1 gives poor intraorbital contrast (note: subacute blood >5 days appear bright).

   T_2-weighted images give very poor intraocular contrast.
4. Fat suppression: on T_1-weighted images, gives ability to find white-appearing orbital pathology on noncontrast MRI that is not caused by fat. White-colored pathology may be subacute blood, melanin, or high-protein fluid.
5. Gadolinium-diethylene-triamine-pentaacetic acid (Gd-DTPA) is a contrast agent for MRI that distributes in the extracellular space and does not cross intact blood–brain barriers. Gd-DTPA is best for T_1 fat-suppressed images. It is useless on T_2 images. The lacrimal gland and extraocular muscles enhance with Gd-DTPA. The optic nerve does NOT normally enhance.
6. Once you have the images, how to tell T_1 from T_2 image
   a. Looking at the image

      T_1: fat looks bright (i.e., high signal intensity); vitreous and intracranial ventricles are dark.

      T_2: vitreous is bright.
   b. Looking at the radiographic parameters

      T_1: TR (time to repeat) usually <1,000; TE (time to echo) usually low (<100).

      T_2: TR usually >1,000; TE usually high.

Uses in Ophthalmology

1. Excellent for defining extent of orbital/central nervous system (CNS) masses.
2. Excellent for suspected intracranial lesions affecting neuro-ophthalmic pathways.
3. Very poor for defining bone or acute blood.
4. Excellent for diagnosing intracranial masses.
5. Useful for characterization of intraocular mass lesion in an eye with opaque media.

Hints for Ordering the Study

1. When looking for ocular or orbital pathologic condition, should request an orbital surface coil; if the lesion or process is suspected to

extend posterior to the orbital apex (i.e., optic chiasm), request a head coil.
2. Must order fat suppression for T_1-weighted images when using contrast (Gd-DTPA).
3. When attempting to visualize lacrimal gland pathologic conditions, it is best to order a fat-suppressed T_1 with Gd-DTPA. Unenhanced T_1 and T_2 images are poor for lacrimal gland visualization.
4. Contraindications to MRI: Cardiac pacemaker, suspected magnetic intraocular/intraorbital foreign bodies, metal surgical clips.

16.6 MAGNETIC RESONANCE ANGIOGRAPHY (MRA)

Description
Special application of MRI technology in which the region of interest is imaged repeatedly at short intervals after intravenous injection of paramagnetic contrast agent to evaluate blood flow in the regional vasculature.

Uses in Ophthalmology
1. Suspected carotid or ophthalmic artery stenosis/occlusion.
2. Suspected intracranial and orbital arterial aneurysms (e.g., pupil involving third cranial nerve palsy), arteriovenous malformations, and acquired arteriovenous communications.
3. Suspected orbital or intracranial vascular mass (hemangioma, varix).

Hints for Ordering the Study
1. Cerebral arteriography remains the gold standard for diagnosis of vascular lesions. Currently, the limit of MRA is an aneurysm larger than 2 mm.

16.7 CEREBRAL ARTERIOGRAPHY

Description
This interventional radiologic examination entails intraarterial injection of radiopaque contrast followed by a rapid sequence of x-ray imaging of the region of interest to evaluate the transit of blood through the regional vasculature.

Uses in Ophthalmology
1. It is the gold standard for intracranial aneurysms. Can also be used to diagnose arteriovenous malformations and cavernous sinus thrombosis. Used for suspected vascular masses (e.g., hemangioma, varix).
2. Ocular ischemic syndrome or amaurosis fugax due to suspected atherosclerotic carotid or ophthalmic artery occlusive disease.

Specialized Ophthalmologic Imaging Studies

16.8 PHOTOGRAPHIC IMAGING STUDIES

Description
Various methods of imaging the appearance of the eyes or selected regions of the eye, using white light or various spectral wavelengths of light.

Types of Ophthalmic Photographic Imaging Studies
1. Documentary photography: color pictures of face, external eye, anterior segment, fundus (white light or red-free lighting).
2. Specular microscopy: contact and noncontact photographic techniques used to image the corneal endothelium. The images can then be used to determine endothelial cell counts.

16.9 FLUORESCEIN ANGIOGRAPHY (IVFA)

Description
Photographic method of angiography that does not rely on ionizing radiation. After intravenous injection of fluorescein solution (usually in hand or arm vein), rapid-sequence photography is performed by using a camera with spectrally appropriate excitation and barrier filters.

Uses in Ophthalmology
1. Used to image retinal, choroidal, optic disc, or iris vasculature, or a combination of these. It is used diagnostically as well as in planning for many retinal laser procedures.
2. Transit times between injection and appearance of dye in the choroid, retinal arteries, and veins also can be used to implicate flow through the imaged vessels.

3. Suspected retinal hypoxia (capillary nonperfusion) and neovascularization from various conditions [e.g., diabetes, familial exudative vitreoretinopathy (FEVR)].
4. Suspected choroidal neovascularization from various diseases (e.g., age-related macular degeneration, ocular histoplasmosis, conditions associated with angioid streaks).

Hints for Ordering a Study

1. Side effects of intravenous fluorescein are nausea (less than 10%), vomiting (usually less than 2%), hives, pruritis, vasovagal response. True anaphylaxis is very rare. Extravasation into extracellular space at the injections site can produce local necrosis.
2. Because it is a photographic method, somewhat clear media is required for visualization.

16.10 INDOCYANINE GREEN ANGIOGRAPHY (ICG)

Description

Photographic method of ocular angiography similar to fluorescein angiography; however, the contrast agent is indocyanine green rather than fluorescein. Used for imaging choroidal and retinal blood vessels. Compared with fluorescein angiography, ICG provides better resolution of choroidal vasculature, but lesser resolution of retinal blood vessels.

Uses in Ophthalmology

1. Suspected occult choroidal neovascular membranes (CNVMs), and can also be used to identify recurrence of CNVM after treatment.
2. Suspected retinal pigment epithelial detachment.

Hints for Ordering a Study

1. ICG contains iodine.
2. Most common side effect of ICG is vasovagal response.

16.11 OPHTHALMIC ULTRASONOGRAPHY

Ophthalmic ultrasonography is a diagnostic-imaging technique that uses relatively high-frequency sound waves to generate either cross-sectional imaging (B-scan) or amplitude of reflectivity curves (A-scan) of ocular or orbital tissues.

A-Scan

Description

Uses ultrasound waves to generate linear distance versus amplitude of reflectivity curves of the evaluated ocular and orbital tissues. A-scans do not really create images but are used for taking measurements and characterization of the composition of tissues based on the reflectivity curves. Not all A-scan instruments are standardized. Standardization means that the linear curve generated by testing the probe against gelatin standard has a defined shape at a particular gain setting of the instrument. Both contact and water-bath techniques may be used.

Use in Ophthalmology

1. Primary use in ophthalmology is measurement of axial length of the globe. This information is critical for intraocular lens (IOL) power calculations for cataract surgery. Axial-length information can also be used to identify certain congenital disorders such as microphthalmos, nanophthalmos, and congenital glaucoma.
2. Diagnostic identification of consistency of masses within the globe or orbit.
3. Specialized A-mode ultrasound can be used for corneal pachymetry (measurement of corneal thickness).

Hints for Ordering a Study

1. When used for IOL power calculations, make sure to check both eyes. Both eyes should be within 0.3 mm.

B-Mode

Description

Gives real-time two-dimensional (cross-sectional) image of the eye posterior to the iris to immediately posterior to the globe; does not visualize the anterior chamber well. Both contact and water-bath techniques may be used.

Use in Ophthalmology

1. Define ocular anatomy when media opacities are too great to visualize directly.
2. In setting of trauma, can be used to diagnosis scleral rupture posterior to the muscle insertions or when media opacities prevent direct visualization.

3. Identify intraocular foreign bodies especially if made of metal or glass (spherical objects have a specific echo shadow); wood or vegetable matter has variable echodensity signal; can also give a more precise location if the foreign body is next to the scleral wall.
4. Evaluation of intraocular tumor/mass consistency, retinal detachment, choroidal detachment (serous vs. hemorrhagic), and optic disc abnormalities (e.g., optic disc drusen, coloboma).
5. Can be used for lacrimal gland and anterior orbital pathologic conditions, but this has largely been replaced by magnetic resonance imaging (MRI) or computed tomography (CT).

Hints for Ordering a Study

1. If used in setting of trauma to determine unknown scleral rupture, can be used over closed eyelids with immersion in copious amounts of sterile methylcellulose, such that no pressure is placed on the globe. The gain must be set very high to overcome the sound attenuation of the eyelids. Known ruptured globe is a contraindication to B-scan ultrasonography.
2. When scleral integrity is not in question, B-scan ultrasound should be performed dynamically. The movement of the globe can help differentiate between different structures, such as with retinal detachment versus posterior vitreous detachment.
3. Limitations of B-scan ultrasonography include low cross-sectional resolution; contact techniques do not image anterior segment well.
4. Dense intraocular calcifications (such as occurs in many eyes with phthisis bulbi) result in images that are of poor quality and usually are uninterpretable.

Ultrasound Biomicroscopy

Description

Uses B-mode ultrasound of the anterior one fifth of the globe to give cross sections at near-microscopic resolution. Uses a water bath lid speculum with viscous liquid in bowl of the speculum.

Uses in Ophthalmology

1. Excellent for defining corneoscleral limbal pathologic conditions, anterior-chamber angle, ciliary body, iris pathologic conditions (e.g., ciliary body masses/cysts, plateau iris), and anteriorly located small foreign bodies.
2. Unexplained unilateral angle narrowing or closure.
3. Suspected cyclodialysis.

Hints for Ordering the Study

1. Known ruptured globe is a contraindication to the study.

Orbital Ultrasound/Doppler

Description

Uses B-mode coupled with Doppler technology to visualize flow in the vessels in the orbit.

Use in Ophthalmology

1. Superior ophthalmic vein pathology: high-flow cavernous sinus fistulae, superior ophthalmic vein thrombosis.
2. Orbital varix.
3. Arteriovenous malformations.

DILATING DROPS
Mydriatic and Cycloplegic Agents

Drops	Approximate Maximal Effect	Approximate Duration of Action
MYDRIATIC		
Phenylephrine 2.5, 10%	20 min	3 h
CYCLOPLEGIC/MYDRIATIC		
Tropicamide 0.5%, 1%	20–30 min	3–6 h
Cyclopentolate 0.5%, 1%, 2%	20–45 min	24 h
Homatropine 2%, 5%	20–90 min	2–3 days
Scopolamine 0.25%	20–45 min	4–7 days
Atropine 0.5%, 1%, 2%	30–40 min	1–2 wk

The usual regimen for a dilated examination is:

Adults Phenylephrine 2.5% and tropicamide 1%. Repeat these drops in 15–30 minutes if the eye is not dilated.

Children Phenylephrine 2.5%, tropicamide 1%, and cyclopentolate 1–2%. Repeat these drops in 25–35 minutes if the eye is not dilated.

Infants Phenylephrine 2.5% and tropicamide 0.5%. Homatropine 2% or cyclopentolate 0.5% (generally reserved for infants older than 1–2 months of age) may also be used. The drops can be repeated in 35–45 minutes if the eye is not dilated.

❖ Notes

1. *Dilating drops are contraindicated in most types of angle-closure glaucoma and in eyes with severely narrow anterior-chamber angles.*
2. *Dilating drops tend to be less effective at the same concentration in darkly pigmented eyes.*

COVER/UNCOVER AND ALTERNATE COVER TESTS

Cover/Uncover Test

Differentiates a phoria (the eyes are straight when fixating on a target, but misaligned when tired or not focusing) from a tropia (the eyes are misaligned at all times).

Requirements

Full range of ocular motility, vision adequate to see the target of fixation, foveal fixation in each eye, attention, and patient cooperation. This test should be performed before the alternate cover test.

1. The patient is asked to fixate on an accommodative target at distance (e.g., a letter on the vision chart).
2. Cover one of the patient's eyes while observing the uncovered eye. A refixation movement of the uncovered eye suggests the presence of a tropia.
3. Remove the cover. A phoria is identified by refixation of the eye now being uncovered while the contralateral eye maintains its position and fixation.
4. Repeat the procedure, covering the opposite eye.

❖ **Note** *A tropia may be unilateral, the same eye may be always turned in or out, or it may alternate between eyes. In an alternating tropia, the contralateral eye is sometimes deviated after the cover/uncover test.*

5. The patient is asked to fixate on an accommodative target at near. Both eyes are tested at near in the manner described previously.

❖ **Note** *An esodeviation is detected by a refixation movement temporally (the eye being observed turns away from the nose). An exodeviation is detected* *by a refixation movement nasally (the eye being observed turns toward the nose). A hyperdeviation is detected by a refixation movement inferiorly.*

Alternate Cover Test (Prism and Cover Test)

Measures the total deviation: phoria combined with tropia.

Requirements

Same as for the cover/uncover test.

1. The patient is asked to fixate on an accommodative target at distance.
2. An occluder is held over one eye for a few seconds, and then quickly switched to the other eye. As the occluder alternately covers each eye for a few seconds, the eye being uncovered may be noted to swing into position to refixate on the target. Such eye movement indicates the presence of a deviation.
3. To measure the deviation, prisms are placed in front of one eye until eye movement ceases as the cover is alternated from eye to eye. The base of the prism is placed in the direction of eye movement. The strength of the weakest prism that eliminates eye movement during the alternate cover test is the amount of the deviation.
4. Measurements may be done for any direction of gaze by turning the patient's head away from the target while asking him or her to maintain fixation on it (i.e., right gaze is measured by turning the patient's head toward his or her left shoulder and asking the patient to look at the target).
5. In general, measurements are taken in the straight-ahead position (both at distance and near), in right gaze, left gaze, downgaze (the chin is tilted up while the patient focuses on the target), upgaze (the chin is tilted down while the patient focuses on the target), and with the patient's head tilted toward his or her left shoulder and then toward his or her right shoulder. Measurements are taken both with and without glasses in the straight-ahead position.

AMSLER'S GRID

Used to test macular function or to detect a central or paracentral scotoma.

1. Have the patient wear his or her glasses and occlude the left eye while an Amsler's grid is held approximately 12 inches in front of the right eye (Fig. A-1).
2. The patient is asked what is in the center of the page. Failure to see the central dot may indicate a central scotoma.
3. Have the patient fixate on the central dot (or the center of the page if he or she cannot see the dot), and ask if all four corners of the diagram are visible. Are any of the boxes missing?
4. Again, while staring at the central dot, the patient is asked if all of the lines are straight and continuous or if some are distorted and broken.
5. The patient is asked to outline any missing or distorted areas on the grid with a pencil.
6. Repeat the procedure, covering the right eye and testing the left.

❖ **Notes**
1. *It is very important to monitor the patient's eye for movement away from the central dot.*
2. *A red Amsler's grid may define more subtle defects.*

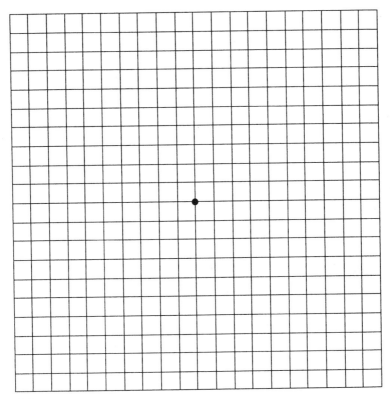

Figure A-1
Amsler's grid.

SEIDEL'S TEST TO DETECT A WOUND LEAK

Concentrated fluorescein dye (from a moistened fluorescein strip) is applied directly over the potential site of perforation while observing the site with the slit lamp (by using the white light; Fig. A-2). If a perforation and leak exist, the fluorescein dye will be diluted by the aqueous and will appear as a green (dilute) stream within the dark orange (concentrated) dye. The stream of aqueous is best be seen with the blue light of the slit lamp.

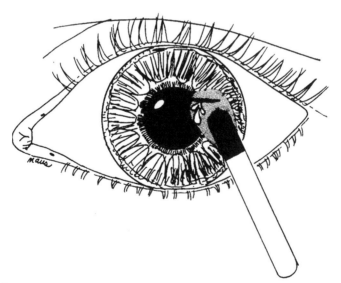

Figure A-2
Seidel's test.

FORCED-DUCTION TEST AND ACTIVE FORCE-GENERATION TEST

Forced-Duction Test

This test distinguishes restrictive causes of decreased ocular motility from other motility disorders. One technique is the following:

1. Place a drop of topical anesthetic (e.g., proparacaine) into the eye.
2. Place a cotton-tipped applicator soaked with cocaine, 10%, on the muscle to be grasped (i.e., the muscle away from the "paretic" field) for about 1 minute.
3. The anesthetized muscle is grasped firmly with toothed forceps (e.g., Graefe's fixation forceps), and the eye is rotated in the "paretic" direction (Fig. A-3). If there is resistance to passive rotation of the eye, a restrictive disorder is diagnosed.

Active Force-Generation Test

The patient is asked to look in the "paretic" direction while a sterile cotton swab is held just beneath the limbus on that same side. The amount of force generated by the "paretic" muscle is compared with that generated in the normal contralateral eye.

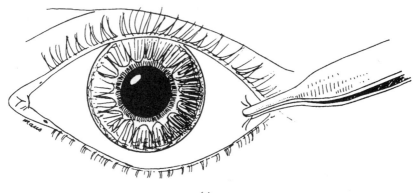

(a)

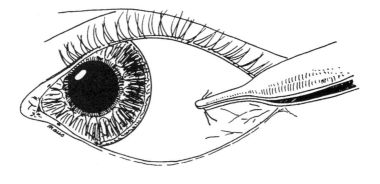

(b)

Figure A-3

Forced ductions. In the case illustrated, the left eye could not look inward. **(a)** The lateral rectus muscle is grasped with forceps. **(b)** The eye can be moved in the paretic direction (inward in this case) without resistance, ruling out a restrictive muscle condition.

TECHNIQUE FOR DIAGNOSTIC PROBING AND IRRIGATION OF THE LACRIMAL SYSTEM

1. Anesthetize the eye with a drop of topical anesthetic (e.g., propara-caine) and hold a cotton-tipped applicator soaked in the topical anes-thetic on the involved punctum for several minutes.
2. Dilate the punctum with a punctum dilator.
3. Gently insert a small Bowman's probe into the punctum 2 mm verti-cally, and then 8 mm horizontally, toward the nose (Fig. A-4). Pull the involved eyelid laterally while slowly moving the probe horizontally to facilitate the procedure and to avoid creating a false passageway.
4. In the presence of an eyelid laceration, a torn canaliculus may be diag-nosed by the appearance of the probe in the site of the eyelid laceration.
5. Irrigation of the lacrimal system is performed after removing the probe and inserting an irrigation canula in the same manner in which the probe was inserted. Five to 10 mL of saline is gently pushed into the system. Leakage through a torn eyelid also diagnoses a severed canaliculus. Resistance to injection of the saline, ballooning of the lacrimal sac, or leakage of the saline out of either punctum may be the result of a lacrimal-system obstruction. A patent lacrimal system usu-ally drains into the throat quite readily, and the arrival of saline there may be noted by the patient.

❖ **Note** *If evaluating solely the patency of the lacrimal system, and not ruling out a laceration, the system can be irrigated as described previously, right after punctum dilatation.*

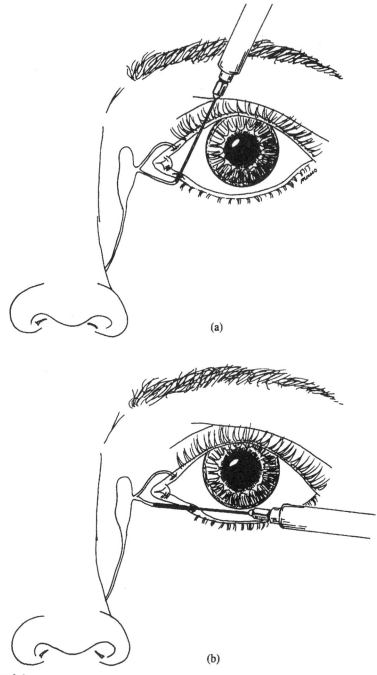

Figure A-4

Diagnostic probing of the lacrimal system. (a) After punctum dilatation, the probe or irrigation needle is directed inferiorly for 2 mm. **(b)** The instrument is rotated horizontally, and with the eyelid stretched laterally, is inserted toward the nose.

TECHNIQUE FOR SUBTENONS AND SUBCONJUNCTIVAL INJECTIONS

Technique for Subtenons Injection

1. Topical anesthesia is applied to the area to be injected (e.g., topical proparacaine or a cotton-tipped applicator soaked in proparacaine or both held on the area for 1 to 2 minutes). If subtenons steroids are to be injected, then 0.1 ml of lidocaine may be injected in the same manner as described next, several minutes before the steroids. The inferotemporal quadrant is usually the easiest location for injection.
2. With the aperture of a 25-gauge, 5/8-inch needle facing the sclera, the bulbar conjunctiva is penetrated 2 to 3 mm from the fornix, avoiding the conjunctival blood vessels (Fig. A-5).
3. As the needle is inserted, lateral motions of the needle are made to ensure that the needle has not penetrated the sclera (at which point, lateral motion would be inhibited).
4. The curvature of the eyeball is followed, attempting to place the aperture of the needle near the posterior sclera.
5. When the needle has been pushed in to the hilt, the stopper of the syringe is pulled back to ensure against intravascular penetration.
6. The contents of the syringe are injected, and the needle is removed.

Technique for Subconjunctival Injection

1. Topical anesthesia is applied as described previously.
2. Forceps are used to tent the conjunctiva, allowing the tip of a 25-gauge, 3/8-inch needle to penetrate the subconjunctival space. The needle is placed several millimeters below the limbus at the 4- or 8-o'clock position, with the aperture facing the sclera and the needle pointed inferiorly toward the fornix (Fig. A-6).

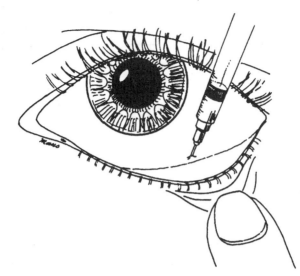

Figure A-5
Subtenons injection. The needle is placed 2 to 3 mm from the fornix, through conjunctiva and Tenon's capsule. If possible, angle the injection so the syringe does not lie over the cornea.

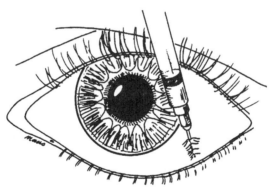

Figure A-6
Subconjunctival injection. The tip of the needle is placed into the subconjunctival space.

3. When the entire tip of the needle is beneath the conjunctiva, the stopper of the syringe is withdrawn to ensure against intravascular penetration.
4. The contents of the syringe are injected, and the needle is removed.

❖ **Note** *An eyelid speculum may be helpful in keeping the eyelids open during these procedures.*

VITREOUS EXAMINATION FOR CELLS

1. Best performed in a completely darkened room with the patient's pupil widely dilated.
2. *Anterior vitreous*   Use the high-power magnification of the slit lamp, reduce the beam height to less than the pupil diameter, and narrow the beam width to focus through the pupil. Set the illumination to the brightest setting. Move the slit lamp forward with the joystick, angling the beam of light until the anterior vitreous can be seen posterior to the lens. By moving the joystick, several optical sections can be sampled. Patients are sometimes asked to move their eyes from left to right, facilitating the recognition of vitreous cells as they float by.
3. *Middle and posterior vitreous*   By using a Hruby (first choice), fundus contact, or 60-diopter lens, the slit beam is initially focused on the disc. The joystick is then used to slowly pull the slit lamp away from the eye, refocusing the light on the posterior vitreous. Again, patients may be asked to look toward their left and right and then to resume primary position to produce movement of cells and to facilitate their recognition.

MAKING FORTIFIED TOPICAL ANTIBIOTICS

Fortified Tobramycin (or Gentamicin)

With a syringe, inject 2 ml of tobramycin, 40 mg/ml, directly into a 5-ml bottle of tobramycin, 0.3%, ophthalmic solution (e.g., Tobrex). This gives a 7-ml solution of fortified tobramycin (approximately 15 mg/ml). Refrigerate. Expires after 14 days.

Fortified Cefazolin

Add enough sterile water (without preservative) to 500 mg of cefazolin dry powder to form 10 ml of solution. This provides a strength of 50 mg/ml. Refrigerate. Expires after 7 days.

Fortified Vancomycin

Add enough sterile water (without preservative) to 500 mg of vancomycin dry powder to form 10 ml of solution. This provides a strength of 50 mg/ml. To achieve a 25-mg/ml concentration, take 5 ml of 50-mg/ml solution and add 5 ml sterile water. Refrigerate. Expires after 4 days.

Fortified Bacitracin

Add enough sterile water (without preservative) to 50,000 U bacitracin dry powder to form 5 ml of solution. This provides a strength of 10,000 U/ml. Refrigerate. Expires after 7 days.

TETANUS PROPHYLAXIS

History of Tetanus Immunization (doses)	Clean Minor Wounds		All Other Wounds	
	Tetanus Toxoid	Immune Globulin	Tetanus Toxoid	Immune Globulin
Uncertain	Yes	No	Yes	Yes
0–1	Yes	No	Yes	Yes
2	Yes	No	Yes	No*
3 or more	No†	No	No‡	No

Dose of tetanus toxoid is 0.5 ml i.m.
*Unless wound is more than 24 hours old.
†Unless more than 10 years since last dose.
‡Unless more than 5 years since last dose.
From U.S. Public Health Service, Advisory Committee on Immunization Practices. *Morbidity and Mortality Weekly Report*, Supplement. vol. 21, no. 25, June 24, 1972. Atlanta, Center for Disease Control.

ANGLE CLASSIFICATION

Spaeth's Classification (See Fig. A-7)

Iris Insertion

A. *Above Schwalbe's line* Schwalbe's line is not visible.

B. *Below Schwalbe's line* Schwalbe's line is visible, but the trabeculum is not.

C. *Scleral spur* Part of the scleral spur is visible. Usually seen in patients of African or Asian descent.

D. *Deep* The anterior ciliary body is visible. Usually seen in white patients.

E. *Extremely deep* An unusually large part of the ciliary body is visible. Indentation gonioscopy may be necessary to differentiate false opposition of the iris against structures in the iridocorneal angle (letters put in parentheses; see Fig. A-7) from the true iris insertion (letters without parentheses; see Fig. A-7).

Curvature of the Peripheral Iris

R. *Regular* Slight anterior bowing of the iris.

S. *Steep* Steep convex curvature of the iris (increased risk of developing angle-closure glaucoma).

Q. *Queer* Marked posterior concavity of the peripheral iris (may be seen in patients with high myopia or lens subluxation).

Angular Approach

The subjective measure of the angle between Schwalbe's line and the peripheral one third of the iris.

For example, on initial gonioscopy (without indentation) of a (B)C30R angle, Schwalbe's line, but not the trabeculum, is visible, yet on indentation,

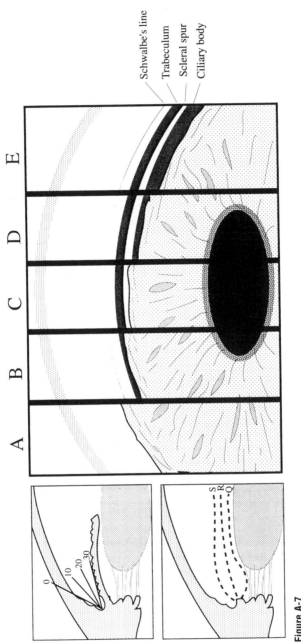

Schwalbe's line
Trabeculum
Scleral spur
Ciliary body

Figure A-7
Spaeth's classification of the anterior-chamber angle.

the scleral spur comes into view. The angle formed by Schwalbe's line and the peripheral one third of the iris is subjectively measured to be 30 degrees, and there is a normal degree of anterior bowing to the iris.

Angle Occluded

A or B iris insertion.

Angle Potentially Occludable

C or D iris insertion (without indentation), R iris curvature, angle 5 degrees or less.

C or D iris insertion (without indentation), S iris curvature, angle 20 degrees or less.

Shaffer's Classification (See Fig. A-8)

Grade 0   The angle is closed.

Grade 1   Extremely narrow angle (10 degrees). Only Schwalbe's line, and perhaps also the top of the trabeculum, can be visualized. Closure is probable.

Grade 2   Moderately narrow angle (20 degrees). Only the trabeculum can be seen. Closure is possible.

Grade 3   Moderately open angle (20 to 35 degrees). The scleral spur can be seen. Closure is not possible.

Grade 4   Angle wide open (35 to 45 degrees). The ciliary body can be visualized with ease. Closure is not possible.

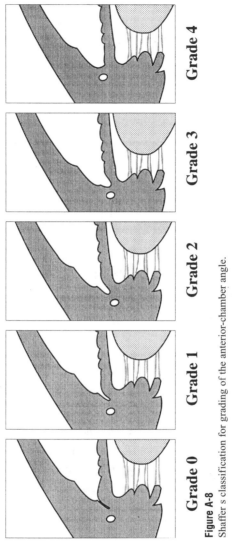

Figure A-8

Shaffer's classification for grading of the anterior-chamber angle.

TUBERCULIN SKIN TEST GUIDELINES*

Description

The intracutaneous (Mantoux) test is the best means of detecting infection with *Mycobacterium tuberculosis*. This test involves injecting 0.1 mL [5 tuberculin units (TU)] purified protein derivative (PPD) antigen into the forearm just beneath the surface of the skin by using a 1/4 to 1/2-inch 27-gauge needle on a tuberculin syringe. A wheal 6 to 10 mm in diameter should be produced when the test is performed correctly. The test should be read 48 to 72 hours after injection by measuring the diameter in millimeters of the area of induration (determined both by inspection and palpation).

Interpretation†

A reaction of greater than 5 mm is considered positive in the following groups:

1. Human immunodeficiency virus (HIV)-infected patients or those with risk factors for HIV and unknown HIV status,
2. Patients with recent close contact to infectious tuberculosis (TB) cases, and
3. Patients with evidence of old healed TB on chest radiograph.

A reaction of ≥10 mm is considered positive in patients not meeting these criteria, but with other risk factors for TB, including:

1. Foreign-born patients from high-prevalence countries in Asia, Africa, and Latin America,
2. Intravenous drug users,

---

*MMWR, Vol. 46, RR-15, 9/5/97.

†For the most current guidelines, consult the CDC Internet website at http://www.cdc.gov/nchstp/tb/default.htm

3. Patients from medically underserved areas or populations, including high-risk ethnic minorities and low-income groups,
4. Residents of long-term care facilities (e.g., nursing homes, prisons),
5. Patients with medical comorbid risk factors (e.g., immunosuppression, chronic renal failure, malignancy),
6. Employees in certain health-care facilities (dependent on local considerations, including prevalence of TB in community).

For all other persons, a reaction of ≥ 15 mm is considered positive.

❖ **Notes**

- *There is no reliable way to distinguish PPD test reactions caused by prior bacille Calmette–Guérin (BCG) vaccination from those of TB infection, so vaccinated persons with significant reactions (>10 mm) must be evaluated for evidence of disease.*
- *A booster effect is sometimes seen in patients with prior TB infection or BCG vaccination, most commonly in those older than 55 years. This may cause an initial PPD skin test to be negative, but a repeated test up to 1 year later may be positive. Therefore, for adults who will be tested periodically, an initial test followed by a repeated test 1 week later is recommended. Both should be negative to rule out prior TB infection. Thereafter, any subsequent positive PPD test indicates a new exposure.*

SELECTED OPHTHALMOLOGY RESOURCES ON THE INTERNET*

American Academy of Ophthalmology (AAO)

http://www.eyenet.org

Presents Academy news and services, patient-education materials, and links to noncommercial academic, medical, governmental, and research information sources.

Centers for Disease Control and Prevention (CDC)

http://www.cdc.gov

Includes access to *Morbidity and Mortality Weekly Report* (*MMWR*), CDC statistical reports, guidelines for infectious disease screening, and travelers' health information.

Wills Eye Hospital

http://jeffline.tju.edu/wills

Includes information about the hospital, medical staff, services and departments, training programs, case reports, and medical library holdings.

Eye Diseases Links

http://www.mic.ki.se/Diseases/c11.html

An extensive list developed by Karolinska Institute Library. Arranged by eye disorder, the list includes links to international associations, patient-education resources, publications, and drug information.

*Originally compiled by Judith Schaeffer Young, M.S.L.S., AHIP, Director, Medical Library, Wills Eye Hospital. Used by permission.

Eye Resources on the Internet

http://webeye.ophth.uiowa.edu/dept/websites/eyeres.htm
Maintained by the Association of Vision Science Librarians. Includes associations, patient-education materials, and support groups.

Eyes on the Net

http://www.hesp.it/hesp/cso/links.html
An alphabetic compilation of eye care–related resources from Italy, including international organizations, universities, publications, support groups, equipment and drug vendors, and bulletin-board–type listserves.

National Eye Institute

http://www.nei.nih.gov
Lists clinical trials, funding information, publications, and a staff directory.

Digital Journal of Ophthalmology

http://www.djo.harvard.edu/meei
Online journal produced by the Massachusetts Eye and Ear Infirmary and Harvard University Department of Ophthalmology.

Macular Degeneration Fact Sheet

http://www.eri.harvard.edu/Documentation/md.html

Ophthalmology News

http://www.vol.it/OCULISTICA/indexgb.html

National Association for the Visually Handicapped

http://www.navh.org

University of Iowa Department of Ophthalmology

http://webeye.ophth.uiowa.edu

Vitreous Society

http://www.vitreoussociety.org

Wills Eye Hospital Glaucoma Foundation

http://www.wills-glaucoma.org

Resource for patients and physicians interested in glaucoma.

Wills Eye Hospital Vision Research

http://www.vision-research.org

A resource guide for patients and health care professionals interested in retinal disease.

DRUG GLOSSARY
Contraindications and Side Effects

The following is a list of drugs commonly used in ophthalmology along with some of their contraindications and side effects that have clinical importance. Most of these drugs should not be used in pregnant or breast-feeding women, in infants, in those with significant renal or hepatic disease, or in patients in whom an allergy to the drug is suspected or known (therefore, these contraindications are not listed separately for each drug, and should be investigated further if therapy is desired for a patient who is in one of these circumstances).

Acetazolamide (e.g., Diamox) Contraindicated in patients with sulfa allergy, metabolic acidosis, adrenal insufficiency, and a history of kidney stones (a relative contraindication). Be careful in patients taking another diuretic, a systemic steroid, or digoxin, because their potassium level may be reduced to a dangerous level. Side effects: Blood dyscrasias, kidney stones, others.

Acyclovir (e.g., Zovirax) Contraindicated in renal failure, adjust dose for chronic renal insufficiency. Side effects: Gastrointestinal (GI) disturbance, rash, renal toxicity.

Aminocaproic acid (e.g., Amicar) Contraindicated in patients with an intravascular clotting disorder. Side effects: Hypotension (particularly postural), nausea, vomiting, others.

Amphotericin B Highly toxic when used systemically. Side effects: Fever, chills, dyspnea, hypotension, renal failure, electrolyte abnormalities, bone marrow suppression, nausea/vomiting, phlebitis at infusion site.

Apraclonidine (e.g., Iopidine; topical) Contraindicated in patients taking monoamine oxidase inhibitors. Side effects: Allergy, mydriasis, dry mouth, dry eye, hypotension, lethargy.

Atropine (topical) Contraindicated in most angle-closure situations, infants, albinos, and Down's syndrome patients. Use cautiously in pediatric patients as the margin for toxicity is low. Side effects: Urinary retention, tachycardia, delirium, others. *Treatment of anticholinergic (e.g., atropine) overdose* Physostigmine, 1 to 4 mg, i.v., repeating 0.5 to 1.0 mg, i.v., q 15 minutes until the symptoms improve.

Brimonidine (e.g., Alphagan; topical) See Apraclonidine.

Brinzolamide (e.g., Azopt; topical) See Acetozolamide.

Carbachol (topical)   See Pilocarpine.

Carbogen (95% O_2, 5% CO_2)   Contraindicated in patients with pulmonary disease or an electrolyte disorder.

Clindamycin Side effects: Pseudomembranous colitis, others.

Cocaine (topical)   Contraindicated with compromised cardiovascular or cerebrovascular status.

Cyclopentolate (topical)   See Atropine.

Dipivefrin (e.g., Propine; topical)   See Epinephrine.

Dorzolamide (e.g., Trusopt; topical)   See Acetazolamide.

Doxycycline   See Tetracycline.

Echothiophate iodide (e.g., Phospholine iodide; topical)   See Pilocarpine. Patients (or parents) are told that succinylcholine should never be given for general anesthesia (the combination of the two drugs can be lethal).
Treatment of anticholinesterase overdose Atropine, 2 mg, i.v., q 5 minutes until relief of symptoms, or pralidoxime, 25 mg/kg, i.v., in 500 mL of 5% D_5W over 2 hours (do not use in overdose of neostigmine and physostigmine).

Epinephrine (topical)   Contraindicated in patients with severe cardiovascular disease. Side effects: Macular edema in aphakic patients, conjunctival reaction, precipitation of narrow-angle glaucoma, others. Allergic conjunctivitis is common.

Fluorometholone (topical)   See Prednisolone acetate.

Gentamicin Side effects: Nephrotoxicity, ototoxicity, neuromuscular blockade (myasthenia-like syndrome), others.

Homatropine (topical)   See Atropine.

Isosorbide   See Mannitol.

Itraconazole (e.g., Sporanox)   See Ketoconazole. Less hepatotoxic than ketoconazole.

Ketoconazole   Contraindicated with certain medications metabolized by the hepatic cytochrome P-450 system, including terfenadine, astemizole, cisapride, triazolam. Side effects: GI distress, rash, pruritus, peripheral edema, hepatotoxicity [monitor liver-function tests (LFTs), discontinue if anorexia, nausea/vomiting, or signs of jaundice occur].

Latanoprost (e.g., Xalatan; topical)   Increase in melanin pigmentation in iris, blurred vision, eyelid redness; cystoid macular edema and anterior uveitis has been reported, systemic upper respiratory infection symptoms, backache, chest pain, myalgia. Contraindicated in pregnancy.

Levobunolol (e.g., Betagan; topical)   See Timolol.

Mannitol   Contraindicated in patients with hypotension, cardiovascular compromise, or concomitant administration of another osmotic agent. Side effects: Congestive heart failure, subarachnoid or subdural hemorrhage, mental confusion, others.

Methazolamide (e.g., Neptazane)   See Acetazolamide.

Natamycin (topical)   Side effects: mild conjunctival irritation, corneal epithelial toxicity, allergy.

Neomycin (topical) Side effects: Superficial punctate keratitis and allergic conjunctivitis are common.

Phenylephrine (e.g., Neo-Synephrine; topical)   Contraindicated in patients with significant cardiac disease, sympathetic denervation (i.e., those taking monoamine oxidase inhibitors and diabetics with neuropathy), most angle-closure glaucomas, and in the presence of occludable anterior-chamber angles.

Physostigmine (e.g., Esserine; topical)   Miotic agent. Contraindicated with succinyl-choline. See Echothiophate iodide and Pilocarpine.

Pilocarpine (topical) Side effects: Exacerbates iritis, can precipitate or exacerbate angle-closure glaucoma when used in high concentrations (usually 4% to 6% or greater), retinal detachment (with especially high concentrations, or other strong miotic agents such as echothiophate), brow ache, others.

Prednisolone acetate (topical)   Often contraindicated in patients with herpes simplex or fungal keratitis. Side effects: Increased intraocular pressure, cataract, increased susceptibility to infectious organisms, others.

Prednisone   Contraindicated in patients with peptic ulcer disease, tuberculosis, active infection, psychosis, or pregnancy. Workup includes complete blood count, glucose tolerance test, pregnancy test, purified protein derivative (PPD), anergy panel, chest radiograph, stool guaiac test. Side effects: Hyperglycemia, hypokalemia, hypertension, peptic ulcer, increased intraocular pressure, cataract, pseudotumor cerebri, mental status changes, aseptic necrosis of bone, osteoporosis, decreased wound healing, growth suppression in children, fluid retention, others.

Proparacaine (topical) Side effects: Corneal epithelial erosions and ulcers with repeated and prolonged use.

Pyridostigmine (e.g., Mestinon)   Contraindicated in patients with urinary or intestinal obstruction; use with caution in asthmatics. Side effects: GI distress, rash, muscle cramps. Overdose may lead to cholinergic crisis.

Scopolamine (topical)   See Atropine.

Steroids   See Prednisone.

Sulfacetamide (topical) Side effects: Stevens–Johnson syndrome, bone-marrow suppression, others.

Sulfadiazine   See Sulfacetamide.

Tetracycline   Contraindicated in children younger than 8 years (tooth discoloration). Side effects: GI upset, pseudotumor cerebri, hepatotoxicity, skin sensitivity to sunlight (patients are told on starting the drug to avoid sunlight if possible), others.

Timolol (e.g., Timoptic; topical)   Contraindicated in patients with asthma or other breathing problems, bradycardia (the patient's pulse is checked before administering a β-blocker), arrhythmias, congestive heart failure, hypotension, others.

Tobramycin   See Gentamicin.

Tropicamide (topical)   See Atropine.

Valacyclovir (e.g., Valtrex)   Associated with thrombotic thrombocytopenic purpura/hemolytic uremic syndrome (TTP/HUS) in immunocompromised patients. See also Acyclovir.

Vancomycin Side effects: Nephrotoxicity, ototoxicity, others.

GENERAL GLOSSARY

Accommodation   an increase in the refractive power of the natural lens of the eye; it is generally employed while doing near work (e.g., reading).

Amaurosis fugax   monocular blurring of vision developing completely by 30 seconds and lasting from 10 minutes to 2 hours. It may be associated with visible emboli in the retinal vessels.

Amblyopia   a unilateral or bilateral reduction of best-corrected central visual acuity in the absence of a visible organic lesion corresponding to the degree of visual loss.

Anisocoria   a difference in size between the two pupils.

Anisometropia   a difference in refractive error between the two eyes (e.g., one eye may be farsighted and one nearsighted, one eye may be relatively normal and the other very nearsighted).

Anterior chamber   the space in the eye bordered anteriorly by the cornea and posteriorly by the iris and the pupil.

Applanation tonometer   an instrument that measures intraocular pressure.

Astigmatism   the refracting power of the eye is not the same in all meridians (e.g., more hyperopic vertically than horizontally).

Bell's phenomenon   reflex upturning of the eye with active lid closure.

Bulbar conjunctiva   a freely movable tissue which forms the most superficial covering of the globe from the limbus to the fornices.

Buphthalmos   distention of the globe in response to elevated intraocular pressure; seen in patients with congenital glaucoma.

Chemosis   edema of the conjunctiva.

Coloboma   congenital absence of any eye structure.

Conjunctivitis   inflammation of the conjunctiva.

Cotton-wool spot   a superficial retinal infarction appearing as a fluffy white lesion, sometimes obscuring retinal vessels.

Crowding phenomenon   individual letters can be read better than a whole line; most commonly seen in amblyopic patients.

Cycloplegic   anything that causes paralysis of the ciliary muscle and therefore paralysis of accommodation.

Descemet's membrane   an inner (posterior) corneal layer.

Diplopia   double vision.

Ectopia lentis   dislocated lens.

Ectropion iridis (ectropion uveae)   eversion of the iris at the pupillary rim such that the pigmented posterior aspect of the iris is visualized.

Enophthalmos   a measurable depression of the globe within the bony orbit.

Enucleation   removal of the eye.

Episcleritis   inflammation of the external surface of the sclera (beneath the bulbar conjunctiva).

Esophoria   the eyes are aligned during binocular vision, but have a latent tendency to cross (e.g., while not focusing).

Esotropia   ocular misalignment in which the nonfixating eye is turned inward ("cross-eyed").

Exenteration   removal of the eye and orbital contents.

Exophoria the eyes are aligned during binocular vision, but have a latent tendency to turn away from one another.

Exophthalmos   a measurable protrusion of the globe from the bony orbit.

Exotropia   ocular misalignment in which the nonfixating eye is turned outward ("wall-eyed").

Flare   increased protein in the anterior-chamber fluid, permitting visualization of the slit-lamp beam.

Floaters   visual perception of dots or spots which may seem to "swim" or shift location when the position of gaze is shifted.

Fluorescein angiography   a diagnostic test utilizing intravenously injected fluorescein to highlight vascular abnormalities in the eye, most commonly in the fundus.

Fovea   an area of the retina corresponding to central vision, approximately 1.5 mm in diameter, located temporal and slightly inferior to the center of the optic disc.

Foveola   the center of the fovea, 0.5 mm in diameter.

Ghost vessels   corneal stromal blood vessels containing no blood.

Gonioscopy   examination of the anterior-chamber angle structures of the eye, including the trabecular meshwork.

Guttata (corneal)   dropletlike excrescences on the posterior surface of Descemet's membrane.

Hard exudates   deep retinal lipid, often glistening yellow in appearance.

Heterochromia   a difference in coloration, especially between the two irides in a given patient.

Hyperopia (farsightedness)   a condition in which the eye is too short or the refractive power too weak to bring objects at distance or near into clear focus (without the use of accommodation).

Hyphema   blood in the anterior chamber; when layering or clotting of the blood is present, the term hyphema is used; when only suspended red blood cells are present, the term microhyphema is employed.

Hypopyon   layering of white blood cells inferiorly in the anterior chamber.

Hypotony   abnormally low intraocular pressure, usually below 6 mm Hg.

Indirect ophthalmoscopy   the use of a relatively large lens located between the patient and the observer, in combination with a light source, to view the fundus.

Intraretinal microvascular abnormalities   dilated, often telangiectatic, retinal capillaries that act as shunts between arterioles and venules.

Iritis (anterior uveitis, iridocyclitis, cyclitis)   inflammation of the iris, ciliary body, or both.

Keratic precipitates cellular aggregates that form on the corneal endothelium, often inferiorly, in a base-down triangular pattern.

Krukenberg's spindle a narrow, vertically oriented band of pigment located along the central corneal endothelium.

LASIK (Laser In-situ Keratomileusis) type of refractive surgery in which an excimer laser is used to reshape the corneal stromal bed beneath a corneal flap created by a microkeratome.

Leukocoria a grossly visible white pupil.

Macula an area 3-4 disc diameters in size centered at the posterior part of the retina.

Meibomianitis inflamed, inspissated oil glands along the eyelid margins, reflecting inflammation of the meibomian glands.

Metamorphopsia abnormal visual perception causing objects to appear distorted or variable in size/shape.

Microkeratome suction ring with moving blade used to create partial-thickness corneal flap for LASIK refractive surgery.

Microphthalmia a congenitally small, disorganized eye.

Micropsia abnormal visual perception causing objects to appear smaller than normal.

Miosis constriction of the pupil.

Mydriasis dilatation of the pupil.

Myopia (nearsightedness) a condition in which the eye is too long or the refractive power too great to bring objects at a distance clearly into focus.

Nanophthalmos a congenitally small but otherwise normal eye.

Neovascularization growth of abnormal new blood vessels.

Nystagmus rhythmic oscillations or tremors of the eyes that occur independently of normal movements.

Ophthalmoplegia (internal) paralysis of the pupil.

Ophthalmoplegia (external) paralysis of the extraocular muscles.

Optic neuritis inflammation of the optic nerve.

Ora serrata the most peripheral portion of the retina.

Oscillopsia the perception that the environment is moving back and forth.

Palpebral conjunctiva the most superficial covering of the underside of the eyelids from the fornices to the eyelid margins.

Papilledema optic-disc swelling produced by increased intracranial pressure.

Peripapillary surrounding the optic disc.

Peripheral anterior synechiae adhesions between the peripheral iris and anterior-chamber angle or peripheral cornea.

Peripheral iridectomy removal of a portion of the peripheral iris.

Phoria the eyes remain well aligned under conditions of normal binocular vision but have a latent tendency to become misaligned (e.g., when not focusing).

Photophobia ocular pain on exposure to light.

Photopsia a sensation of instantaneous flashes of light; most commonly indicative of retinal traction.

Photorefractive Keratectomy (PRK) type of refractive surgery in which an excimer laser is used to ablate thin layers of the anterior corneal surface to induce refractive changes.

Phototherapeutic Keratectomy (PTK) type of surgery in which an excimer laser is used to ablate anterior corneal opacities or abnormalities.

Polycoria presence of many openings in the iris.

Posterior synechiae   adhesions between the iris and the anterior lens capsule, most commonly at the pupillary border.

Proptosis   protrusion of the globe from the bony orbit.

Pseudohypopon   a layered collection of noninflammatory cells in the anterior chamber, usually associated with neoplastic conditions.

Ptosis (blepharoptosis)   drooping of the upper eyelid.

Punctum   the opening of the tear drainage system in the eyelid margin.

Pupillary block   aqueous humor is prevented from flowing from the posterior chamber into the anterior chamber between the iris and lens.

Radial keratotomy   a surgical technique in which radial incisions are made into the superficial cornea in an effort to change the corneal topography and therefore the patient's refractive error.

Relative afferent pupillary defect   a decreased pupillary constriction to light in one eye as compared with the other eye, using the swinging-flashlight test.

Retinitis   inflammation of the retina.

Retinoscopy   a technique by which the reflex from a streak of light shined on the retina is used to estimate the refractive error of the eye.

Rhegmatogenous retinal detachment   detachment of the retina as a result of a retinal break (hole).

Scleral depression   a technique by which indentation of the peripheral retina is combined with indirect ophthalmoscopy in order to view the peripheral retina.

Scleritis   inflammation of the sclera.

Scotoma   an area of loss of sensitivity in the visual field.

Staphyloma   an outpouching of the sclera that involves the uvea.

Strabismus   ocular misalignment.

Tarsorrhaphy   a surgical technique by which the margins of the upper and lower eyelids of an eye are joined together, either partially or completely.

Trabeculectomy   a surgical technique used to improve aqueous outflow in glaucoma patients.

Tropia   ocular misalignment.

Vitritis   inflammation of the vitreous.

BIBLIOGRAPHY

American Academy of Ophthalmology. *Basic and Clinical Science Course.* Sections 1–12, 1997–1998. San Francisco: American Academy of Ophthalmology, 1998.

Benson WE. *Retinal Detachment:* Diagnosis and Management. 2nd ed. Philadelphia: JB Lippincott, 1988.

Benson WE, Brown GC, Tasman W, eds. *Diabetes and Its Ocular Complications.* Philadelphia: WB Saunders, 1988.

Burde RM, Savino PJ, Trobe JD, eds. *Clinical Decisions in Neuro-ophthalmology.* 2nd ed. St. Louis: CV Mosby, 1992.

Cohen E. Contact lenses and external disease. *Int Ophthalmol Clin* 1988;26:1.

Deutsch TA, Feller DB, eds. *Paton and Goldberg's Management of Ocular Injuries.* 2nd ed. Philadelphia: WB Saunders, 1985.

Gass JDM. *Stereoscopic Atlas of Macular Diseases:* Diagnosis and Treatment. 3rd ed. St. Louis: CV Mosby, 1987.

Kanski JJ. *Uveitis:* A Colour Manual of Diagnosis and Treatment. London: Butterworth, 1987.

Kaufman HE, Barron BA, McDonald MB, Waltman SST, eds. *The Cornea.* New York: Churchill Livingstone, 1988.

Reynolds LA, Closson RG, eds. *Extemporaneous Ophthalmic Preparations.* Vancouver, WA: Applied Therapeutics, 1993.

Roy FH. *Ocular Differential Diagnosis.* 5th ed. Philadelphia: Lea & Febiger, 1992.

Shields JA. *Diagnosis and Management of Intraocular Tumors.* St. Louis: CV Mosby, 1983.

Shields JA. *Diagnosis and Management of Orbital Tumors.* Philadelphia: WB Saunders, 1989.

Shields JA, Shields CL. *Intraocular Tumors:* A Text and Atlas. Philadelphia: WB Saunders, 1992.

Shields MB. *Textbook of Glaucoma.* 3rd ed. Baltimore: Williams & Wilkins, 1991.

Smolin G, Thoft RA, eds. *The Cornea:* Scientific Foundations and Clinical Practice. 3rd ed. Boston: Little, Brown, 1994.

Spoor TC, Nesi GA, eds. *Management of Ocular, Orbital and Adnexal Trauma.* New York: Raven Press, 1988.

Tasman W, Jaeger EA, eds. *Duane's Clinical Ophthalmology.* Rev. ed. Philadelphia: JB Lippincott, 1993.

Tasman WS, ed. *Clinical Decisions in Medical Retinal Disease.* St. Louis: Mosby-Year Book, 1994.

Walsh TJ. *Neuro-ophthalmology:* Clinical Signs and Symptoms. 3rd ed. Philadelphia: Lea & Febiger, 1991.

SUBJECT INDEX

SUBJECT INDEX